PROGRESS IN BRAIN RESEARCH

VOLUME 81

THE CENTRAL NEURAL ORGANIZATION
OF CARDIOVASCULAR CONTROL

PROGRESS IN BRAIN RESEARCH

VOLUME 81

THE CENTRAL NEURAL ORGANIZATION OF CARDIOVASCULAR CONTROL

EDITED BY

JOHN CIRIELLO

Department of Physiology, Health Sciences Centre, The University of Western Ontario, London, Canada, N6A 5C1

MONICA M. CAVERSON

Department of Anatomy, Health Sciences Centre, The University of Western Ontario, London, Canada, N6A 5C1

and

CANIO POLOSA

Department of Physiology, McIntyre Medical Sciences Bldg., McGill University, Montreal, Canada, H3G 1Y6

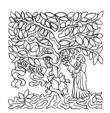

ELSEVIER
AMSTERDAM – NEW YORK – OXFORD
1989

Published by:
Elsevier Science Publishers B.V. (Biomedical Division)
P.O. Box 211
1000 AE Amsterdam
The Netherlands

Sole distributors for the USA and Canada:
Elsevier Science Publishing Company, Inc.
655 Avenue of the Americas
New York, NY 10010
USA

Printed in The Netherlands

List of Contributors

E.M. Adams, Case Western Reserve University, School of Medicine, 2119 Abington Road, Cleveland, OH 44106, U.S.A.

V. Arango, Division of Neurobiology, Cornell University Medical College, 411 East 69th Street, New York, NY 10021, U.S.A.

S. Baradziej, Department of Physiology, Medical Academy, 00 325 Warsaw, Poland

S.M. Barman, Departments of Pharmacology and Toxicology, Michigan State University, East Lansing, MI 48824, U.S.A.

R.M. Bauer, Departments of Veterinary Biosciences, Physiology and Biophysics, University of Illinois, Urbana-Champaign, IL 61801, U.S.A.

T.G. Bedford, Department of Physiology and Biophysics, University of Oklahoma Health Sciences Center, P.O. Box 26901, Oklahoma City, OK 73190, U.S.A.

W.W. Blessing, Department of Medicine, Flinders Medical Centre, Bedford Park, 5042 S.A., Australia

M.J. Brody, Department of Pharmacology and Cardiovascular Center, University of Iowa, Iowa City, IA 52242, U.S.A.

J. Callaway, Division of Neurobiology, Department of Neurology and Neuroscience, Cornell University Medical College, 411 East 69th Street, New York, NY 10021, U.S.A.

R.R. Campos Jr., Departamento de Fisiologia, Escola Paulista de Medicina, Cx. Postal 20.393 (04034), São Paulo, SP, Brazil

M.M. Caverson, Department of Anatomy, Health Sciences Centre, The University of Western Ontario, London, Ontario, N6A 5C1, Canada

N.S. Cherniack, Case Western Reserve University, School of Medicine, 2119 Abington Road, Cleveland, OH 44106, U.S.A.

J. Ciriello, Department of Physiology, Health Sciences Centre, The University of Western Ontario, London, Ontario, N6A 5C1, Canada

B.F. Cox, Department of Pharmacology and Cardiovascular Center, University of Iowa, Iowa City, IA 52242, U.S.A.

S.L. Cravo, Division of Neurobiology, Cornell University Medical College, 411 East 69th Street, New York, NY 10021, U.S.A.

J. Czachurski, I. Physiologisches Institut, Universität Heidelberg, Im Neuenheimer Feld 325, 6900 Heidelberg, F.R.G.

R.A.L. Dampney, Department of Physiology, University of Sydney, Sydney, N.S.W. 2006, Australia

T.A. Day, Department of Physiology and the Neuroscience Centre, University of Otago Medical School, Dunedin, New Zealand

K. Dembowsky, I. Physiologisches Institut, Universität Heidelberg, Im Neuenheimer Feld 326, 6900 Heidelberg, F.R.G.

K.J. Dormer, Department of Physiology and Biophysics, University of Oklahoma Health Sciences Center, P.O. Box 26901, Oklahoma City, OK 73190, U.S.A.

P. Ernsberger, Division of Neurobiology, Department of Neurology and Neuroscience, Cornell University Medical College, 411 East 69th Street, New York, NY 10021, U.S.A.

G.L. Gebber, Department of Pharmacology and Toxicology, and Physiology, Michigan State University, East Lansing, MI 48824, U.S.A.

A. Gong, Division of Neurobiology, Department of Neurology and Neuroscience, Cornell University Medical College, 411 East 69th Street, New York, NY 10021, U.S.A.

C.L. Grosskreutz, Department of Pharmacology and Cardiovascular Center, University of Iowa, Iowa City, IA 52242, U.S.A.

P.G. Guertzenstein, Departamento de Fisiologia, Escola Paulista de Medicina, Cx. Postal 20.393 (04034), São Paulo, SP, Brazil

P.G. Guyenet, Department of Pharmacology, University of Virginia School of Medicine, Charlottesville, VA 22908, U.S.A.

J.R. Haselton, Department of Pharmacology, University of Virginia, School of Medicine, Charlottesville, VA 22908, U.S.A.

M. Haxhiu, Case Western Reserve University, School of Medicine, 2119 Abington Road, Cleveland, OH 44106, U.S.A.

C.J. Helke, Department of Pharmacology, Uniformed Services University of the Health Sciences, 4301 Jones Bridge Road, Bethesda, MD 20814-4799, U.S.A.

G.A. Iwamoto, Department of Cell Biology, University of Texas Southwestern Medical Center, 5323 Harry Hines Boulevard, Dallas, TX 75235, U.S.A.

H. Kannan, Department of Physiology, School of Medicine, University of Occupational and Environmental Health, Yahatanishi-ku, Kitakyushu, 807 Japan

P. Li, Department of Physiology, Shanghai Medical University, Shanghai 200032, People's Republic of China

Y.-W. Li, Departments of Medicine and Physiology, Centre for Neuroscience, Flinders University of South Australia, Bedford Park, 5042 S.A., Australia

F. Lioy, Department of Physiology, University of British Columbia, Vancouver, B.C., Canada V5T 1W5

T.A. Lovick, Department of Physiology, University of Birmingham, Birmingham B15 2TJ, U.K.

R.M. McAllen, Howard Florey Institute of Experimental Physiology and Medicine, University of Melbourne, Victoria 3052, Australia

T.A. Milner, Division of Neurobiology, Department of Neurology and Neuroscience, Cornell University Medical College, 411 East 69th Street, New York, NY 10021, U.S.A.

J.H. Mitchell, Harry S. Moss Heart Center, University of Texas Southwestern Medical Center, Dallas, TX 75235, U.S.A.

J. Mitra, Case Western Reserve University, School of Medicine, 2119 Abington Road, Cleveland, OH 44106, U.S.A.

S.F. Morrison, Division of Neurobiology, Department of Neurology and Neuroscience, Cornell University Medical College, 411 East 69th Street, New York, NY 10021, U.S.A.

S. Nishi, Department of Physiology, Kurume University School of Medicine, Kurume, Japan

V.M. Pickel, Division of Neurobiology, Cornell University Medical College, 411 East 69th Street, New York, NY 10021, U.S.A.

C. Polosa, Department of Physiology, McGill University, McIntyre Medical Sciences Building, 3655 Drummond Street, Montreal, Quebec H3G 1Y6, Canada

N.R. Prabhakar, Case Western Reserve University, School of Medicine, 2119 Abington Road, Cleveland, OH 44106, U.S.A.

W.N. Raby, Neurosciences Unit, Montreal General Hospital Research Institute and McGill University, 1650 Cedar Avenue, Montreal, Quebec, Canada H3G 1A4

D.J. Reis, Division of Neurobiology, Department of Neurology and Neuroscience, Cornell University Medical College, 411 East 69th Street, New York, NY 10021, U.S.A.

L.P. Renaud, Neurosciences Unit, Montreal General Hospital Research Institute and McGill University, 1650 Cedar Avenue, Montreal, Quebec, Canada H3G 1A4

D.A. Ruggiero, Division of Neurobiology, Cornell University Medical College, 411 East 69th Street, New York, NY 10021, U.S.A.

H.N. Sapru, Section of Neurosurgery, New Jersey Medical School, Medical Sciences Building, Room H529, 185 South Orange Ave., Newark, NJ 07103, U.S.A.

C.A. Sasek, Department of Pharmacology, Uniformed Services University of the Health Sciences, 4301 Jones Bridge Road, Bethesda, MD 20814-4799, U.S.A.

H. Seller, I. Physiologisches Institut, Universität Heidelberg, Im Neuenheimer Feld 326, 6900 Heidelberg, F.R.G.

M.-K. Sun, Department of Pharmacology, University of Virginia, School of Medicine, Charlottesville, VA 22908, U.S.A.

K.B. Thor, Department of Pharmacology, Uniformed Services University of the Health Sciences, 4301 Jones Bridge Road, Bethesda, MD 20814-4799, U.S.A.

A. Trzebski, Department of Physiology, Medical Academy, 00 325 Warsaw, Poland

Y. Ueta, Department opf Physiology, School of Medicine, University of Occupational and Environmental Health, Yahatanishi-ku, Kitakyushu, 807 Japan

K.J. Varner, Department of Pharmacology and Cardiovascular Center, University of Iowa, Iowa City, IA 52242, U.S.A.

T.G. Waldrop, Departments of Veterinary Biosciences, Physiology and Biophysics, University of Illinois, Urbana-Champaign, IL 61801, U.S.A.

H. Yamashita, Department of Physiology, School of Medicine, University of Occupational and Environmental Health, Yahatanishi-ku, Kitakyushu, 807 Japan

M. Yoshimura, Department of Physiology, Kurume University School of Medicine, Kurume, Japan

Preface

A Satellite Symposium of the 18th Annual Meeting of the Society for Neuroscience entitled '*Function of the Ventrolateral Medulla in the Control of the Circulation*' was held in London, Ontario, Canada, on the 11th and 12th of November 1988. This volume contains the papers presented by the participants to that Symposium.

The main theme of this volume is the central neural organization of cardiovascular control. The central nervous system plays a critical role in this control by regulating the activity level of the autonomic innervation of heart and blood vessels, by controlling the release of the hormones that regulate the circulation and by coupling the circulatory system to different behaviours. During recent years, due to the explosive progress in the neurosciences, the evolution of thinking in this field has led to the gradual obsolescence of the concept of a medullary vasomotor center, i.e. of a medullary 'final common path' for cardiovascular control. Instead, the more recent experimental evidence suggests that this role is played by the preganglionic neurons. Of the discrete neural pathways converging onto these neurons, those originating from the ventrolateral medulla are of the greatest significance. These ventrolateral medullary pathways have been implicated in the generation of basal sympathetic tone as well as in the mediation of the cerebral ischaemic response, and of the responses evoked by arterial baroreceptors or chemoreceptors. In addition, they are involved in the humoral regulation of the cardiovascular system by controlling the activity of hypothalamic magnocellular neurosecretory (vasopressin) neurons.

The various contributions to this volume represent a sample of current work on topics related to the control of the cardiovascular system by the central nervous system, with emphasis on the prominent role the ventrolateral medulla has in this control. The number of contributions devoted to the issue of the identification and characteristics of the neural circuitry antecedent to the sympathetic preganglionic neuron demonstrates the intense activity in this area. Considerable ingenuity is required in arriving at the identification of neurons as antecedent to the sympathetic preganglionic neurons. This contrasts with the ease with which the preganglionic neuron itself is identified and accounts for the slower rate at which questions about the antecedent neurons are answered.

A related topic concerns the transmitters by means of which the antecedent brainstem neurons communicate with the preganglionic neurons. The immunohistochemical data presented provide a number of possibilities. In attempts to interpret this data it must be remembered that transmitters can produce fast or slow synaptic responses, that a particular chemical is often associated with only one type of response and finally that the two types of response have a different influence on the activity of neurons. Of considerable interest is the discovery of several types of neuropeptides associated with the ventrolateral medullary neurons. In this context, whatever physiological role is hypothesized for the neuropeptides, it must be a role compatible with the constraints imposed by the biology of these substances, in particular the somatic site of synthesis and the slow transport to the axon terminals. Possibly the generalization will emerge that monoamines and peptides have a role in regulating the gain of a transmission system rather than in producing transmission.

Another interesting issue brought into focus by some of the contributions is that of the criteria for deciding whether or not a given area of the central nervous system is involved in a particular cardiovascular behaviour. Many other issues of outstanding interest, but which would take too long to review, were brought up by the contributors. As the purpose of the Editors in assembling this volume was not only to survey current research but also to provide a stimulus for further focused work in this area, this volume proves that the contributors have achieved both aims admirably.

Acknowledgements

The Editors would like to thank the colleagues at the University of Western Ontario who assisted with the scientific, social and administrative work of the Symposium. The Editors are also grateful to all participants for making the Symposium successful and to Elsevier Science Publishers for undertaking the publication of this volume. Finally, the Editors acknowledge the financial support to the Symposium by the following bodies:

Ayerst, McKenna and Harrison (Canada), Inc.
Department of Physiology, The University of Western Ontario
Faculty of Graduate Studies, The University of Western Ontario
Faculty of Medicine, The University of Western Ontario
Fisher Scientific (Canada)
Medical Research Council of Canada
Ontario Ministry of Health
Smith, Kline and French Canada Ltd.
UpJohn Company of Canada
Wild Leitz Canada Ltd.

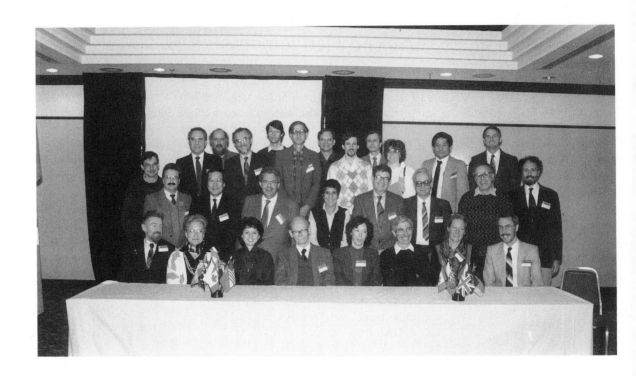

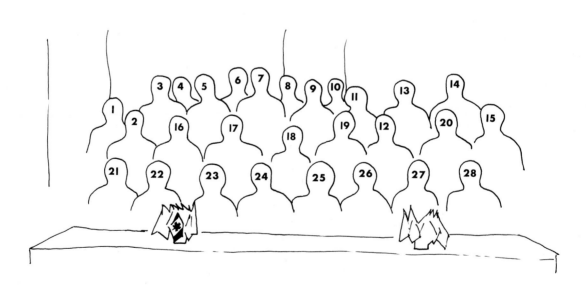

List of Chairmen and Speakers

Symposium on Function of the Ventrolateral Medulla in the Control of the Circulation
London, Ontario, Canada, November 11 – 12, 1988

1	K. Dembowsky	15	D.A. Ruggiero
2	J. Ciriello	16	H. Yamashita
3	L.P. Renaud	17	P.G. Guertzenstein
4	W.W. Blessing	18	M. Kalia
5	F. Lioy	19	N.S. Cherniack
6	R.M. McAllen	20	D.J. Reis
7	H.N. Sapru	21	A. Trzebski
8	G.L. Gebber	22	P.M. Gootman
9	S.F. Morrison	23	M.M. Caverson
10	P.G. Guyenet	24	H.P. Koepchen
11	S.M. Barman	25	C.J. Helke
12	V.P. Lebedev	26	C. Polosa
13	G.A. Iwamoto	27	T.A. Lovick
14	K.J. Dormer	28	T.A. Day

Absent: M.J. Brody

Contents

INTRODUCTION

Thirty years of research on the ventral medulla: the way from Hans Loeschcke's first discovery to modern concepts of ventral medullary function in cardiorespiratory control*

H.-P. Koepchen

Berlin, Germany

In 1958, the first full paper published in this field was entitled: '*Versuch zur Lokalisation des Angriffsortes der Atmungs- und Kreislaufwirkung von Novocain im Liquor cerebrospinalis*' (Attempt to localize the site of action of procaine in the cerebrospinal fluid on respiration and circulation). Although at that time the location of the site of action was still uncertain, three points were already emphasized: (1) the responsible structures must be localized near the ventral surface of the lower brainstem; (2) the central H^+ chemosensitivity of respiration is affected, but not the rhythmogenic apparatus itself; (3) there must exist a similar central site as the source of drive for the cardiovascular system.

Following further developments in the field, the same basic questions remained: (a) The question of localization: What is the neuronal substrate and its precise site below the ventral medullary surface? (b) The question of specificity: Is there a common system in the ventral medulla that drives the circulation and respiration or are the common effects simply the expression of two separate structures in close vicinity to each other? It can now be assumed that: (A) Central H^+ chemosensitivity for respiration is concentrated in three superficial areas identified by Loeschcke and his school, known as rostral (area M), intermediate (area S) and caudal (area L), where area S is considered the most crucial one. (B) From a similar site, approximately corresponding to area S, important descending bulbospinal pathways mediating sympathetic vasoconstrictor resting tone and vasoconstrictor reactions take their origin. In spite of the precise identification of the responsible neurons the question that remains to be answered is whether these ventral medullary neurons produce or only mediate the resting vasomotor tone.

Most of the remaining unsolved or controversial questions appear to be the result of the specialization of the laboratories studying either respiratory or cardiovascular

---

* Modified from author's Abstract submitted for presentation at the symposium by the author — The Editors.

physiology, whereby the attempts to correlate both together are relatively few. For example, the first discovery was made by the attempt to define the adequate central stimulus for respiration. As a result, central chemosensitivity was described by Loeschcke and his school under the main heading of a respiratory regulatory system for the H^+ ion concentration in the extracellular fluid of the brain. The cardiovascular effects observed during activation of the respiratory system were mentioned, but not thoroughly analyzed.

The second root of research on the ventral medulla started with the observation of Feldberg and Guertzenstein that drugs applied at the ventral medullary surface elicited changes in blood pressure. Most of these studies and those which followed investigating the cardiovascular effects were performed in animals under artificial ventilation without monitoring phrenic activity. The first localization of bulbospinal neurons near the ventral surface projecting to the intermediolateral column of the spinal cord in Seller's laboratory was performed with reference to the similar localization of central chemosensitivity and the involvement of blood pressure in the experience of Loeschcke's group. The blocking agents applied to the ventral medullary surface had affected at the same time, but independently, afferent projections to respiratory neurons and efferent projections to spinal sympathetic neurons. This is still the main opinion of investigators studying the cardiovascular functions of the ventral medulla. The central chemosensitivity of sympathetic tone was shown by the laboratories of Trzebski and Polosa to originate, at least in part, from superficially located structures on the ventral medulla. However, the question that remains is whether there is a common source of central chemosensitivity for respiration *and* the circulation, or whether both systems are controlled independently. Irrespective of chemosensitivity the question of a common drive for respiration and the circulation in alerting reactions with relay stations near the ventral medullary surface was raised by Hilton and remains a controversial topic. In this respect the last hypothesis of Loeschcke, after more than two decades of a vain search for the histologically identifiable chemoreceptor, that H^+ ions act on synapses near the surface, should be taken into consideration.

Thus many questions exist with respect to the interaction between the control systems for respiration and the circulation, and remain an on-going challenge that will require the cooperation between the different specialized groups!

SECTION I

Central Projections and Neurochemistry of Ventrolateral Medullary Neurons

J. Ciriello, M.M. Caverson and C. Polosa (Eds.)
Progress in Brain Research, Vol. 81
© 1989 Elsevier Science Publishers B.V. (Biomedical Division)

CHAPTER I

Relation of enkephalin-like immunoreactive neurons to other neuropeptide and monoamine-containing neurons in the ventrolateral medulla

John Ciriello and Monica M. Caverson

Department of Physiology, Health Sciences Centre, University of Western Ontario, London, Ontario, Canada, N6A 5C1

Introduction

There is now a considerable amount of experimental evidence suggesting that neurons in the ventrolateral medulla (VLM) are involved in the maintenance and reflex regulation of systemic arterial pressure (for a review see Ciriello et al., 1986b). Although the descending pathways from VLM neurons to spinal sympathetic centers that may be involved in mediating these functions have been investigated in the cat (Amendt et al., 1979; Caverson et al., 1983,1984; Caverson and Ciriello, 1984), surprisingly little is known about the neurotransmitter content of the pathways. In the rat, it has been suggested that monoamine and substance P containing fibers are involved in mediating the circulatory responses elicited by VLM stimulation (Helke et al., 1982; Howe et al., 1983; Ross et al., 1984; Takano et al., 1984).

Recently it has been shown in the rat that microinjections of an enkephalin analogue into the rostral VLM elicit decreases in arterial pressure, whereas microinjections into the caudal VLM elicit increases in arterial pressure (Punnen et al., 1984; Willette et al., 1984). These data suggested that an enkephalinergic system in the VLM may be involved in controlling the circulation. In support of this suggestion, the rat VLM has been shown to contain neurons that are immunoreactive to methionine (Met)-enkephalin (Hokfelt et al., 1979; Finley et al., 1981) and β-endorphin (Leibstein et

al., 1985). In addition, opiates have been shown to inhibit central adrenergic neurons (Aghajanian, 1978). C1 adrenergic neurons in the VLM are thought to be involved in cardiovascular regulation (Ross et al., 1984). Furthermore, Met-enkephalin neurons in the VLM of the rat have been shown to project to the spinal cord (Hokfelt et al., 1979). Finally, experimental evidence in the cat indicates that enkephalinergic pathways may be involved in the control of the cardiovascular system as leucine-enkephalin (Leu-ENK) immunoreactive fibers and terminals have been shown to form a dense plexus around sympathetic preganglionic neurons in the intermediolateral nucleus of the thoracolumbar cord (Krukoff et al., 1985).

In the present study, a series of experiments was done to map the presence of neuronal perikarya containing Leu-ENK and Met-ENK in the cat VLM. ENK immunoreactive neurons were identified in animals after the administration of colchicine into the cisterna magna and in animals that did not receive colchicine. Colchicine is known to disrupt axonal transport (Hokfelt and Dahlstrom, 1971) and result in the accumulation of peptides in neuronal perikarya.

Methods

Experiments were done in adult male cats weighing 2.5 – 3.5 kg. In the colchicine-treated animals, the cats were anesthetized with ketamine (35 mg/kg i.m.; Rogarsetic, Roger/STB Inc., Montreal, Canada) and placed in a Kopf stereotaxic frame. The head was flexed approximately 30° forward and the atlanto-occipital membrane was exposed and pierced with a 26-gauge hypodermic needle. A PE-10 polyethylene cannula attached to a 20 μl Hamilton syringe containing colchicine (20 μg/ml saline; Sigma Chemical Co., St. Louis, MO, U.S.A.) was inserted into the subarachnoid space and 300 – 400 μg of colchicine per cat were injected. Animals were given postoperative care.

After a survival period of 27 – 48 h the animals were deeply anesthetized with pentobarbital sodium (50 mg/kg i.p.: Somnotol, M.T.C. Pharmaceuticals, Hamilton, Canada), and perfused transcardially with 500 ml of 0.9% physiological saline followed by 2 l of Zamboni's fixative (Ciriello et al., 1986a). The animals which did not receive colchicine were perfused similarly. The brainstem from the level of the spino-medullary junction to the inferior colliculi was removed and placed in Zamboni's fixative at 4°C for 4 – 6 h and then transferred to 10% sucrose in phosphate-buffered saline (PBS; pH 7.2). At approximately 24 h intervals the brainstem was transferred sequentially to 20% and 30% sucrose-PBS. Serial transverse, sagittal or horizontal sections were cut in a cryostat (−17°C) at a thickness of 50 μm, collected in PBS and treated with antisera for Leu-ENK or Met-ENK (Immuno Nuclear Corp., Stillwater, MN, U.S.A.). The Leu-ENK and Met-ENK antibodies were produced against synthetic Leu-ENK and Met-ENK conjugated to bovine serum albumin. In each cat, one in every three sections was treated with the antisera.

The immunohistochemical procedure of Hsu et al. (1981) was used. These procedures have been summarized in other publications from this laboratory (Ciriello et al., 1986a,1988). Alternate sections were counterstained with either thionin or neutral red to visualize cell bodies and aid in the identification of cytoarchitectonically defined nuclei in the brainstem.

The antiserum produced against Leu-ENK showed approximately 5% cross-reactivity with Met-ENK, but did not significantly cross-react with bombesin, calcitonin, vasoactive intestine peptide, substance P, gastrin, somatostatin and dynorphin peptides (Gall and Moore, 1984; Reiner et al., 1984; Griesler et al., 1985).

Two types of control experiments were done in the present study for immunospecificity of the antiserum. Representative sections from the medulla were placed in the diluted primary antiserum which had been preadsorbed with an excess (10 μg/ml) of the respective synthetic peptide (Sigma and Immuno Nuclear), and in the second group, reaction of the tissue sections with the primary antisera was omitted (Krukoff et al., 1985; Ciriello et al., 1986a). Under these conditions no immunoreactive perikarya could be demonstrated.

All sections were examined systematically with a Nikon Optiphot light microscope, and the distribution of immunoreactive cell bodies was mapped on a representative series of projection drawings of the entire brainstem from each animal. The atlases and nomenclature of Taber (1961) and Berman (1968) were used for the identification of brainstem structures. Projection drawings of immunoreactive perikarya were made with a Nikon camera lucida attachment.

Results

In the cats without colchicine treatment, small numbers of cell bodies containing ENK-like immunoreactivity were observed throughout the intermediate and rostral extent of the VLM. In contrast, in cats treated with colchicine, the numbers of neurons which exhibited ENK immunoreactivity greatly increased throughout the rostrocaudal extent of the VLM.

A large number of perikarya containing Leu-ENK-like immunoreactivity was observed in the VLM of colchicine-treated cats (approximately 30 – 65 Leu-ENK cells/section throughout the rostrocaudal extent of the VLM). The distribution in the VLM of perikarya containing Leu-ENK is

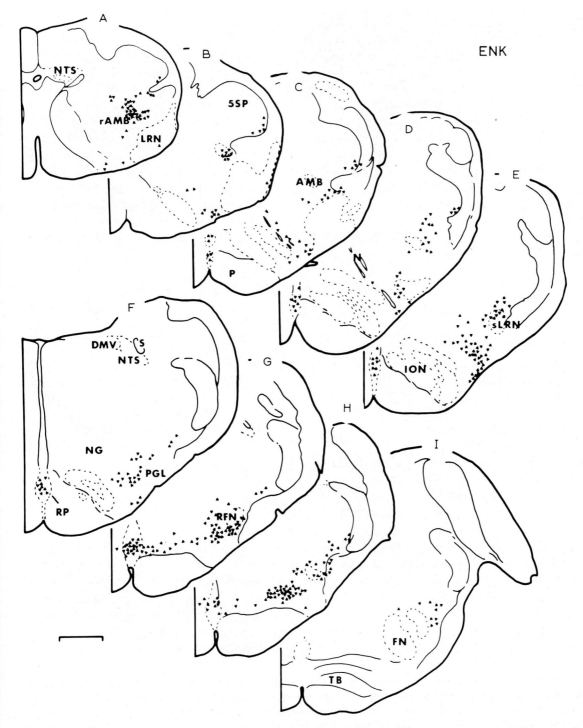

Fig. 1. Series of projection drawings of transverse hemi-sections of the brainstem of the cat at approximately 0.9 mm intervals extending from approximately 1.8 mm (A) caudal to 5.4 mm (I) rostral to the obex showing the location of Leu-ENK immunoreactive perikarya (triangles). Section B corresponds approximately to frontal plane P15.0 (Berman, 1968). Each triangle represents one Leu-ENK immunoreactive cell body found in the section drawn. Calibration mark = 1 mm.

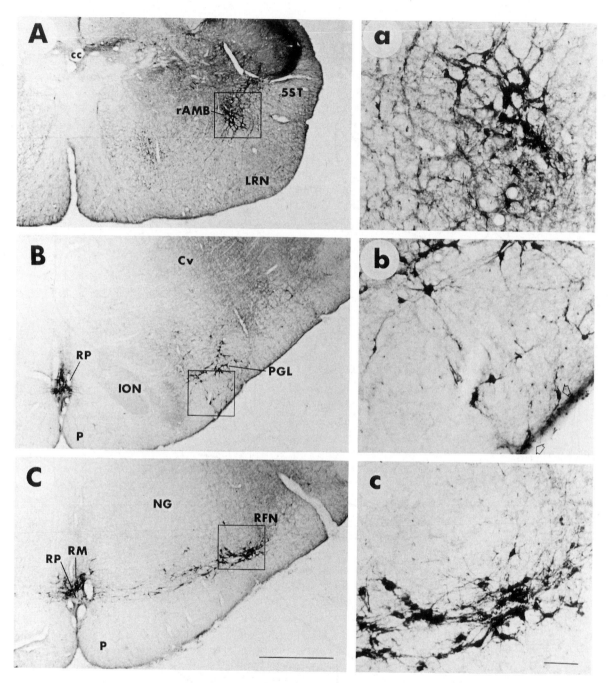

Fig. 2. Brightfield photomicrographs of unstained transverse sections of the cat brainstem showing Leu-ENK-like immunoreactive perikarya in different regions of the VLM. (A) Dense cluster of Leu-ENK cells in the rAMB in the caudal medulla. Note the dense network of intertwining processes from the cells. (B) Leu-ENK cells in the PGL near the ventral surface of the medulla (arrows in b). (C) Dense cluster of Leu-ENK cells near the ventromedial border of the RFN. Note the extensive, branching processes of the cells and that these processes were in close association with other immunoreactive cells. In addition, note the many Leu-ENK cells spanning the area between the raphe nuclei and RFN. a, b and c correspond to areas outlined by rectangle in A, B and C, respectively. Calibration mark in C of 1 mm also applies to A and B. Similarly, calibration mark in c of 100 μm also applies to a and b.

shown in Fig. 1. Two distinct continuous columns of Leu-ENK cells were observed to extend from the caudal pole of the lateral reticular nucleus (LRN) to the caudal extent of the superior olivary nucleus, bilaterally: a dorsolateral and a ventrolateral column. A small number of cells were also observed spanning these two columns. In the caudal VLM, the dorsolateral column appeared to originate as a dense cluster of cells in and around the caudal aspects of the nucleus retroambiguus (Figs. 1A and 2A-a). As this dorsolateral column coursed rostrally, through the region between the nucleus ambiguus and the LRN (Fig. 1B–D), towards the lateral aspects of the retrofacial nucleus (RFN) and facial nucleus (FN) (Fig. 1E–I), the number of immunoreactive neurons progressively decreased. A few scattered cells were also observed as far rostrally as the superior olivary nucleus, along its lateral border.

In contrast, in the caudal medulla the ventrolateral column of Leu-ENK cells appeared to begin as a sparse collection of neurons in the region ventromedial to the LRN and lateral to the exiting intramedullary rootlets of the hypoglossal nerve (12 N), near the ventral surface. A dense cluster of cells in this column were first encountered at the level of the rostral extent of the LRN (Figs. 1H and 2B). At more rostral levels a few cells from both columns appeared to encircle the RFN (Fig. 1H, C and 2C). In addition, a continuous band of Leu-ENK cells was observed to span the region dorsal to the pyramidal tract between the nucleus raphe pallidus and the spinal trigeminal tract (Figs. 1G, H and 2C). Although a few cells were found within a few microns from the ventral surface of the medulla in the nucleus paragigantocellularis lateralis (PGL) (Fig. 2B), the majority of cells were found 0.8–1 mm away from the ventral surface. In addition to the VLM, Leu-ENK cells were also observed throughout the nucleus raphe pallidus and magnus (Fig. 1C–H and 2B,C). Although perikarya in the VLM containing Met-ENK-like immunoreactivity had a similar distribution (Fig. 3) to that observed for Leu-ENK cells (Fig. 1), several differences were

apparent. First, the number of Met-ENK cells in the VLM was approximately half of that for Leu-ENK. Second, the dorsolateral column of Met-ENK cells was only observed in the caudal VLM and restricted to the region in and around the nucleus retroambiguus (Fig. 3A,B). Third, a considerable number of cells were observed along the ventral portion of the parvicellular component of the LRN (Figs. 3A–D and 4A). Finally, although Met-ENK and Leu-ENK containing cells had overlapping dorsoventral distributions with regard to their location near the ventrolateral surface of the medulla, most of the Met-ENK immunoreactive cells were found to occupy the area immediately ventral to that containing Leu-ENK cells (Figs. 3 and 4).

Some of the morphological characteristics of the Leu-ENK and Met-ENK immunoreactive cells are shown in Fig. 5. Throughout the rostrocaudal extent of the VLM, ENK cells were observed to be multipolar with two to four major dendritic processes, which branched frequently, emanating from the cell bodies, often in more than one direction (Fig. 5). In horizontal and sagittal sections dendritic processes were observed to extend rostrocaudally. In the rostral VLM Leu-ENK neurons in and around the RFN formed compact clusters (Fig. 2C). The dendrites of cells in these clusters extended in all directions and intertwined with each other in the clusters. The long axes of ENK immunoreactive cells did not appear to have any specific orientation in the VLM, except for cells near the ventrolateral surface of the medulla that had their long axes parallel to the surface. In addition, cells which were located in the rostral VLM dorsal to the pyramidal tract and spanning the region between the raphe nuclei and RFN had long axes which were preferentially in the mediolateral direction.

Discussion

The present study has provided a map of the location and a description of some of the morphological characteristics of neuronal perikarya

8

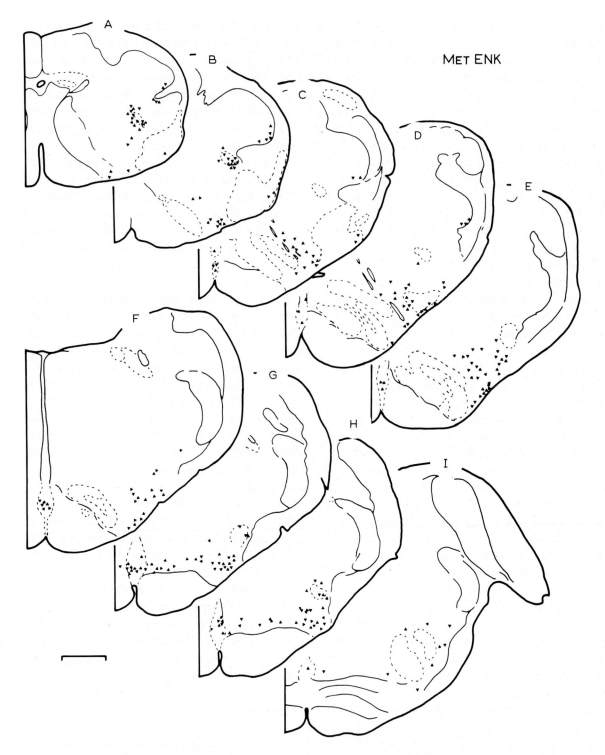

MET ENK

Fig. 3. Series of projection drawings of transverse hemi-sections of the cat brainstem showing the location of Met-ENK immunoreactive perikarya (triangles) in the VLM. Note that there are considerably fewer (approximately half) Met-ENK cells compared to Leu-ENK cells (Fig. 1) at similar rostrocaudal levels and that they generally occupy the region immediately ventral to that occupied by Leu-ENK cells. Refer to Fig. 1 for additional details.

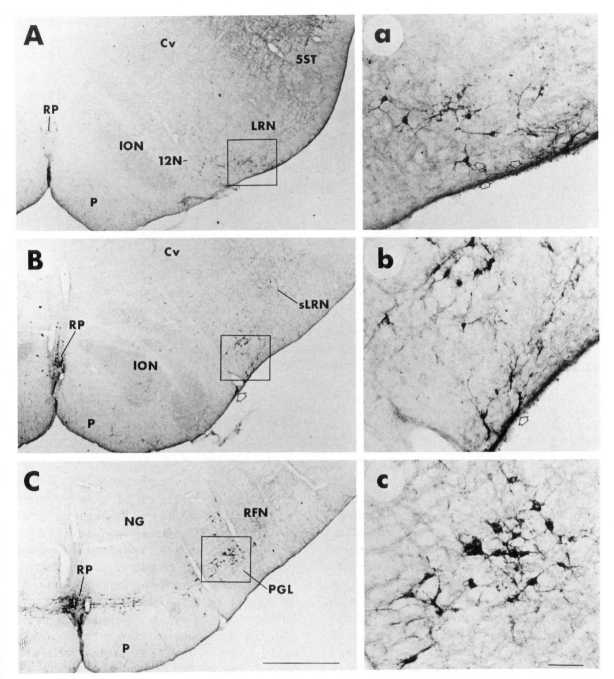

Fig. 4. Brightfield photomicrographs of unstained transverse sections of the cat brainstem showing the location of Met-ENK immunoreactive perikarya. (A) Dense cluster of Met-ENK cells along the medial aspect of the parvicellular component of the LRN, and lateral to the 12 N. Note that some these cells send dendritic processes towards the pial surface and that some turn and course parallel to the surface (arrows in a and b). (B) Met-ENK cells in the PGL near ventrolateral surface of the medulla. Arrow points to labelled perikarya adjacent pial surface near point of exit of intramedullary rootlet of 12 N. (C) Dense cluster of Met-ENK cells in rostral PGL, near RFN. Note the fewer number of Met-ENK cells in the region compared to Leu-ENK cells (Fig. 2c). Refer to Fig. 2 for additional details.

A

B

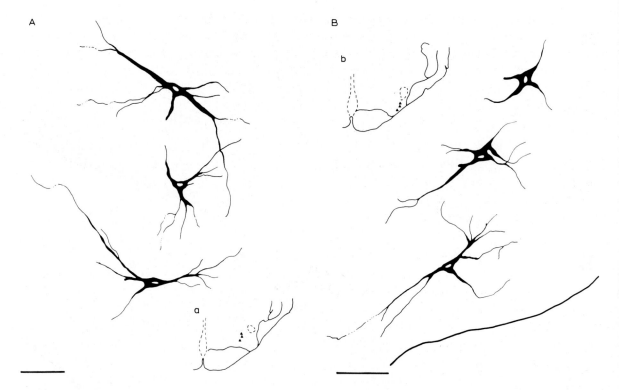

b

a

Fig. 5. Camera lucida projection drawings showing some of the morphological characteristics of Leu- (A) and Met-ENK (B) cells in the VLM. Note that cells near the ventral surface send dendritic processes towards the pial surface. a and b show the location of cell bodies (triangles) in A and B, respectively. Refer to Fig. 1H and 1G for identification of structures in a and b, respectively. Calibration mark = 100 μm.

containing ENK-like immunoreactivity in the VLM of the cat. These data generally confirm and extend previous immunohistochemical studies on the location of Met-ENK containing cell bodies in the cat (Hunt and Lovick, 1982) and rat (Finley et al., 1981) VLM and Leu-ENK immunoreactive cells in the cat (Glazer et al., 1981).

Dense clusters of ENK cells were found in and around the nucleus retroambiguus, in the regions ventromedial and dorsolateral to the LRN, in the PGL near the ventral surface of the medulla and in a region ventrolateral to the RFN. The finding of ENK immunoreactive cells in the cat VLM confirms the finding of a few scattered Leu-ENK cells that have been described in the region medial and dorsal to the LRN in the caudal medulla and in the region of the PGL in the rat (Finley et al., 1981) and cat (Glazer et al., 1981). In addition, a brief

report describing the location of Met-ENK cells in the rostral VLM of the cat has been previously published (Hunt and Lovick, 1982). In this latter study Met-ENK cells were observed to extend from the PGL caudally into the rostral part of the LRN in the VLM region. Few cells immunoreactive for Met-ENK were observed below the rostral third of the inferior olivary nucleus (ION) (Hunt and Lovick, 1982). In contrast, in the present study, ENK cells were observed throughout the rostro-caudal extent of the VLM, around the region located ventromedial to the LRN, and in the nucleus retroambiguus. The reasons for these differences are not clear, but they may reflect the different sensitivities of the immunohistochemical techniques used (Van Den Pol, 1984) and the different amounts and locations of the colchicine administered in the two studies. In the rat, Met-ENK cells have been described in the VLM (Finley et al., 1981). The distribution pattern of these cells is similar to that of Leu-ENK (Finley et al., 1981) and β-endorphin immunoreactive cells (Leibstein et al., 1985) in the VLM of the rat.

The functional role of these ENK containing cells in the VLM of the cat is not known as their connections have not been studied. However, there are a considerable number of anatomical and electrophysiological studies in the cat which have identified the functional characteristics and projections of cells in the VLM which overlap those containing ENK immunoreactive cells in the present study. The likelihood that the groups of VLM cells

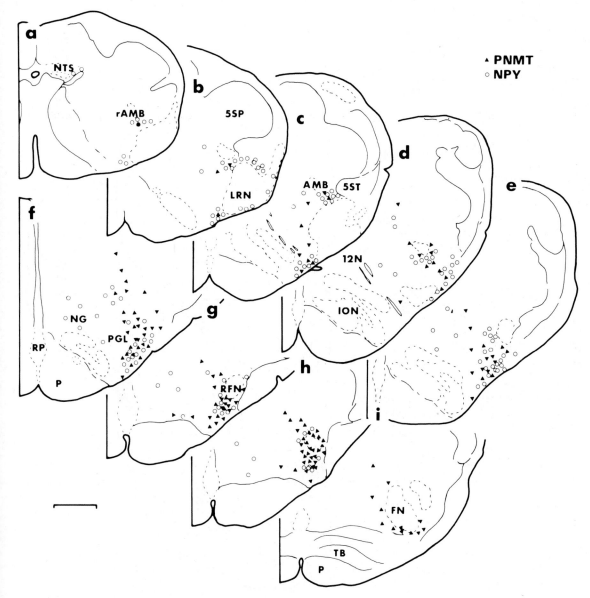

Fig. 6. Series of projection drawings of transverse hemi-sections of the brainstem of the cat showing the location of phenylethanolamine N-methytransferase (PNMT) and neuropeptide Y (NPY) immunoreactive perikarya. Refer to Fig. 1 for additional details.

described in this report were involved in these earlier neuroanatomical and physiological studies, suggests that they are likely components of neuronal circuits involved in autonomic regulation. In the cat and rat it has been demonstrated that injections of tritiated amino acids into regions of the VLM shown in the present study to contain

the cells immunoreactive for ENK results in anterograde labelling throughout the intermediate gray region of the thoracolumbar cord (Basbaum and Fields, 1979; Holstage and Kuypers, 1982; Caverson and Ciriello, 1984; Ross et al., 1984). In addition, horseradish peroxidase injections into the region of the intermediolateral nucleus in the

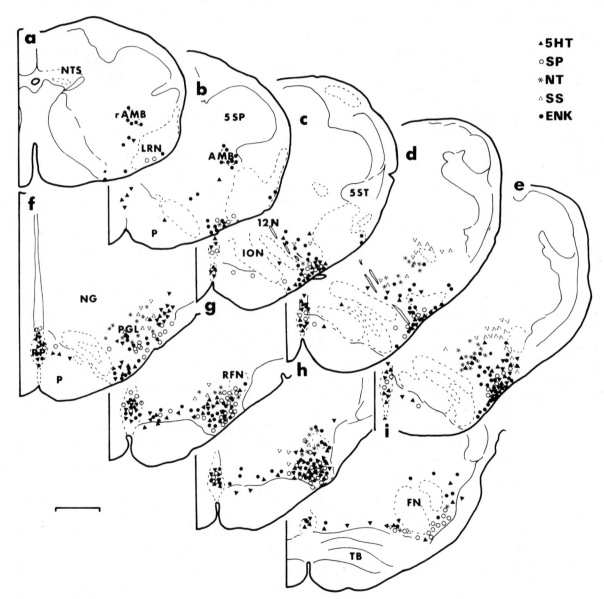

Fig. 7. Series of projection drawings of transverse hemi-sections of the cat brainstem showing relation of ENK immunoreactive perikarya to those containing substance P, serotonin, neurotensin, and somatostatin in the ventrolateral medulla. Refer to Fig. 1 for additional details.

cat result in the retrograde labelling of cells in the VLM (Amendt et al., 1979; Caverson et al., 1983). The location of these retrogradely labelled cells overlaps considerably with that area of the VLM shown in this study to contain ENK immunoreactive cells. These observations, combined with the observations of ENK immunoreactivity in fibers and terminals around sympathetic preganglionic neurons in the intermediolateral nucleus and central autonomic area in the thoracolumbar cord (Krukoff et al., 1985) suggests that these ENK VLM cells make synaptic contacts with sympathetic preganglionic neurons. This suggestion is supported by the finding in the rat that cells retrogradely labelled after spinal cord injections of tracers are immunoreactive for Met-ENK (Hokfelt et al., 1979). This evidence, taken together with the finding of neurons in the region of the cat VLM, where ENK immunoreactive cells were found in this study, that receive and relay baroreceptor and chemoreceptor afferent inputs directly to the intermediolateral nucleus and central autonomic area (Caverson et al., 1983,1984) strongly suggests that ENK containing cells in the VLM are involved in the reflex regulation of arterial pressure and heart rate. It is interesting to note that ENK cells were found close to the ventral surface of the brainstem in regions from which topical application of the putative inhibitory neurotransmitter glycine and/or bilateral lesions has been shown to result in systemic arterial hypotension (Guertzenstein and Silver, 1974) and to alter vascular tone (Hanna et al., 1979; McAllen et al., 1982) and the baroreceptor reflex (McAllen et al., 1982).

The distribution of ENK cells in the rostral VLM overlaps that of phenylethanolamine N-methyltransferase and neuropeptide Y-containing cells in the cat (Fig. 6; Ciriello et al., 1986a). As one of the morphological features of ENK cells is that they have several frequently branching processes suggests that these cells make synaptic contacts with neighboring cells. Therefore, the possibility exists that ENK cells functionally contact and inhibit adrenaline containing cells in the

rostral VLM. This suggestion is supported by the demonstration that opiates inhibit central adrenergic cells (Aghajanian, 1978). In addition, microinjections of enkephalin analogues into the rostral VLM elicit decreases in systemic arterial pressure (Punnen et al., 1984). On the other hand, stimulation of the rostral VLM elicits increases in sympathetic activity and arterial pressure (Ciriello et al., 1986b).

Finally, these data, combined with those of previous studies (Ciriello et al., 1986a; 1988) summarized in Figs. 6 and 7 indicate that the VLM can be subdivided on the basis of the relative distribution of immunocytochemically identified neurons. However, some overlap in the distribution of neurons containing different peptides and monoamines is present, suggesting that more than one of the neuroactive substances may be co-localized in the same neuron. These monoamines and neuropeptides have also been localized immunocytochemically in fibers and terminals around sympathetic preganglionic neurons of the thoracolumbar cord and magnocellular neurosecretory neurons in the hypothalamus. In addition, this distribution in the spinal cord and hypothalamus overlap those areas that receive projections from VLM neurons. Taken together, the results suggest that these neuroactive substances are likely to play an important role in the control of sympathetic preganglionic and hypothalamic magnocellular neurosecretory neurons.

Acknowledgements

The technical assistance of L. D'Ippolito and J.A. Nichols is appreciated. This work was supported by the Medical Research Council of Canada and the Heart and Stroke Foundation of Ontario. Dr. J. Ciriello is a Heart and Stroke Foundation of Ontario Career Investigator and Dr. M.M. Caverson is a Canadian Heart Foundation Scholar. Dr. Caverson's present address is the Department of Anatomy, at The University of Western Ontario, London, Ontario, Canada, N6A 5C1.

14

References

Aghajanian, G.K. (1978) Tolerance of locus coeruleus neurons to morphine and suppression of withdrawal response by clonidine. *Nature*, 276: 186 – 188.

Amendt, K., Czachurski, J., Dembowsky, K. and Seller, H. (1979) Bulbospinal projections to the intermediolateral cell column; a neuroanatomical study. *J. Auton. Nerv. Syst.*, 1: 103 – 117.

Basbaum, A.I. and Fields, H.L. (1979) The origin of descending pathways in the dorsolateral funiculus of the spinal cord of the cat and rat: pain modulation. *J. Comp. Neurol.*, 187: 513 – 532.

Berman, A.L. (1968) *The Brain Stem of the Cat*, The University of Wisconsin Press, Madison, Wisconsin.

Caverson, M.M. and Ciriello, J. (1984) Direct projections from ventrolateral medullary pressor regions to thoracolumbar sympathetic areas in the cat. *Soc. Neurosci. Abstr.*, 10: 32.

Caverson, M.M., Ciriello, J. and Calaresu, F.R. (1983) Direct pathway from cardiovascular neurons in the ventrolateral medulla to the region of the intermediolateral nucleus of the upper thoracic cord: an anatomical and electrophysiological investigation in the cat. *J. Auton. Nerv. Syst.*, 9: 451 – 475.

Caverson, M.M., Ciriello, J. and Calaresu, F.R. (1984) Chemoreceptor and baroreceptor inputs to ventrolateral medullary neurons. *Am. J. Physiol.*, 247: R872 – R879.

Ciriello, J. and Caverson, M.M. (1984a) Ventrolateral medullary neurons relay cardiovascular inputs to the paraventricular nucleus. *Am. J. Physiol.*, 246: R968 – R978.

Ciriello, J. and Caverson, M.M. (1984b) Direct pathway from neurons in the ventrolateral medulla relaying cardiovascular afferent information to the supraoptic nucleus of the cat. *Brain Res.*, 292: 221 – 228.

Ciriello, J. and Caverson, M.M. (1984c) Organization of ventrolateral medullary (VLM) afferents to the paraventricular (PVH) and supraoptic (SON) nuclei in the cat. *Fed. Proc.*, 43: 401.

Ciriello, J. and Caverson, M.M. (1986) Bidirectional cardiovascular connections between ventrolateral medulla and nucleus of the solitary tract. *Brain Res.*, 367: 273 – 281.

Ciriello, J., Caverson, M.M., Krukoff, T.L. and Calaresu, F.R. (1985) Distribution of neuropeptide and serotonin immunoreactive neurons in the ventrolateral medulla of the cat. *Anat. Rec.*, 211: 41A.

Ciriello, J., Caverson, M.M. and Park, D.H. (1986a) Immunohistochemical identification of noradrenaline- and adrenaline-synthesizing neurons in the cat ventrolateral medulla. *J. Comp. Neurol.*, 253: 216 – 230.

Ciriello, J., Caverson, M.M. and Polosa, C. (1986b) Function of the ventrolateral medulla in the control of the circulation. *Brain Res. Rev.*, 11: 359 – 391.

Ciriello, J., Caverson, M.M., Calaresu, F.R. and Krukoff, T.L. (1988) Neuropeptide and serotonin immunoreactive neurons in the cat ventrolateral medulla. *Brain Res.*, 440: 53 – 66.

Duncan, D.B. (1955) Multiple range and multiple F tests. *Biometrics*, 11: 1 – 42.

Finley, J.C., Maderdrut, J.L. and Petrusz, P. (1981) The immunocytochemical localization of enkephalin in the central nervous system of the rat. *J. Comp. Neurol.*, 198: 541 – 565.

Gall, C. and Moore, R.Y. (1984) Distribution of enkephalin, substance P, tyrosine hydroxylase, and 5-hydroxytryptamine immunoreactivity in the septal region of the rat. *J. Comp. Neurol.*, 225: 212 – 227.

Giesler, G.J. and Elde, R.P. (1985) Immunocytochemical studies of the peptidergic content of fibers and terminals within the lateral spinal and lateral cervical nuclei. *J. Neurosci.*, 5: 1833 – 1841.

Glazer, E.J., Steinbusch, H., Verhofstad, A. and Basbaum, A.I. (1981) Serotonin neurons in nucleus raphe dorsalis and paragigantocellularis of the cat contain enkephalin. *J. Physiol. (Paris)*, 77: 241 – 245.

Guertzenstein, P.G. and Silver, A. (1974) Fall in blood pressure produced from discrete regions of the ventral surface of the medulla by glycine and lesions. *J. Physiol. (Lond.)*, 242: 489 – 503.

Hanna, B.D., Lioy, F. and Polosa, C. (1979) The effect of cold blockade of the medullary chemoreceptors on the CO_2 modulation of the vascular tone and heart rate. *Can. J. Physiol. Pharmacol.*, 57: 461 – 468.

Helke, C.J., Neil, J.J., Massari, V.J. and Loewy, A.D. (1982) Substance P neurons project from the ventral medulla to the intermediolateral cell column and ventral horn in the rat. *Brain Res.*, 243: 147 – 152.

Hokfelt, T. and Dahlstrom, A. (1971) Effects of two mitosis inhibitors (colchicine and vinblastine) on the distribution and axonal transport of noradrenaline storage particles, studied by fluorescence and electron microscopy. *Z. Zellforsch.*, 119: 460 – 482.

Hokfelt, T., Terenius, L., Kuypers, H.G.J.M. and Dann, O. (1979) Evidence for enkephalin immunoreactive neurons in the medulla oblongata projecting to the spinal cord. *Neurosci. Lett.*, 14: 55 – 60.

Holstege, G. and Kuypers, H.G.J.M. (1982) The anatomy of brain stem pathways to the spinal cord in cat. A labeled amino acid tracing study. In H.G.J.M. Kuypers and G.F. Martin (Eds.), *Descending Pathways to the Spinal Cord, Progress in Brain Research, Vol. 57*, Elsevier, Amsterdam, pp. 145 – 175.

Howe, P.R.C., Kuhn, D.M., Minson, J.B., Stead, B.H. and Chalmers, J.P. (1983) Evidence for a bulbospinal serotonergic pressor pathway in the rat brain. *Brain Res.*, 270: 29 – 36.

Hsu, S., Raine, L. and Fanger, H. (1981) Use of avidin-biotin-peroxidase complex (ABC) in immunoperoxidase technique: a comparison between ABC and unlabeled antibody (PAP) procedures. *J. Histochem. Cytochem.*, 29: 577 – 580.

Hunt, S.P. and Lovick, T.A. (1982) The distribution of

serotonin, met-enkephalin and β-lipotropin-like immunoreactivity in neuronal perikarya of the cat brainstem. *Neurosci. Lett.*, 30: 139 – 145.

Krukoff, T.L., Ciriello, J. and Calaresu, F.R. (1985) Segmental distribution of peptide- and 5HT-like immunoreactivity in nerve terminals and fibers of the thoraco-lumbar sympathetic nuclei of the cat. *J. Comp. Neurol.*, 240: 103 – 116.

Leibstein, A.G., Dermietzel, R., Willenberg, I.M. and Pauschert, R. (1985) Mapping of different neuropeptides in the lower brainstem of the rat: with special reference to the ventral surface. *J. Auton. Nerv. Syst.*, 14: 299 – 313.

McAllen, R.M., Neil, J.J. and Loewy, A.D. (1982) Effect of kainic acid applied to the ventral surface of the medulla oblongata on vasomotor tone, the baroreceptor reflex and hypothalamic autonomic responses. *Brain Res.*, 238: 65 – 76.

Punnen, S., Willette, R.N., Krieger, A.J. and Sapru, H.N. (1984) Cardiovascular response to injections of enkephalin in the pressor area of the ventrolateral medulla. *Neuropharmacology*, 23: 939 – 946.

Reiner, A., Davis, B.M., Brecha, N.C. and Karten, H.J. (1984) The distribution of enkephalin-like immunoreactivity in the telencephalon of the adult and developing domestic chicken. *J. Comp. Neurol.*, 228: 245 – 262.

Ross, C.A., Ruggiero, D.A., Joh, T.H., Park, D.H. and Reis, D.J. (1984) Rostral ventrolateral medulla: selective projections to the thoracic autonomic cell column from the region containing Cl adrenaline neurons. *J. Comp. Neurol.*, 228: 168 – 185.

Taber, E. (1961) The cytoarchitecture of the brain stem of the cat. 1. Brain stem nuclei of cat. *J. Comp. Neurol.*, 116: 27 – 69.

Takano, Y., Martin, J.E., Leeman, S.E. and Loewy, A.D. (1984) Substance P immunoreactivity released from rat spinal cord after kainic acid excitation of the ventral medulla oblongata: a correlation with increases in blood pressure. *Brain Res.*, 291: 168 – 172.

Van Den Pol, A.N. (1984) Colloidal gold and biotin-avidin conjugates as ultrastructural markers for neural antigens. *Q. J. Exp. Physiol.*, 69: 1 – 33.

Willette, R.N., Punnen, S., Krieger, A.J. and Sapru, H.N. (1984) Hypertensive responses following stimulation of opiate receptors in the caudal ventrolateral medulla. *Neuropharmacology*, 23: 401 – 406.

J. Ciriello, M.M. Caverson and C. Polosa (Eds.)
Progress in Brain Research, Vol. 81
© 1989 Elsevier Science Publishers B.V. (Biomedical Division)

CHAPTER 2

Chemical neuroanatomy of the parapyramidal region of the ventral medulla in the rat

C.J. Helke, K.B. Thor and C.A. Sasek

Department of Pharmacology, Uniformed Services University of the Health Sciences, 4301 Jones Bridge Rd., Bethesda, MD 20814 – 4799, U.S.A.

Introduction

Anatomical, neurochemical and functional evidence showed that several regions of the ventral medulla are involved in cardiovascular control (Loeschke et al., 1970; Keeler et al., 1984; Ross et al., 1984a; McCall and Clements, 1988). One of these regions, an area which will be referred to as the parapyramidal region, consists of neurons located close to the ventral surface and lateral to the pyramidal tract (Fig. 1). The cells of the parapyramidal region have variably been referred to in the literature as the nucleus interfascicularis hypoglossi, nucleus paragigantocellularis pars alpha, medial aspect of the nucleus paragigantocellularis lateralis, parapyramidal nucleus, paraolivary nucleus, arcuate nucleus, and the lateral portions of B1 and B3 (Chan-Palay et al., 1978; Hökfelt et al., 1978; Johansson et al., 1981; Newman, 1985; Ciriello et al., 1988). Neurons of the parapyramidal region of the ventral medulla project to the intermediolateral cell column (IML) of the thoracic spinal cord (Loewy et al., 1981; Charlton and Helke, 1987; Hirsch and Helke, 1988) and to the nucleus of the solitary tract (NTS) (Loewy et al., 1981; Thor and Helke, 1987; Millhorn et al., 1987a). Activation of the parapyramidal region increases mean arterial blood pressure (Howe et al., 1983; Pilowsky et al., 1986b; Minson et al., 1987), an effect which is independent of the more laterally located C1 (rostral ventrolateral medulla) region (Minson et al., 1987).

Putative transmitters

Several putative neurotransmitter systems were demonstrated in the parapyramidal region of the ventral medulla. Many of the neurons contained serotonin (5-HT) and thus have been considered lateral extensions of B1 (and B3) neurons (Steinbusch, 1981; Loewy and McKellar, 1981; Skagerberg and Bjorklund, 1985). In addition, many of the neurons of the region contained immunoreactivity (ir) for neuropeptides, e.g. substance P (SP) (Ljungdahl et al., 1978; Marson and Loewy, 1985; Charlton and Helke, 1987), thyrotropin-releasing hormone (TRH) (Johansson et al., 1981; Bowker et al., 1982; Lechan et al., 1983; Hirsch and Helke, 1988), enkephalin (ENK) (Leger et al., 1986; Bowker et al., 1987; Millhorn et al., 1987a), cholecystokinin (Mantyh and Hunt, 1984), somatostatin (Bowker et al., 1987; Millhorn et al., 1987a), galanin (Skoftisch and Jacobowitz, 1985), proctolin (Holets et al., 1987), β-lipotropin (Hunt and Lovick, 1982), and human growth hormone (Lechan et al., 1983).

Transmitter-identified projections

For some transmitter-identified (SP, TRH, 5-HT, ENK) neurons, projections to the IML were

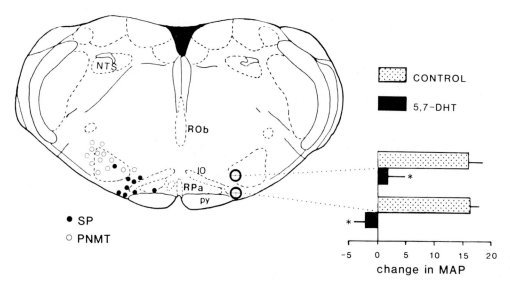

Fig. 1. Schematic of rat medulla oblongata. Left side of the medulla shows the distribution of SP-ir neurons in the parapyramidal region and PNMT-ir neurons in the RVL (Ross et al., 1984b; Charlton and Helke, 1987; Thor and Helke, 1987, 1988a; Milner et al., 1988). Serotonin-ir neurons have the same distribution as shown for SP. Right side of the medulla and the bar graph are adapted from the work of Minson and colleagues (1987). The sites of injection of L-glutamate (10 nmol) into the parapyramidal region of the ventral medulla are shown. The changes in MAP (mmHg) elicited at each injection site in both control and 5,7-DHT-treated rats are demonstrated in the bar graphs to the right. * Indicates statistically significant change in the MAP response in 5,7-DHT-treated rats compared to control rats. Abbreviations: 5,7-DHT = 5,7-dihydroxytryptamine; IO = inferior olive; PNMT = phenylethanolamine N-methyltransferase-ir (i.e. epinephrine-containing); py = pyramidal tract; MAP = mean arterial pressure; NTS = nucleus of the solitary tract; ROb = raphe obscurus; RPa = raphe pallidus.

demonstrated (Loewy and McKellar, 1981; Charlton and Helke, 1987; Hirsch and Helke, 1988; Sasek and Helke, 1989a; Sasek et al., 1988). Other transmitter-specific (e.g. proctolin, somatostatin, cholecystokinin) projections from the parapyramidal region to the spinal cord were demonstrated but specific termination sites were not determined (Mantyh and Hunt, 1984; Holets et al., 1987; Millhorn et al., 1987a,b). In addition, SP- and 5-HT-ir neurons projected from the parapyramidal region to the NTS (Thor and Helke, 1987, 1988; Thor et al., 1988b). Other transmitter-specific projections from the parapyramidal region are relatively unexplored.

SP- and TRH-ir projections to the IML
Ventral medullary SP- and TRH-ir projections to the IML were investigated using multiple approaches. Projections were initially studied using electrolytic lesions of the ventral medulla and

subsequent RIA of SP and TRH in microdissected IML (Helke et al., 1982, 1986). Changes in the SP and TRH content of the microdissected IML were determined following unilateral (left) lesions of the parapyramidal region at the level of the nucleus paragigantocellularis lateralis (PGCL) and at the level of the nucleus interfascicularis hypoglossi (NIH). Lesions of the left parapyramidal region, at either level (PGCL or NIH), reduced the TRH and SP contents of the left IML (Fig. 2). Lesions of the rostral midline raphe magnus did not significantly alter the IML content of SP or TRH (Fig. 2) (Helke et al., 1986).

Subsequently, bulbospinal SP- and TRH-ir projections to the IML were more directly studied using the retrograde transport of rhodamine-labelled latex microspheres (rhodamine beads) from the T3 IML combined with immunohistochemistry (Charlton and Helke, 1987; Hirsch and Helke, 1988). IML-projecting neurons which contained

SP- and TRH-ir (Fig. 3) were primarily found in the parapyramidal region, and in the midline medullary raphe pallidus and magnus (Charlton and Helke, 1987; Hirsch and Helke, 1988). There is also evidence for IML-projecting serotonergic neurons in the parapyramidal region. The loss of anterograde transport from the ventral medulla to the IML subsequent to destruction of serotonergic neurons with a neurotoxin suggested a ventral medullary serotonergic projection to the IML (Loewy and McKellar, 1981). Recently, we confirmed this finding and mapped the location of the cells in the parapyramidal region and the midline medullary raphe (Fig. 5B) by using retrograde transport of rhodamine beads from the IML combined with 5-HT immunocytochemistry. The IML-projecting 5-HT-ir neurons were found in the same sites as the IML-projecting SP-ir and TRH-ir neurons (Sasek et al., 1989).

ENK projections to the IML

Bulbospinal ENK-ir cells were previously demonstrated in the parapyramidal region and midline raphe pallidus (Hökfelt et al., 1979; Bowker et al., 1987; Menetery and Basbaum, 1987; Millhorn et al., 1987a). In addition, ENK-ir terminals were detected in the IML (Holets and Elde, 1982; Romagnano and Hamill, 1984; Krukoff, 1987). It was not known whether the ventral medullary or intraspinal neurons (Romagnano and Hamill, 1984) provided ENK-ir innervation of the IML. By combining retrograde transport of rhodamine beads and immunocytochemistry, we recently found that parapyramidal and midline raphe ENK-ir cells project to the IML (Sasek and Helke, 1989a).

SP and 5-HT projections to the NTS

Neurons of the parapyramidal region were also shown to project to the medial NTS (Thor and Helke, 1987). In addition, many of these projection neurons were SP-ir or 5-HT-ir (Fig. 4) (Thor and Helke, 1987). Thus, cells in the ventral medulla project to the NTS as well as to the IML, and the cells that project to each region are neurochemically similar.

Coexistence of putative neurotransmitters

Given the multiplicity of putative transmitters in cells of the parapyramidal region, it is not surprising that certain of the agents were colocalized in the same neuron. SP, TRH, ENK, and cholecystokinin were each found in ventral medullary serotonergic neurons (Johansson et al., 1981; Hunt

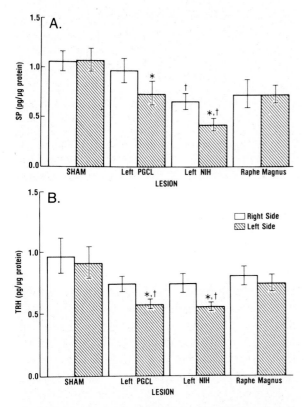

Fig. 2. Effect of ventral medullary lesions on the (A) substance P (SP) and (B) thyrotropin-releasing hormone (TRH) content of the IML. Electrolytic lesions were made in the left parapyramidal region at the level of the nucleus paragigantocellularis lateralis (PGCL), left parapyramidal region at the level of the nucleus interfascicularis hypoglossi (NIH), and in the midline raphe magnus of anesthetized rats. Two weeks later the rats were sacrificed and the content of SP and TRH determined in micropunch dissected samples of thoracic IML by RIA. * = $p < 0.05$ for paired comparisons with the right side of the same rats. † = $p < 0.05$ for grouped comparisons with the left side of sham-lesioned rats. (Adapted from Helke et al., 1986.)

and Lovick, 1982; Mantyh and Hunt, 1984; Sasek et al., 1989; Thor et al., 1988b). SP and TRH, and ENK and somatostatin were also colocalized (Johansson et al., 1981; Bowker, 1987; Millhorn et al., 1987a). However, there appears to be some heterogeneity in combinations of colocalized neurotransmitters. For example, SP was frequent-ly colocalized with 5-HT and TRH but was infre-quently colocalized with enkephalin (Johansson et al., 1981; Bowker, 1987; Sasek and Helke, 1989a). Thus, there may be multiple populations of 5-HT-ir cells (in addition to non-5-HT neurons) which colocalize SP and/or TRH, or ENK.

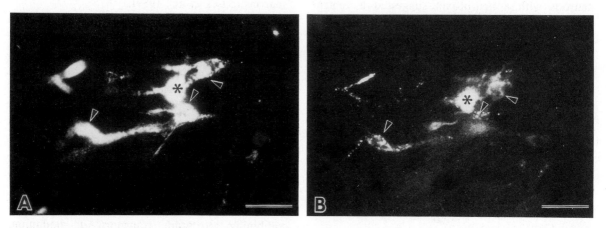

Fig. 3. Paired photomicrographs of neurons in the parapyramidal region at the level of the PGCL. Individual cells which are double labelled with rhodamine-labelled microspheres retrogradely transported from the IML (A) and with TRH immunocytochemistry (B) are indicated by single arrow heads. Asterisk in (B) indicates yellow "crossover" fluorescence from the extremely heavy rhodamine labelling seen in (A). Calibration bar = 50 μm. (Adapted from Hirsch and Helke, 1988.)

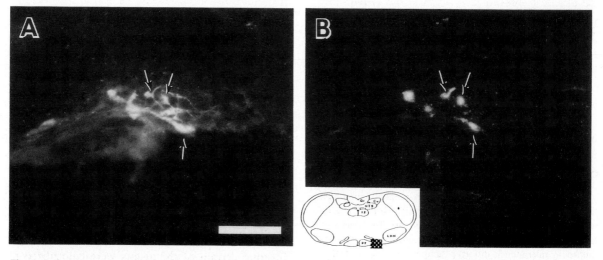

Fig. 4. Paired photomicrographs of neurons in the parapyramidal region at the level of the NIH. Individual cells which are double labelled with rhodamine-labelled microspheres retrogradely transported from the NTS (B) and with serotonin immunocytochemistry (A) are indicated by arrows. Field of view in (A) and (B) corresponds to the shaded area in inset of panel (B). Calibration bar = 150 μm. (Taken from Thor and Helke, 1987.)

Transmitter coexistence in parapyramidal neurons which project to the IML

Our initial work on coexistence of SP or TRH with serotonin in bulbospinal projections to the IML employed the approaches of serotonin neurotoxin-induced lesions and RIA of microdissected IML (Helke et al., 1982, 1986). The serotonin neurotoxin, 5,7-dihydroxytryptamine (5,7-DHT), depleted the serotonin content of the spinal cord, and reduced the TRH content of the IML by 45%. It did not significantly alter the SP content of the IML. However, the ventral horn content of TRH and SP was reduced by 92% and 42%, respectively, in 5,7-DHT-treated rats (Helke et al., 1986). Although indirect, these data suggested that whereas TRH co-exists with 5-HT in IML projections, SP may not. The question of TRH co-existence with SP could not be addressed by this approach.

More recently, co-existence in IML projections from the ventral medulla was studied with dual color immunohistochemistry combined with retrograde tracing. Multiple antigens were viewed in individual IML projecting cells (i.e. containing rhodamine beads retrogradely transported from T3-4 IML) by dual color immunofluorescence. Using primary antibodies from different species and secondary antisera coupled with either FITC (green) or 7-amino-4-methyl-coumarin-3-acetic acid (AMCA, blue), two antigens could be seen in a single projection specific neuron. A third antigen could be identified in the same neuron by comparing adjacent 4 μm sections.

Several combinations were found in IML-projecting neurons, i.e. SP and TRH; SP and 5-HT; SP, TRH and 5-HT (Sasek et al., 1989). These cells were found in the parapyramidal region and in the midline medullary raphe nuclei. Of the ventral medullary IML-projecting cells, the majority of SP- or TRH-ir neurons contained both peptides, many were also serotonergic. In addition, immunocytochemical studies of SP and TRH colocalization in terminals in the IML clearly showed their presence in both serotonergic and non-serotonergic terminals (Appel et al., 1986, 1987;

Wessendorf and Elde, 1987; Sasek and Helke, unpublished). Thus, the SP RIA data of microdissected IML following serotonin neurotoxin lesions were misleading. The RIA studies showed that the content of SP did not significantly decline in the IML following destruction of serotonin nerve terminals (Helke et al., 1982, 1986). We interpreted those data to suggest that SP was not present in serotonergic projections to the IML. However, the SP content of the IML arises from several sources besides ventral medullary neurons (some of which also contain 5-HT, some of which do not). SP-ir is also present in terminals of intraspinal neurons (Davis et al., 1984) and in SP-ir cell bodies in the IML (Krukoff et al., 1985). Thus, the SP-ir terminals and the cell bodies in the IML which remain after a 5,7-DHT lesion are likely to contribute to the SP content. Sprouting of remaining terminals may further maintain the SP content of the nucleus (Davis et al., 1984). In contrast, the TRH content of the IML, and both the SP and TRH contents of the ventral horn which arise largely from medullary sources, were significantly reduced after serotonin neurotoxin treatment (Helke et al., 1982, 1986).

Because of the similar localization of ENK cells with cells containing SP and/or 5-HT, coexistence of ENK with SP or 5-HT was of interest. However, we found that ENK rarely coexisted with SP in IML-projecting neurons of the ventral medulla or in terminals in the IML (Sasek and Helke, 1989a, unpublished). In addition, although ENK was occasionally colocalized with 5-HT (Leger et al., 1986; Sasek and Helke, unpublished), our preliminary studies suggest that the proportion of non-serotonergic ENK-ir cells was considerably higher (Sasek and Helke, unpublished). Thus, it appears that SP and ENK-ir projections to the IML from the ventral medulla are largely from separate groups of neurons.

Transmitter coexistence in parapyramidal neurons which project to the NTS

In the medial NTS, another nucleus that receives projections from the ventral medulla, we demonstrated the coexistence of SP and 5-HT in terminals (Thor et al., 1988a). The presence of both SP and 5-HT neuronal projections to the NTS from the parapyramidal region and from the midline raphe (Thor and Helke, 1987) prompted studies of the coexistence of SP and 5-HT in these NTS projections. 5-HT and SP-ir were visualized using dual color immunocytochemistry with AMCA- and FITC-conjugated secondary antibodies. NTS-projecting neurons were visualized in the ventral medulla by retrograde labelling with rhodamine beads following injection into the NTS. Extensive colocalization of 5-HT and SP-ir was seen in NTS projection neurons located in the parapyramidal region and the midline medullary raphe nuclei (Thor et al., 1988b).

Transmitter coexistence in RVL neurons which project to the IML

Although the primary focus of this work was not the more laterally located C1 area of the rostral ventrolateral medulla (RVL) (Ross et al., 1984a,b), the relationship to the more medially located IML-projecting neurons of the parapyramidal region was investigated. In retrograde transport and immunocytochemical studies, we found IML-projecting RVL cells which were ir for phenylethanolamine *N*-methyltransferase (PNMT) (presumably epinephrine-containing), neuropeptide Y, and much less frequently for ENK and SP (Sasek and Helke, 1989b). Whereas PNMT and neuropeptide Y were generally colocalized in IML-projecting neurons in the C1 area, neuropeptide Y-ir neurons of the C1 area only rarely colocalized SP (Sasek and Helke, 1989b). In addition, although an early study (Lorenz et al., 1985) suggested extensive colocalization of SP and PNMT in spinal cord-projecting neurons of the ventral medulla, subsequent studies (Pilowsky et al., 1986a; Milner et al., 1988) did not substantiate this coexistence.

These data suggest that IML-projecting ventral medullary neurons can be subdivided based on both their relative anatomic location (e.g. medially located SP/TRH/5-HT cells vs. laterally located

PNMT/neuropeptide Y cells), and within a region, by their putative neurotransmitters and patterns of coexistence (e.g. enkephalin vs. SP/TRH/5-HT).

Serotonin binding sites in the parapyramidal region

Central administration (including ventral medullary application) of serotonergic drugs produced significant cardiovascular effects (Fozard et al., 1987; McCall et al., 1987; Yoshioka et al., 1987; Gillis et al., 1989). In addition, activation of the 5-HT$_{1A}$ somatic autoreceptors suppressed the firing of ventral medullary sympathoexcitatory 5-HT neurons but did not affect non-5-HT neurons in the same region (McCall and Clement, 1989). Thus, we studied the presence, localization and subtypes of serotonin receptors in the ventral medulla (Thor et al., 1987).

In vitro light microscopic receptor autoradiography was used. Frozen sections of rat medulla were incubated with ^{3}H-5-HT (5 nM) to label 5-HT$_1$ sites, ^{3}H-8-OH-dipropyl-aminotetralin (^{3}H-8-OH-DPAT, 2 nM) to label 5-HT$_{1A}$ sites, ^{125}I-cyanopindolol (^{125}I-CYP) with 30 μM isoproterenol to label 5-HT$_{1B}$ sites, and ^{125}I-lysergic acid diethylamide (^{125}I-LSD, 1 nM) with domperidone to label 5-HT$_2$ sites. Non-specific binding of 5-HT$_1$ sites was assessed by adding 1 μM 5-HT to incubation buffers whereas non-specific binding of 5-HT$_2$ sites was assessed by adding 10 μM ketanserin to incubation buffers. Blocking experiments were conducted with 1 μM cold 8-OH-DPAT, 10 μM propranolol, or 10 μM chlorimipramine. Slides were apposed to ^{3}H-sensitive Ultrofilm.

High densities of serotonin binding sites were present in the ventral medulla. Dense and discretely localized 5-HT$_{1A}$ binding was present in the rostral (but not caudal) extent of the parapyramidal region and the midline raphe pallidus (Fig. 5A). 5-HT$_{1B}$ binding sites were present in the ventral medulla but their localization showed no particular association with the parapyramidal region (Fig. 5D). Very little 5-HT$_2$ binding was present in

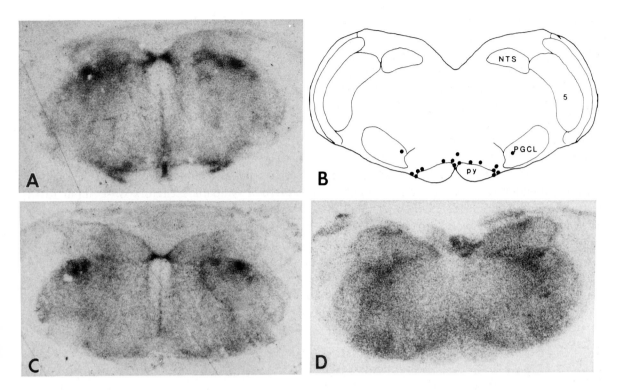

Fig. 5. (A) Autoradiogram of 5-HT$_{1A}$ binding sites in the rat medulla labelled with ^{3}H-8-OH-DPAT (2 nM). (B) Schematic of the same level of the rat medulla shown in (A) (C) and (D). Dots represent location of 5-HT-ir cells which project to the IML. The IML-projecting cells were retrogradely labelled with rhodamine beads (40 nl) and stained for 5-HT-ir (Sasek et al., 1989). (C) Autoradiogram of 5-HT$_{1A}$ binding sites in the medulla of a rat pretreated with 5,7-DHT 2 weeks prior to sacrifice (200 μg i.c.v. followed in 2 days with 200 μg i.c.). (D) Autoradiogram of 5-HT$_{1B}$ binding sites in rat medulla labelled with ^{125}I-CYP (50 pM plus 30 μM isoproterenol). Abbreviations: 5 = spinal trigeminal nucleus; NTS = nucleus of the solitary tract; PGCL = nucleus paragigantocellularis lateralis; py = pyramidal tract. (From Thor et al., 1989.)

the medulla.

Because the 5-HT$_{1A}$ labelling was coincident with the distribution of serotonergic neurons and because of evidence for 5-HT$_{1A}$ somatic autoreceptors in the ventral medulla (McCall and Clement, 1989), we evaluated the effect of the serotonin neurotoxin, 5,7-DHT, on serotonin binding in the medulla. Desmethylimipramine-pretreated rats were injected twice with 5,7-DHT (200 μg free base in 0.01% ascorbic acid) or vehicle. The first injection was i.c.v., the second was intracisternal two days later. As shown in Fig. 5A,C, the 5-HT$_{1A}$ binding sites in the ventral medulla were significantly reduced in animals treated with 5,7-DHT. The anatomic association

of these sites with serotonergic cell body areas and the reduction seen with the serotonin neurotoxin are consistent with the hypothesis that these sites are somatic autoreceptors.

Discussion

These studies on the chemical neuroanatomy of the neurons of the parapyramidal region provide further evidence for the significance of the region in neural regulation of the cardiovascular system. Neurons of the parapyramidal region project to two cardiovascular control sites, the IML and the NTS. In addition, the neurons contain various putative neurotransmitters (e.g. SP, TRH, 5-HT,

24

ENK) that were shown to alter preganglionic neuronal activity (Gilbey et al., 1983; McCall, 1983; Backman and Henry, 1984; Ma and Dun, 1986; Dun and Mo, 1988) and cardiovascular function (Howe et al., 1983; Keeler et al., 1985; Helke et al., 1987b; Helke and Phillips, 1988; Li et al., 1988; Solomon and Gebhart, 1988).

Classical studies by several investigators (reviewed by Ciriello et al., 1986) showed that exposure of the ventral surface of the medulla to various excitatory and inhibitory drugs, alterations in pCO_2, electrical stimulation or focal cooling, resulted in marked changes in cardiovascular function. These perturbations, no doubt, affected the parapyrami-

dal neurons since they are superficially located on or near the ventral surface of the medulla at the appropriate rostrocaudal level of the medulla. Furthermore, based upon their location, their direct projections to the thoracic IML and NTS, and their content of putative sympathoregulatory transmitters, it is likely that many of the cardiovascular effects elicited from ventral medullary surface perturbations are mediated by the parapyramidal region neurons. Evidence in support of a sympathoexcitatory SP-ir input to the IML from the parapyramidal region was provided by the finding that sympathoexcitatory responses elicited from ventral medulla application of

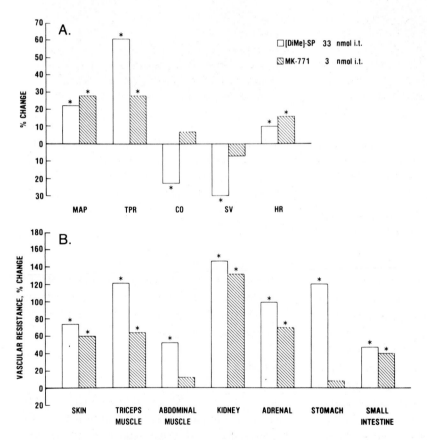

Fig. 6. Comparison of (A) cardiovascular responses and (B) regional vascular resistance responses to intrathecal injection of similar pressor doses of a SP agonist [pGlu[5], MePhe[8], MeGly[9]]-substance $P_{(5-11)}$ ([DiMe]-SP) (33 nmol), and a TRH agonist, MK-771 (3 nmol, 1 μg). Data are presented as percent change, actual values and S.E.M. are presented for each agonist in separate publications (Helke et al., 1987b; Helke and Phillips, 1988). * = $p < 0.05$ comparing agonist response to vehicle-control response. Abbreviations: CO = cardiac output; HR = heart rate; MAP = mean arterial pressure; SV = stroke volume; TPR = total peripheral resistance.

bicuculline or kainic acid (Loewy and Sawyer, 1982; Keeler and Helke, 1985) were attenuated by the application to the spinal cord of substance P antagonists. However, because intrathecal administration of SP antagonists did not reduce total peripheral resistance (Helke et al., 1987a), the SP input to the IML appears not to be involved in tonic maintenance of arterial vasomotor tone. The parapyramidal region also appears to be important in mediating the hypotensive effects of $5\text{-}HT_{1A}$ agonist drugs at the ventral surface of the medulla (Gillis et al., 1989), as indicated by the extremely dense concentration of $5\text{-}HT_{1A}$ sites associated with parapyramidal neurons (Fig. 5). The IML- and/or NTS-projecting parapyramidal neurons containing $5\text{-}HT_{1A}$ binding sites may be clinically important as sites of action for the antihypertensive effects of $5\text{-}HT_{1A}$ agonists (Fozard et al., 1987; McCall et al., 1987). Thus, although the parapyramidal region probably plays a modulatory role in cardiovascular regulation [in contrast to the tonic sympathoexcitatory pacemaker role of the RVL (Ross et al., 1984a; Sun et al., 1981)], it is nonetheless of considerable importance in the neural regulation of the cardiovascular system.

When the numerous putative neurotransmitters and combinations of transmitters in IML- and NTS-projecting neurons are considered, it becomes apparent that the modulation of sympathetic activity by the parapyramidal region may be quite complex. Considering the subtle differences found between the cardiovascular and regional hemodynamic effects of SP and TRH when each is administered intrathecally (Fig. 6), the possibility of intricate and selective modulatory influences becomes likely. Furthermore, frequency-dependent differential release of colocalized transmitters (Lundberg and Hökfelt, 1983) and differences in afferent and/or efferent connections of specific parapyramidal neurons would allow for a very sophisticated level of modulation of sympathetic activity.

In summary, the parapyramidal region of the ventral medulla is a neurochemically complex group of cells which projects to cardiovascular-related CNS nuclei and which affects sympathetic activity to the cardiovascular system. The importance of this neurochemical complexity in either discrete regulation or refinement of sympathetic activity to specific vascular beds and/or the heart remains to be determined.

Acknowledgements

This work was supported by NIH grants NS24876 and NS20991 to C.J.H. NRSA fellowship awards supported K.B.T. (NS08084) and C.A.S. (HL07565).

References

Appel, N.M., Wessendorf, M.W. and Elde, R. (1986) Coexistence of serotonin- and substance P-like immunoreactivity in nerve fibers apposing identified sympathoadrenal preganglionic neurons in the intermediolateral cell column. *Neurosci. Lett.*, 65: 241–246.

Appel, N.M., Wessendorf, M.W. and Elde, R. (1987) Thyrotropin-releasing hormone in spinal cord: coexistence with serotonin and with substance P in fibers and terminals apposing identified preganglionic sympathetic neurons. *Brain Res.*, 415: 137–143.

Backman, S.B. and Henry, J.L. (1984) Effects of substance P and thyrotropin-releasing hormone on sympathetic neurons in the upper thoracic intermediolateral nucleus of the cat. *Can. J. Physiol. Pharmacol.*, 62: 248–251.

Bowker, R.M. (1987) Evidence for the co-localization of somatostatin- and methionine-enkephalin-like immunoreactivities in raphe and gigantocellularis nuclei. *Neurosci. Lett.*, 81: 75–81.

Bowker, R.M., Westlund, K.N., Sullivan, M.C., Welber, J.F. and Coulter, J.D. (1982) Transmitters of the raphe-spinal complex: immunocytochemical studies. *Peptides*, 3: 291–298.

Bowker, R.M., Reddy, V.K., Fung, S.J., Chan, J.Y.H. and Barnes, C.D. (1987) Serotonergic and non-serotonergic raphe neurons projecting to the feline lumbar and cervical spinal cord: a quantitative horseradish peroxidase-immunohistochemical study. *Neurosci. Lett.*, 75: 31–37.

Chan-Palay, V., Jonsson, G. and Palay, S.L. (1978) Serotonin and substance P coexist in neurons of the cat's central nervous system. *Proc. Natl. Acad. Sci. U.S.A.*, 75: 1582–1586.

Charlton, C.G. and Helke, C.J. (1987) Substance P-containing medullary projections to the intermediolateral cell column: identification with retrogradely transported rhodamine-labeled latex microspheres and immunohistochemistry. *Brain*

26

Res., 418: 245 – 254.

Ciriello, J., Caverson, M.M. and Polosa, C. (1986) Function of the ventrolateral medulla in the control of the circulation. Brain Res. Rev., 11: 359 – 391.

Ciriello, J., Caverson, M.M., Calaresu, F.R. and Krukoff, T.L. (1988) Neuropeptide and serotonin immunoreactive neurons in the cat ventrolateral medulla. Brain Res., 440: 53 – 66.

Davis, B.M., Krause, J.E., McKelvy, J.F. and Cabot, J.B. (1984) Effects of spinal lesions on substance P levels in the rat sympathetic preganglionic cell column: evidence for local spinal regulation. Neuroscience, 13: 1311 – 1316.

Dun, N.J. and Mo, N. (1988) In vitro effects of substance P on neonatal rat sympathetic preganglionic neurones. J. Physiol., 399: 321 – 333.

Egan, T.M. and North, R.A. (1981) Both mu and delta opiate receptors exist on the same neuron. Science, 214: 923 – 924.

Fozard, J.R., Mir, A.K. and Middlemiss, D.N. (1987) Cardiovascular responses to 8-hydroxy-2-(di-n-propyl-amino)tetralin (8-OH-DPAT) in the rat: site of action and pharmacologic analysis. J. Cardiovasc. Pharmacol., 9: 328 – 347.

Gilbey, M.P., McKenna, K. and Schramm, L.P. (1983) Effects of substance P on sympathetic preganglionic neurons. Neurosci. Lett., 41: 157 – 159.

Gillis, R.A., Hill, K., Kirby, J.S., Quest, J.A., Hamosh, P., Norman, W.P. and Kellar, K.J. (1989) Effect of activation of CNS serotonin 1A receptors on cardiorespiratory function. J. Pharmacol. Exp. Ther., 248: 851 – 857.

Helke, C.J. and Phillips, E.T. (1988) Thyrotropin-releasing hormone receptor activation in the spinal cord increases blood pressure and sympathetic tone to the vasculature and adrenals. J. Pharmacol. Exp. Ther., 245: 41 – 46.

Helke, C.J., Neil, J.J., Massari, V.J. and Loewy, A.D. (1982) Substance P neurons project from the ventral medulla to the intermediolateral cell column and ventral horn in the rat. Brain Res., 243: 147 – 152.

Helke, C.J., Sayson, S.C., Keeler, J.R. and Charlton, C.G. (1986) Thyrotropin-releasing hormone neurons project from the ventral medulla to the intermediolateral cell column: partial coexistence with serotonin. Brain Res., 381: 1 – 7.

Helke, C.J., Phillips, E.T. and O'Neill, J.T. (1987a) Intrathecal administration of a substance P receptor antagonist: studies on peripheral and CNS hemodynamics and on specificity of action. J. Pharmacol. Exp. Ther., 242: 131 – 136.

Helke, C.J., Phillips, E.T. and O'Neill, J.T. (1987b) Regional peripheral and CNS hemodynamic effects of intrathecal administration of a substance P receptor agonist. J. Auton. Nerv. Syst., 21: 1 – 7.

Hirsch, M.D. and Helke, C.J. (1988) Bulbospinal thyrotropin-releasing hormone projections to the intermediolateral cell column: a double fluorescence immunohistochemical-retrograde tracing study. Neuroscience, 25: 625 – 637.

Hökfelt, T., Ljungdahl, A., Steinbusch, H., Verhofstad, A., Nilsson, G., Brodin, E., Pernow, B. and Goldstein, M. (1978) Immunohistochemical evidence of substance P-like immunoreactivity in some 5-hydroxytryptamine-containing neurons in the rat central nervous system. Neuroscience, 3: 517 – 538.

Hökfelt, T., Terenius, L., Kuypers, H.G.J.M. and Dann, O. (1979) Evidence for enkephalin immunoreactive neurons in the medulla oblongata projecting to the spinal cord. Neurosci. Lett., 14: 55 – 60.

Holets, V. and Elde, R. (1982) The differential relationship of serotonergic and peptidergic fibers to sympathoadrenal neurons in the intermediolateral cell column of the rat: a combined retrograde axonal transport and immunofluorescence study. Neuroscience, 7: 1155 – 1174.

Holets, V., Hökfelt, T., Ude, J., Eckert, M., Penzlin, H., Verhofstad, A.A.J. and Visser, T.J. (1987) A comparative study of the immunohistochemical localization of a presumptive proctolin-like peptide, thyrotropin-releasing hormone and 5-hydroxytryptamine in the rat central nervous system. Brain Res., 408: 141 – 153.

Howe, P.R.C., Kuhn, D.M., Minson, J.B., Stead, B.H. and Chalmers, J.P. (1983) Evidence for a bulbospinal serotonergic pressor pathway in the rat brain. Brain Res., 270: 29 – 36.

Hunt, S.P. and Lovick, T.A. (1982) The distribution of serotonin, met-enkephalin and beta-lipotropin-like immunoreactivity in neuronal perikarya of the cat brain. Neurosci. Lett., 30: 139 – 145.

Johansson, O., Hökfelt, T., Pernow, B., Jeffcoate, S.L., White, N., Steinbusch, H.W.M., Verhofstad, A.A.J., Emson, P.C. and Spindel, E. (1981) Immunohistochemical support for three putative transmitters in one neuron: coexistence of 5-hydroxytryptamine, substance P- and thyrotropin-releasing hormone-like immunoreactivity in medullary neurons projecting to the spinal cord. Neuroscience, 6: 1857 – 1881.

Keeler, J.R. and Helke, C.J. (1985) Spinal cord substance P mediates bicuculline-induced activation of cardiovascular responses from the ventral medulla. J. Auton. Nerv. Syst., 13: 19 – 34.

Keeler, J.R., Shults, C.W., Chase, T.N. and Helke, C.J. (1984) The ventral surface of the medulla in the rat: pharmacologic and autoradiographic localization of GABA-induced cardiovascular effects. Brain Res., 297: 217 – 224.

Keeler, J.R., Charlton, C.G. and Helke, C.J. (1985) Cardiovascular effects of spinal cord substance P: studies with a stable receptor agonist. J. Pharmacol. Exp. Ther., 233: 755 – 760.

Krukoff, T.L. (1987) Peptidergic inputs to sympathetic preganglionic neurons. Can. J. Physiol. Pharmacol., 65: 1619 – 1623.

Krukoff, T.L., Ciriello, J. and Calaresu, F.R. (1985) Segmental distribution of peptide-like immunoreactivity in cell bodies of the thoracolumbar sympathetic nucleus of the cat. *J. Comp. Neurol.*, 240: 90 – 102.

Lechan, R.M., Molitch, M.E. and Jackson, I. (1983) Distribution of immunoreactive human growth hormone-like material and thyrotropin-releasing hormone in the rat central nervous system: evidence for their coexistence in the same neuron. *Endocrinology*, 112: 877 – 884.

Leger, L., Charnay, Y., Dubois, P. and Jouvet, M. (1986) Distribution of enkephalin-immunoreactive cell bodies in relation to serotonin-containing neurons in the raphe nuclei of the cat: immunohistochemical evidence for coexistence of enkephalin and serotonin in certain cells. *Brain Res.*, 362: 63 – 73.

Li, S.-J., Zhang, X. and Ingenito, A.J. (1988) Depressor and bradycardic effects induced by spinal subarachnoid injection of D-Ala^2-D-Leu^5-enkephalin in rats. *Neuropeptides*, 12: 81 – 88.

Ljungdahl, A., Hökfelt, T. and Nilsson, G. (1978) Distribution of substance P-like immunoreactivity in the central nervous system of the rat. I. Cell bodies and nerve terminals. *Neuroscience*, 3: 861 – 944.

Loeschke, H.H., Lattre, J. de, Schlaefke, M.E. and Trouth, C.L. (1970) Effects on respiration and circulation of electrically stimulating the ventral surface of the medulla oblongata. *Respir. Physiol.*, 10: 184 – 197.

Loewy, A.D. and McKellar, S. (1981) Serotonergic projections from the ventral medulla to the intermediolateral cell column in the rat. *Brain Res.*, 211: 146 – 152.

Loewy, A.D. and Sawyer, W.B. (1982) Substance P antagonist inhibits vasomotor responses elicieted from ventral medulla in rat. *Brain Res.*, 245: 379 – 383.

Loewy, A.D., Wallach, J.H. and McKellar, S. (1981) Efferent connections of the ventral medulla oblongata in the rat. *Brain Res. Rev.*, 3: 63 – 80.

Lorenz, R.G., Saper, C.B., Wong, D.L., Ciarenello, R.D. and Loewy, A.D. (1985) Co-localization of substance P and phenylethanolamine-*N*-methyltransferase-like immunoreactivity in neurons of ventrolateral medulla that project to the spinal cord: potential role in control of vasomotor tone. *Neurosci. Lett.*, 55: 255 – 260.

Lundberg, J.M. and Hökfelt, T. (1983) Coexistence of peptides and classical neurotransmitters. *Trends Neurosci.*, 6: 325 – 332.

Ma, R.C. and Dun, N.J. (1986) Excitation of lateral horn neurons of the neonatal spinal cord by 5-hydroxytryptamine. *Dev. Brain Res.*, 24: 89 – 98.

Mantyh, P.W. and Hunt, S.P. (1984) Evidence for cholecystokinin-like immunoreactive neurons in the rat medulla oblongata which project to the spinal cord. *Brain Res.*, 291: 49 – 54.

Marson, L. and Loewy, A.D. (1985) Topographic organization of substance P and monoamine cells in the ventral medulla of the cat. *J. Auton. Nerv. Syst.*, 14: 271 – 285.

McCall, R.B. (1983) Serotonergic excitation of sympathetic

preganglionic neurons: a microiontophoretic study. *Brain Res.*, 289: 121 – 127.

McCall, R.B. and Clement, M.E. (1989) Identification of serotonergic and sympathetic neurons in medullary raphe nuclei. *Brain Res.*, 477: 172 – 182.

McCall, R.B., Patel, B.N. and Harris, L.T. (1987) Effect of serotonin, and serotonin$_2$ receptor agonists and antagonists on blood pressure, heart rate and sympathetic nerve activity. *J. Pharmacol. Exp. Ther.*, 242: 1152 – 1159.

Menetery, D. and Basbaum, A.I. (1987) The distribution of substance P-, enkephalin- and dynorphin-immunoreactive neurons in the medulla of the rat and their contribution to bulbospinal pathways. *Neuroscience*, 23: 173 – 187.

Millhorn, D.E., Seroogy, K., Hökfelt, T., Schmued, L.C., Terenius, L., Buchan, A. and Brown, J.C. (1987a) Neurons of the ventral medulla oblongata that contain both somatostatin and enkephalin immunoreactivities project to nucleus tractus solitarius and spinal cord. *Brain Res.*, 424: 99 – 108.

Millhorn, D.E., Hökfelt, T., Seroogy, K., Oertel, W., Verhofstad, A.A.J. and Wu, J.-Y. (1987b) Immunohistochemical evidence for colocalization of gamma-amino butyric acid and serotonin in neurons of the ventral medulla oblongata projecting to the spinal cord. *Brain Res.*, 410: 179 – 185.

Milner, T.A., Pickel, V.M., Abate, C., Joh, T.H. and Reis, D.J. (1988) Ultrastructural characterization of substance P-like immunoreactive neurons in the rostral ventrolateral medulla in relation to neurons containing catecholamine-synthesizing enzymes. *J. Comp. Neurol.*, 270: 427 – 445.

Minson, J.B., Chalmers, J.P., Caon, A.C. and Renaud, B. (1987) Separate areas of rat medulla oblongata with populations of serotonin- and adrenaline-containing neurons alter blood pressure after L-glutamate stimulation. *J. Auton. Nerv. Syst.*, 19: 39 – 50.

Newman, D.B. (1985) Distinguishing rat brainstem reticulospinal nuclei by their neuronal morphology. I. Medullary nuclei. *J. Hirnforsch.* 26: 187 – 226.

Pilowsky, P., Minson, J., Hodgson, A., Howe, P. and Chalmers, J. (1986a) Does substance P coexist with adrenaline in neurones of the rostral ventrolateral medulla in the rat? *Neurosci. Lett.*, 71: 293 – 298.

Pilowsky, P., Kapoor, V., Minson, J.B., West, M.J. and Chalmers, J.P. (1986b) Spinal cord serotonin release and raised blood pressure after brainstem kainic acid injection. *Brain Res.*, 366: 354 – 357.

Romagnano, M.A. and Hamill, R.W. (1984) Spinal sympathetic pathway: an enkephalin ladder. *Science*, 225: 737 – 739.

Ross, C.A., Ruggiero, D.A., Park, D.H., Joh, T.H., Sved, A.F., Fernandez-Pardal, J., Saavedra, J.M. and Reis, D.J. (1984a) Tonic vasomotor control by the rostral ventrolateral medulla: effect of electrical or chemical stimulation of the area containing C$_1$ adrenaline neurons on arterial pressure, heart rate, and plasma catecholamines and vasopressin. *J.*

Neurosci., 4: 474 – 494.

Ross, C.A., Ruggiero, D.A., Joh, T.H., Park, D.H. and Reis, D.J. (1984b) Rostral ventrolateral medulla: selective projections to the thoracic autonomic cell column from the region containing C_1 adrenaline neurons. *J. Comp. Neurol.*, 228: 168 – 185.

Sasek, C.A. and Helke, C.J. (1989a) Medullary enkephalin-immunoreactive neuronal projections to the intermediolateral cell column: relationship to substance P-immunoreactive neurons. *J. Comp. Neurol.* (in press).

Sasek, C.A. and Helke, C.J. (1989b) Differential coexistence of substance P-immunoreactivity with other neurochemicals in intermediolateral cell column-projecting neurons in the ventral medulla oblongata. *Soc. Neurosci. Abst.* (in press).

Sasek, C.A., Wessendorf, M. and Helke, C.J. (1989) Evidence for coexistence of thyrotropin-releasing hormone, substance P, and serotonin in ventral medullary neurons that project to the intermediolateral cell column in the rat. *Neuroscience* (in press).

Skagerberg, G. and Bjorklund, A. (1985) Topographic principles in the spinal projections of serotonergic and non-serotonergic brainstem neurons in the rat. *Neuroscience*, 15: 445 – 480.

Skoftisch, G. and Jacobowitz, D.M. (1985) Immunohistochemical mapping of galanin-like neurons in the rat central nervous system. *Peptides*, 6: 509 – 546.

Solomon, R.E. and Gebhart, G.F. (1988) Mechanisms of effects of intrathecal serotonin on nociception and blood pressure. *J. Pharmacol. Exp. Ther.*, 245: 905 – 912.

Steinbusch, H.W.M. (1981) Distribution of serotonin-immunoreactivity in the central nervous system of the rat. Cell bodies and terminals. *Neuroscience*, 6: 557 – 618.

Sun, M.K., Young, B.S., Hackett, J.T. and Guyenet, P.G. (1988) Reticulospinal pacemaker neurons of the rat rostral ventrolateral medulla with putative sympathoexcitatory function: an intracellular study in vitro. *Brain Res.*, 442: 229 – 239.

Thor, K.B. and Helke, C.J. (1987) Serotonin and substance P-containing projections to the nucleus tractus solitarii of the rat. *J. Comp. Neurol.*, 265: 275 – 293.

Thor, K.B. and Helke, C.J. (1988) Catecholamine-synthesizing neuronal projections to the nucleus tractus solitarii in the rat. *J. Comp. Neurol.*, 268: 264 – 280.

Thor, K.B., Blitz, A. and Helke, C.J. (1987) Analysis of serotonergic receptor subtypes in autonomic regions of the rat medulla using quantitative autoradiographic techniques. *Soc. Neurosci. Abst.*, 13: 1128.

Thor, K.B., Hill, K.M., Harrod, C. and Helke, C.J. (1988a) Immunohistochemical and biochemical analysis of serotonin and substance P colocalization in the nucleus tractus solitarii and associated afferent ganglia of the rat. *Synapse*, 2: 225 – 231.

Thor, K.B., Hill, K., Harrod, C. and Helke, C.J. (1988b) An immunohistochemical and biochemical analysis of serotonin and substance P colocalization in nucleus tractus solitarius-afferent projections in the rat. *Soc. Neurosci. Abst.*, 14: 356.

Thor, K.B., Blitz-Siebert, A. and Helke, C.J. (1989) Discrete localization of high density 5-HT_{1A} binding sites in the midline raphe and parapyramidal region of the ventral medulla oblongata of the rat. *Neurosci. Lett.* (in press).

Wessendorf, M.W. and Elde, R. (1987) The coexistence of serotonin and substance P-like immunoreactivity in the spinal cord of the rat as shown by immunofluorescent double labeling. *J. Neurosci.*, 7: 2352 – 2363.

Yoshioka, M., Matsumoto, M., Togashi, H., Minami, M. and Saito, H. (1987) Central sympathoinhibitory actions of ketanserin in rats. *J. Pharmacol. Exp. Ther.*, 243: 1174 – 1178.

J. Ciriello, M.M. Caverson and C. Polosa (Eds.)
Progress in Brain Research, Vol. 81
© 1989 Elsevier Science Publishers B.V. (Biomedical Division)

CHAPTER 3

Adrenergic neurons in the rostral ventrolateral medulla: ultrastructure and synaptic relations with other transmitter-identified neurons

Teresa A. Milner, Virginia M. Pickel, Shaun F. Morrison and Donald J. Reis

Division of Neurobiology, Department of Neurology and Neuroscience, Cornell University Medical College, 411 East 69th Street, New York, NY 10021, U.S.A.

Introduction

The adrenergic neurons of the C1 group in the rostral ventrolateral medulla (RVL) have been identified immunocytochemically by the presence of the adrenaline-synthesizing enzyme, phenylethanolamine *N*-methyltransferase (PNMT) (Hökfelt et al., 1974; Kalia et al., 1985a,b; Ruggiero et al., 1985b). Neurons of the C1 area project extensively to the thoracolumbar spinal cord where they terminate exclusively within autonomic nuclei of the intermediolateral (IML) and intermediomedial cell columns (Ross et al., 1981, 1984a). In addition, C1 adrenergic neurons project to the A6 noradrenergic cell group of the locus coeruleus (LC) (Aston-Jones et al., 1986), a region with diverse efferent projections throughout the brain and spinal cord (see Saper, 1987 for review).

Sympathoexcitatory neurons located within the C1 region of the RVL play an essential role in the maintenance of tonic (resting) and reflex control of arterial pressure (AP) and in the initiation of cardiovascular responses to cerebral ischemia (for review see Ciriello et al., 1986). The results of physiological investigations suggest that the adrenergic neurons of the C1 group are among the RVL neurons responsible for mediating vasomotor control (Reis et al., 1988). In particular, the medullary region with the densest population of

adrenergic neurons (1) contains neurons with electrophysiological characteristics of cardiovascular neurons (Brown and Guyenet, 1984; Morrison et al., 1988); (2) is the most sensitive zone within the medulla from which electrical or chemical stimulation elevates AP (Ross et al., 1984b); and (3) is the site wherein electrolytic lesions or chemical inactivation of neurons results in a collapse of AP (Granata et al., 1983; 1985; Ross et al., 1984b).

This hypothesis has been substantiated by recent anatomic experiments (Cravo et al., 1988) involving dual labelling for PNMT and retrogradely transported horseradish peroxidase (HRP) which indicate that approximately two-thirds of the PNMT-containing neurons in the RVL project to the thoracic spinal cord. Furthermore, the subpopulation of C1 adrenergic neurons projecting to the LC is distinct from that innervating the IML (Pieribone et al., 1988). Thus, the majority of adrenergic neurons of the C1 group appear to be involved in either regulation of cardiovascular function through their influence on IML neurons or regulation of arousal or attention (see Saper, 1987 for review) through their projection to LC neurons.

The cellular basis for the complex interactions among adrenergic neurons, non-adrenergic neurons and glia of the RVL that may mediate some of the physiological actions, as well as the influence of

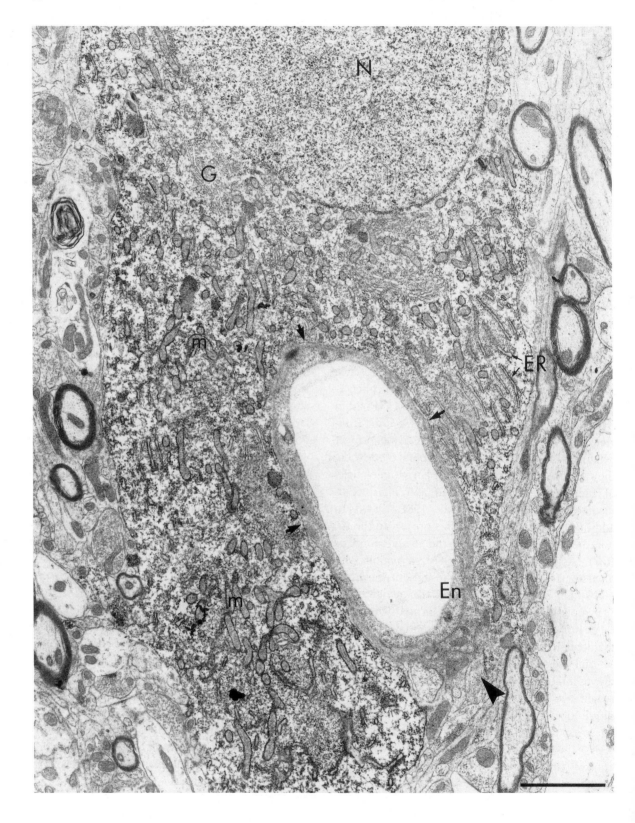

adrenergic projections to the targets of C1 neurons, are now begining to be resolved by electron microscopy using dual labelling immunocytochemical methods. In the first portion of this chapter, we summarize the ultrastructural characteristics of (1) C1 adrenergic neurons in the rostral ventrolateral medulla and (2) adrenergic terminals in their target regions in the IML of the spinal cord and in the locus coeruleus. These studies show that C1 neurons exhibit specialized features such as high mitochondrial content and associations with capillaries and glia. In addition, they suggest a specific functional distribution of adrenergic terminals on sympathetic preganglionic neurons of the IML and on LC neurons. In the second portion of the chapter, we summarize the synaptic relationships within the RVL between axon terminals and perikarya and dendrites containing PNMT, γ-aminobutyric acid, substance P, opiates and acetylcholine. The relevance of the specific transmitters in relation to the C1 neurons is described and correlations with their known cardiovascular effects in the RVL are discussed.

Ultrastructure of C1 adrenergic neurons and their terminals

Adrenergic neurons in the RVL

Several studies have described the topographic distribution of the C1 neurons and their projections (Hökfelt et al., 1974; Kalia et al., 1985a,b; Ruggiero et al., 1985b). Moreover, the ultrastructure and synaptic connections of these cells have recently been examined (Milner et al., 1987a) using the peroxidase-antiperoxidase (PAP) method of Sternberger (1979) as modified by Pickel (1981) to localize a polyclonal antibody to PNMT (Joh and Goldstein, 1973; Joh and Ross, 1983) by electron microscopy. We have shown a characteristic ultrastructure of the PNMT-labelled neurons and particular relationships with the cerebral vasculature consistent with their postulated role in cardiovascular regulation and the cerebral ischemic response.

The PNMT-labelled perikarya are large (20 – 30 μm) and have an indented nucleus with a single nucleolus. Mitochondria are the most numerous organelles within the abundant cytoplasm. The labelled cytoplasm of these perikarya has an average of 136 $\pm$ 11.6 mitochondria per 100 μm^2; this is 38% greater than the number found in the cytoplasm of similarly labelled neurons in the nucleus of the solitary tract. The cytoplasm also contains rough endoplasmic reticulum, Golgi apparatus, lysosomes, dense core and coated vesicles (Fig. 1). PNMT-containing dendrites range from small (0.3 – 0.6 μm) to large (1.0 – 2.4 μm), with the largest lying closest to the somata. The labelled dendrites also contain numerous mitochondria. Only a few axons and axon terminals containing immunoreactivity for PNMT are observed. The axons are both myelinated and unmyelinated. The PNMT-containing terminals are characterized by a few mitochondria, numerous small (25 – 55 nm) clear vesicles and 1 – 10 large dense-core vesicles.

The PNMT-labelled somata and dendrites are often found in direct apposition to the basement membrane of small capillaries. Moreover, the labelled perikarya and dendrites often are closely apposed to satellite cells (supporting astrocytes). In some cases the labelled neuronal perikarya almost completely encapsulate the endothelial cells of the capillaries making the intervening astrocytic processes difficult to differentiate (Fig. 1). Both the PNMT-labelled perikarya and dendrites receive synaptic contacts primarily from unlabelled axon terminals. The terminals form mostly symmetric

Fig. 1. Adrenergic neurons in the RVL. Low magnification electron micrograph of a PNMT-labelled perikarya which almost completely encircles a small capillary (small arrows) except for a small region (arrowhead). The astrocytic processes separating the basement membrane of the endothelial cell (En) from the immunoreactive perikarya are difficult to distinguish. ER = rough endoplasmic reticulum; G = Golgi apparatus; m = mitochondria; N = nucleus. Bar = 2.0 μm. (Reprinted by permission from Milner et al., 1986a.)

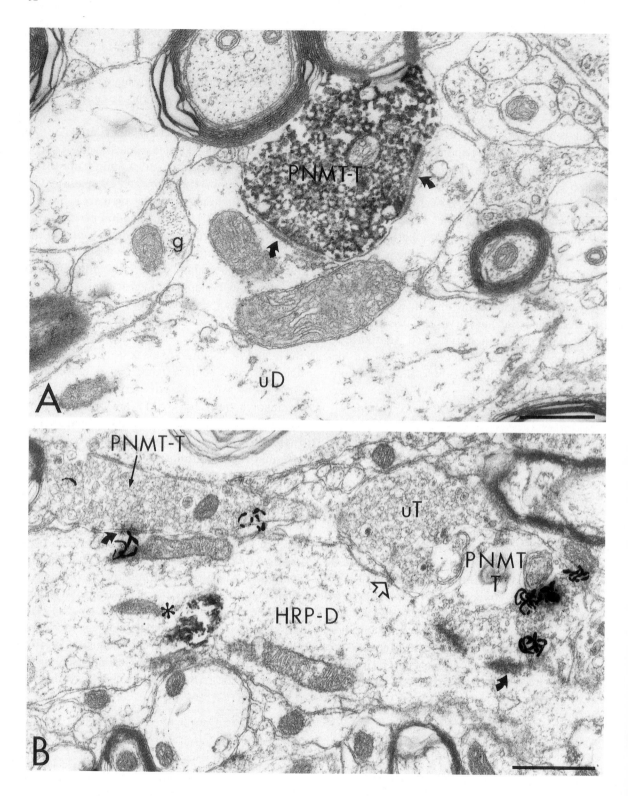

synapses with the somata and both asymmetric and symmetric junctions with the labelled dendrites and dendritic spines. Many times the PNMT-labelled perikarya and dendrites as well as their presynaptic terminals are surrounded by glial processes.

The PNMT-immunoreactive terminals form primarily symmetric synaptic junctions with unlabelled dendrites. Occasionally, PNMT-labelled terminals contact other PNMT-containing perikarya and dendrites. In these instances, the synaptic junctions appear symmetric. Asymmetric (Gray type I) synapses are believed to mediate excitation based largely on the detection of enriched populations of thickened postsynaptic densities in regions of the brain containing higher proportions of excitatory synapses; similarly, symmetric (Gray type II) synapses are believed to mediate inhibition (Uchizono, 1965; Cohen et al., 1982).

Several functional implications can be inferred from these observations. First, the relatively high density of mitochondria and proximity to blood vessels and glia suggest a high metabolic activity and possibly a chemosensory function of PNMT-containing neurons in the RVL. Second, the existence of myelinated and unmyelinated axons could imply that PNMT-containing neurons have different conduction velocities in efferent pathways to the spinal cord or locus coeruleus. Third, the presence of symmetric (inhibitory) and asymmetric (excitatory) synapses from both labelled and unlabelled terminals on PNMT-labelled neurons suggests that the C1 adrenergic neurons are modulated by the same as well as other putative transmitters in the RVL (see schematic Fig. 8). Fourth, the formation of symmetric synapses between PNMT-labelled terminals and unlabelled neurons support the concept that adrenergic terminals in the RVL probably inhibit neurons containing other transmitters.

Adrenergic terminals in the IML

The neural component for the support of resting arterial pressure results from the tonic discharge of sympathetic preganglionic neurons (SPNs) located in the intermediolateral cell column (IML) of the thoracolumbar spinal cord (see Schramm, 1986 for review). The spontaneous activity of SPNs is maintained by a tonic excitatory drive from neurons that project to the IML from the RVL (Ross et al., 1984a; Willette et al., 1984). Overlap between this vasomotor region and the C1 adrenergic cell group has led to the hypothesis that C1 adrenergic neurons projecting to the spinal cord play a role in the regulation of sympathetic tone and AP (Ross et al., 1981, 1984b). This hypothesis is further supported by electron microscopy showing the synaptic associations between adrenergic terminals and neurons in the IML (Milner et al., 1988a). We used the PAP method (Sternberger, 1979) for the single localization of PNMT to study the ultrastructure and synaptic associations of PNMT-containing terminals in the thoracic spinal cord.

The PNMT-labelled terminals ($0.5-1.4$ μm in diameter) contain a few mitochondria, numerous small clear vesicles and from 1 to 6 large dense-core vesicles. The terminals form synapses primarily with dendrites (Fig. 2A). The type of axodendritic association (i.e. symmetric vs. asymmetric) vary with the size of the dendrite, such that the majority of synapses on large dendrites are symmetric (64% of 28) and those on smaller dendrites and dendritic spines are asymmetric (57% of 61). Additionally, most of the synaptic associations of PNMT-containing terminals are with the smaller

Fig. 2. Adrenergic terminals in the IML of the spinal cord. (A) A PNMT-immunoperoxidase labelled terminal (T) forms an asymmetric synapse (arrows) with the spinous portion of a large unlabelled dendrite (uD). (B) Two PNMT-immunoautoradiographically labelled terminals (PNMT-T) form asymmetric junctions (arrows) on a SPN dendrite identified by retrogradely transported HRP (HRP-D). The HRP granule is denoted by an asterisk. The SPN dendrite also receives a synapse (open arrow) from an unlabelled terminal (uT). Autoradiographic exposure time = 20 months. Bars = 0.5 μm. (Reprinted by permission from Milner et al., 1988a.)

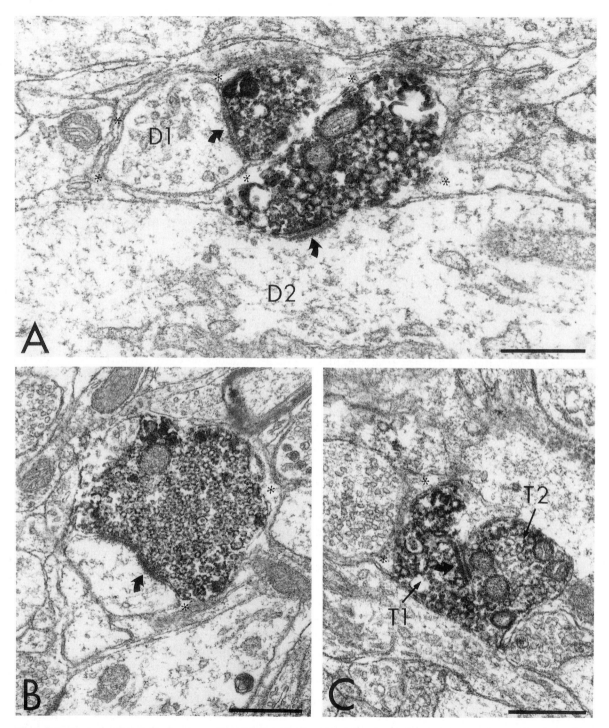

Fig. 3. Adrenergic terminals in the locus coeruleus. (A) Two terminals with PNMT-immunoreactivity form symmetric synapses (arrows) on small (D1) and large (D2) unlabelled dendrites, respectively. (B) A single PNMT-labelled terminal forms an asymmetric synapse (arrow) with a small dendritic spine. (C) Two terminals with PNMT-immunoreactivity (T1 and T2) are adjacent to each other without any apparent glial intervention and the formation of an apparent synaptic density (arrow). Sometimes axons and their postsynaptic targets are separated from the surrounding neuropil by astrocytic processes (asterisks). Bars = 0.5 μm. (Reprinted by permission from Milner et al., 1989a.)

dendritic processes (61 out of 89). Many of the PNMT-labelled terminals, as well as their post-synaptic targets, are surrounded by, or apposed to fibrous astrocytic processes.

In subsequent experiments (Milner et al., 1988a) we combined immunoautoradiographic labelling for PNMT with HRP (Boehringer-Mannheim) retrograde transport identification of SPNs (Pickel and Milner, 1988) to demonstrate that PNMT-containing terminals made direct synaptic contacts with SPN perikarya and dendrites (Fig. 2B). The axosomatic synapses observed between the PNMT-immunoreactive terminals and SPN perikarya are exclusively symmetric; whereas the type of axodendritic association vary depending upon the size of the dendrite such that the majority were asymmetric.

The findings provide ultrastructural evidence that in the rat IML adrenergic terminals can influence sympathetic nerve discharge through a direct effect on the SPN membrane (see schematic Fig. 8). Moreover, adrenergic terminals may be either excitatory (asymmetric) or inhibitory (symmetric) depending on their distribution on the post-synaptic target.

Adrenergic terminals in the locus coeruleus

Noradrenergic neurons of the LC have diverse efferent projections throughout the brain and spinal cord (see Saper, 1987 for review). In contrast, the afferents to the LC are probably more restricted in origin. The two major inputs to the LC arise from the RVL and the rostral dorsal medulla near the prepositus hypoglossus nucleus (Aston-Jones et al., 1986). These two regions contain the adrenergic neurons of the C1 and C2 adrenergic cell groups as identified immunocytochemically by their content of PNMT (Hökfelt et al., 1974; Ruggiero et al., 1985b). That many of the afferent fibers to the LC are adrenergic is supported by the fact that following injections of anterograde tracers into the RVL and rostral dorsal medulla the labelled terminal fields in the LC have a similar

distribution to PNMT-labelled processes (Loewy et al., 1981; Milner et al., 1984; Astier et al., 1987). Moreover, following combined microinfusion of retrograde tracers into the LC and PNMT immunocytochemistry, numerous dually labelled cells are observed in the C1 area (Guyenet and Young, 1987).

By light microscopy, PNMT immunoreactivity in the LC is seen in varicose processes which surround neuronal perikarya throughout the neuropil (Milner et al., 1989a). The majority of these neuronal perikarya contain labelling for the noradrenaline synthesizing enzyme, dopamine-β-hydroxylase (D-β-H) (Olschowka et al., 1981; Pickel and Milner, 1987; Milner et al., 1989a).

Electron microscopy confirms that the PNMT-labelled processes in the LC are primarily axon terminals (Milner et al., 1989a). The immunoreactive axons (0.1 – 0.2 μm in diameter) are exclusively unmyelinated. PNMT-labelled terminals constitute 30% (141 out of 464) of the total identifiable terminals in the LC. The terminals (0.5 – 1.8 μm in diameter) contain many small clear vesicles and from 2 to 10 larger dense-core vesicles (Fig. 3A – C). The targets of the PNMT-containing terminals are principally unlabelled perikarya and dendrites. Synapses on perikarya are rare and exclusively symmetric; those on large (proximal) dendrites are somewhat more numerous and included symmetric as well as asymmetric junctions (Fig. 3A). However, the vast majority (85% from a total of 141) of the terminals with PNMT immunoreactivity form asymmetric junctions on unlabelled small (distal) dendrites and dendritic spines (Fig. 3A,B). Occasionally, the PNMT-labelled terminals form associations with other PNMT-labelled terminals (Fig. 3C).

Overall, our ultrastructural analysis of PNMT-labelled terminals in the LC (Milner et al., 1989a) provides evidence that adrenergic terminals in the LC (1) are one of the more prevalent synaptic inputs to the principally noradrenergic neurons (see schematic Fig. 8); (2) have both symmetric (inhibitory) and asymmetric (excitatory) synaptic membrane specializations; and (3) may modulate other adrenergic terminals through presynaptic mechanisms.

Relationships of C1 adrenergic neurons to other transmitter-identified neurons in RVL

Relationships between adrenergic and GABA-ergic neurons

Neurons in the C1 area are tonically inhibited by γ-aminobutyric acid (GABA). Local application of GABA or its agonist, muscimol, to the ventral surface of the medulla immediately beneath the C1 area or within the RVL reduces AP and heart rate (HR); conversely, application of the GABA antagonist, bicuculline, elevates AP and HR and blocks the baroreceptor reflex (Yamada et al., 1982, 1984; Willette et al., 1983; Ross et al., 1984b; Benarroch et al., 1986). The effects of chemical stimulation of the ventral surface appear to be mediated by vasomotor neurons within the C1 region of the RVL. The immunocytochemical detection of L-glutamic acid decarboxylase (GAD; the synthetic enzyme for GABA), in neurons and processes topographically distributed in regions containing the C1 neurons (Meeley et al., 1985; Ruggiero et al., 1985a,b), suggests that GABA may be synaptically connected to the C1 neurons. Moreover, we have demonstrated the cellular relationships between adrenergic and GABA-ergic neurons in the RVL of the adult rat by electron microscopy (Milner et al., 1987b) utilizing immunoperoxidase labelling for GAD (Oertel et al., 1983) and immunogold labelling for PNMT in single sections.

Ultrastructural analysis of the RVL in non-colchicine-treated animals revealed that peroxidase labelling for GAD is localized primarily to axons and axon terminals. The axons are small and unmyelinated. The GAD-labelled terminals (0.5 – 2.0 μm in diameter) contain a large population of small clear vesicles and a few mitochondria. The GABA-ergic terminals synapse on unlabelled as well as PNMT-containing perikarya and dendrites

(Fig. 4). In all instances, the membrane specializations are symmetric. Both the PNMT-labelled and unlabelled perikarya and dendrites are contacted by more than one GAD-immunoreactive terminal. Moreover, both types of neurons are postsynaptic to unlabelled terminals which formed both symmetric and asymmetric junctions.

These findings indicate that in the RVL, GABA provides a major direct inhibitory (symmetric synapses) input to the C1 adrenergic neurons (see schematic Fig. 8). Additionally, GABA modulates the activity of non-adrenergic neurons in the RVL. These, in turn, may influence C1 neuronal discharge.

Relationships between adrenergic and substance P-containing neurons

The possibility has been raised that substance P (SP)-containing neurons in the RVL may mediate certain of the cardiovascular functions ascribed to the C1 adrenergic neurons (Helke, 1982; Helke et al., 1982; Loewy and Sawyer, 1982). Initially, SP-containing neurons were thought to comprise an anatomical population distinct from the C1 adrenergic neurons (Ljungdahl et al., 1978; Leibstein et al., 1985). However, a subsequent study suggested that SP co-existed with PNMT in a sizable number of C1 adrenergic neurons (Lorenz et al., 1985). Recently, this view has been challenged by Pilowsky et al. (1986) who found, using dual labelling methods, that few neurons of the C1 area contain both SP and PNMT. However, even if SP neurons in the RVL are largely distinct from C1 adrenergic neurons, they still may modulate sympathetic activity through local connections with bulbospinal vasomotor neurons. We examined the relationships between adrenergic and SP-containing neurons in the RVL by light and electron microscopy (Milner et al., 1988b) utilizing immunocytochemical procedures to localize antibodies against substance P (Sera-Lab) and PNMT in single sections (Pickel et al., 1986). We also demonstrated the relationship between SP-labelled neurons and those containing the general catecholamine synthesizing enzyme tyrosine hydroxylase (TH) (Joh and Goldstein, 1973; Joh and Ross, 1983) using the same procedures (Milner et al., 1988b). At this medullary level all of the neurons immunoreactive for TH also contain PNMT and hence correspond to the C1 cell group (Kalia et al., 1985a,b; Ruggiero et al., 1985b).

By light microscopy, the distributions of perikarya containing SP-like immunoreactivity (SPLI) and TH or PNMT (TH/PNMT) are largely topographically distinct. Most of the perikarya with SPLI are located medial and ventral to those labelled with TH/PNMT. However, co-localization of SPLI and TH/PNMT is seen in a few perikarya of colchicine-treated rats; this is confirmed by electron microscopy.

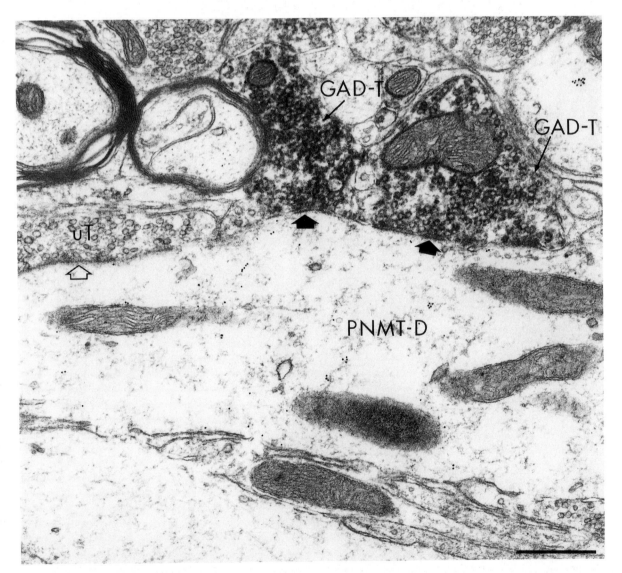

Fig. 4. Relationship between adrenergic and GABA-ergic neurons in the RVL. Two immunoperoxidase GAD-labelled terminals (GAD-T) and one unlabelled terminal (uT) form symmetric synapses (closed and open arrows, respectively) upon a common PNMT-immunogold labelled dendrite (PNMT-D). Bar = 0.5 μm. (Reprinted by permission from Milner et al., 1987b.)

38

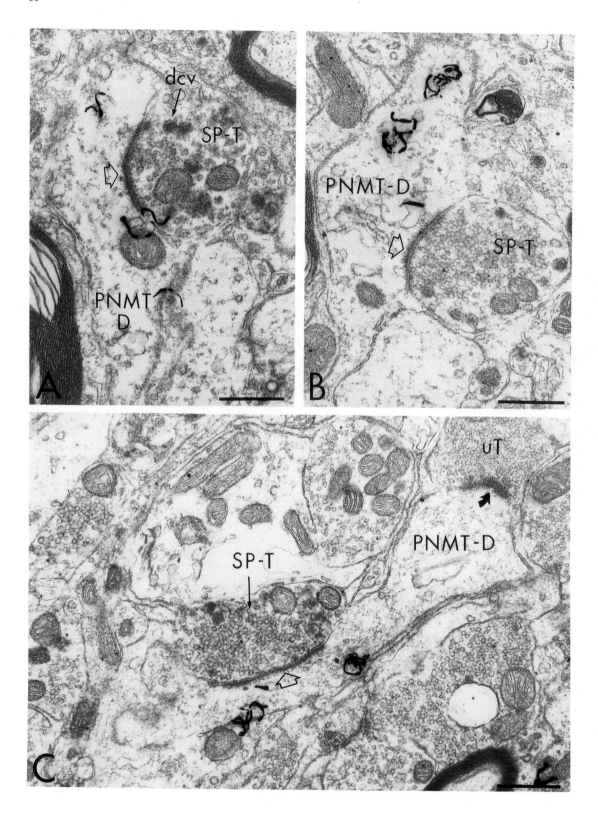

At the ultrastructural level, dense-core vesicles are the most prominent organelles in the cytoplasm of both single- and dual-labelled perikarya. The SP-containing perikarya and dendrites are post-synaptic to primarily unlabelled terminals which formed both symmetric and asymmetric membrane specializations. Sometimes, the SP-immunoreactive perikarya and dendrites are also contacted by similarly labelled terminals.

The terminals with SPLI (0.4–1.4 μm in diameter) contain a few mitochondria, a large population of small clear vesicles and from three to 11 large dense-core vesicles (Fig. 5A–C). In some cases the terminals are continuous with more proximal processes of neurons in the RVL. Terminals with SPLI ($n = 69$) form synaptic junctions primarily (71%) with TH/PNMT-labelled perikarya and dendrites (Fig. 5A–Ĉ). The remainder of the SP-labelled terminals (29%) form synapses with perikarya and dendrites which lack immunoreactivity for TH/PNMT. However, a few of these perikarya and dendrites contain SPLI. In all cases, the axosomatic junctions are primarily asymmetric and often are associated with the spinous portion of the soma. The axodendritic junctions are primarily asymmetric and are found both on the shaft and spinous portion of the dendrites. In addition, both TH- and PNMT-labelled somata and dendrites receive symmetric and asymmetric contacts from terminals lacking SPLI.

These findings provide ultrastructural evidence that in the RVL SP or a closely related neurokinin located in intrinsic neurons or other afferents provides a major direct and probably excitatory (asymmetric synapses) input to C1 adrenergic neurons (see schematic Fig. 8). Additionally, the peptide may modulate the activity of adrenergic neurons through synapses with neurons containing SP or other transmitters.

Relationships between adrenergic and opioid neurons

Local application of several opioid peptides and/or their analogs, including D-Ala^2-D-Leu^5-enkephalin, dynorphin and β-endorphin, to the ventral surface of the medulla lying just beneath the C1 area or microinjections of these agents directly into the C1 area reduces AP and HR; naloxone, an opiate antagonist reverses these responses (Florez et al., 1982; Punnen and Sapru, 1986; Willette et al., 1988). The cardiovascular actions of these opiates and of a number of adrenergic agonists, such as clonidine or α-methyl noradrenaline, when injected into the C1 area are comparable (Bousquet and Schwartz, 1983; Granata et al., 1986). Such observations taken together with the fact that opiate and α_2-adrenergic receptors may be linked (Kunos et al., 1987) raises the prospect that opioid and adrenergic terminals may converge upon common targets in the RVL, conceivably adrenergic neurons of the C1 group.

That opioid and catecholaminergic neurons may interact within the C1 area gains support from the light microscopic immunocytochemical detection of opioid peptides in perikarya and processes topographically distributed in regions containing neurons immunoreactive for PNMT (Williams and Dockray, 1983; Kalia et al., 1985a,b; Ruggiero et al., 1985b; Murakami et al., 1987). We demonstrated the cellular relationships between

---

Fig. 5. Relationships between adrenergic and substance P-containing neurons in the RVL. (A, B) Serial electron micrographs of a SP-immunoperoxidase labelled terminal which forms an asymmetric synapse (open arrow) with a PNMT-immunoautoradiographically labelled dendrite (PNMT-D). (C) An immunoperoxidase terminal with SP-like immunoreactivity (SP-T) forms an asymmetric synapse (open arrow) with the spinous portion of a PNMT-immunoautoradiographically labelled dendrite (PNMT-D). The labelled dendrite also receives an asymmetric synapse (closed arrow) from an unlabelled terminal (uT). Silver grains in lower right corner (asterisk) are in another PNMT-containing dendrite. Autoradiographic exposure = 4 months. Bars = 0.5 μm. (Reprinted by permission from Milner et al., 1988b.)

catecholaminergic and opioid neurons in the RVL of the adult rat by light and electron microscopy (Milner et al., 1989b) utilizing procedures for immunocytochemically localizing a rat monoclonal antibody against Leucine[5] (Leu[5])-enkephalin (Sera-Lab) and a rabbit antiserum against the general catecholamine synthesizing enzyme TH in single sections (Pickel et al., 1986).

By light microscopy, the Leu[5]-enkephalin-like immunoreactivity (LE-LI) is identified by peroxidase reaction product in perikarya and processes. Most of the perikarya containing LE-LI are located dorsolaterally or ventromedially to those showing immunoautoradiographic labelling for TH. However, a few perikarya appear to contain both LE-LI and TH-immunoreactivity (TH-I) which is difficult to differentiate by light microscopy.

By electron microscopy, perikarya and dendrites immunoreactive for LE, TH and both LE and TH are readily discernible. Perikarya and dendrites immunoautoradiographically labelled for TH alone are more numerous than those containing either LE-LI or TH-I and LE-LI. Axon terminals also are immunolabelled either for one or both reaction products.

The perikarya with LE-LI receive synaptic contacts primarily from unlabelled terminals. The junctions formed by these terminals are both symmetric and asymmetric. The LE-labelled dendrites are sometimes contacted by terminals containing LE-LI or TH-I. Both types of terminals form principally symmetric specializations.

The TH-labelled neurons constitute one of the primary (42% from a total of 118) targets of terminals containing LE-LI (Fig. 6). Additionally, some of these terminals containing LE-LI synapse on the same target as TH-labelled terminals. These common target neurons contain either TH-I or TH-I and LE-LI. In most cases the identified junctions are symmetric and the terminals with LE-LI (0.4 – 1.2 μm in diameter) contain either (1) a few small clear vesicles (scv's) and numerous intensely immunoreactive large (100 – 150 nm) dense-core vesicles (dcv's); or (2) many scv's and 0 to 6 dcv's

of a somewhat smaller (80 – 120 nm) diameter. The latter type of terminal is more consistently dually labelled for TH. The remaining terminals containing LE-LI form synaptic junctions with unlabelled perikarya or dendrites (32%), are in apposition to other unlabelled terminals as well as TH or LE- and TH-containing terminals (4%) or are without recognizable associations within the plane of section (22%).

Neurons with TH-I in the RVL are almost exclusively adrenergic (see Milner et al., 1989b). However, axon terminals containing TH-I could either be adrenergic or could arise from noradrenergic neurons of the A1, A2, A5 and A6 cell groups which are known to innervate the RVL (Andrezik et al., 1981). Thus, opioid neurons in the RVL are probably inhibited (symmetric synapses) by other opioid as well as both adrenergic and noradrenergic neurons (see schematic Fig. 8). Moreover, opioid peptides and/or co-existing catecholamines in axon terminals in the RVL directly modulate and probably inhibit (symmetric junctions) the output of adrenergic neurons of the C1 cell group as well as other dually labelled and unlabelled neurons. Inhibition of sympathoexcitatory adrenergic neurons projecting to the intermediolateral cell column of the spinal cord may be the mechanism by which application of opioid transmitters in the RVL produce a depression of cardiovascular activity.

Relationships between adrenergic and cholinergic neurons

Microinjection of cholinergic agents into the C1 area or application onto the surface of the medulla ventral to the RVL produces increases in AP, HR and sympathetic nerve activity (Willette et al., 1984; Benarroch et al., 1986; Giuliano et al., 1988). Enhanced action of acetylcholine released within the RVL may mediate the sympathoexcitation elicited by systemic administration of physostigmine (a cholinesterase inhibitor), since physostigmine-evoked increases in AP and HR can be abolished by electrolytic destruction or chemical

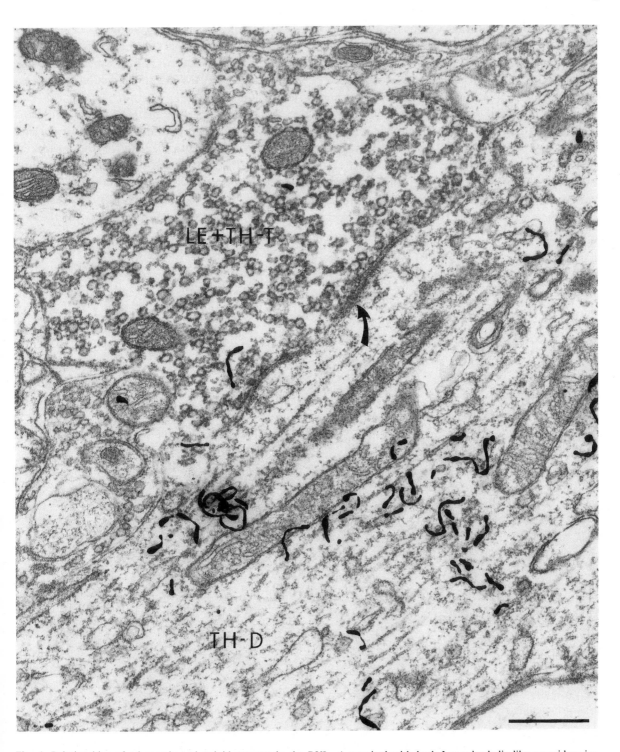

Fig. 6. Relationships of adrenergic and opioid neurons in the RVL. A terminal with both Leu-enkephalin-like peroxidase immunoreactivity and TH-immunoreactivity (LE + TH-T) forms a symmetric synapse (arrow) with a large TH-immunoautoradiographically labelled dendrite (TH-D). A terminal with only LE-LI is found in the same vicinity as the dually labelled terminal. Autoradiographic exposure = 6 months. Bar = 0.5 μm. (Reprinted by permission from Milner et al., 1989b.)

42

inactivation of the RVL, as well as by microinjection of muscarinic antagonists (e.g. atropine, scopolamine) into the region (Punnen et al., 1986; Giuliano et al., 1989). The light microscopic detection of an overlapping distribution of neurons and processes immunoreactive for choline acetyltransferase (CAT) and those containing PNMT in the RVL (Jones and Beaudet, 1987; Ruggiero et al., 1988) suggests that cholinergic and adrenergic neurons may be synaptically connected. We examined the relationships between adrenergic and cholinergic neurons in the RVL (Milner et al.,

1989c) using dual labelling methods for detection of a rat monoclonal antibody against CAT (Boehringer-Mannheim) and a rabbit antiserum against TH or PNMT in single sections (Pickel et al., 1986).

By light microscopy, the CAT-immunoreactive neurons are located both dorsally (i.e. the nucleus ambiguus) and ventromedially to those labelled with TH/PNMT. A few CAT-labelled neurons and processes are dispersed among TH/PNMT-containing neurons and processes in the RVL. However, the majority of overlap between the two

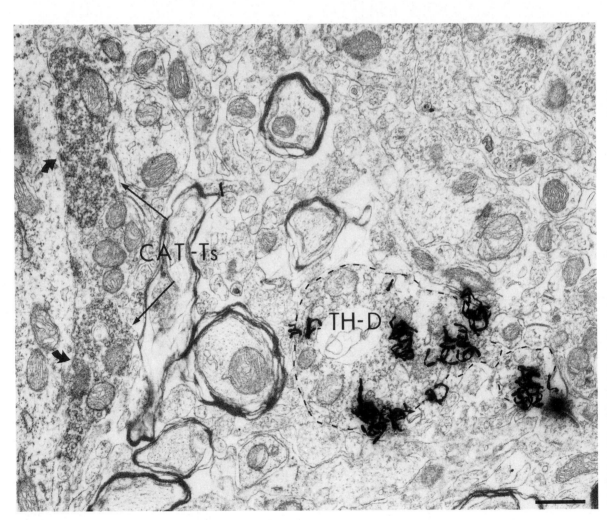

Fig. 7. Relationships of adrenergic and cholinergic neurons in the RVL. Two immunoperoxidase CAT-labelled terminals (CAT-Ts) form symmetric synapses (arrows) with an unlabelled perikarya in a region which also contains a TH-immunoreactive dendrite (TH-D). Autoradiographic exposure = 14 months. Bar = 0.5 µm. (From Milner et al., 1989c.)

cell types is immediately ventral to the nucleus ambiguus.

By electron microscopy, CAT-immunoreactivity (CAT-I) is detected in neuronal perikarya, dendrites, axons and axon terminals. The CAT-labelled perikarya in the ventromedial RVL (15 – 25 μm) are elongated, contain abundant cytoplasm and have slightly indented nuclei. Many CAT-containing dendrites of labelled neurons in the nucleus ambiguus are oriented dorsoventrally toward the RVL. However, the cellular origin (i.e. from CAT-labelled neurons in the RVL vs. nucleus ambiguus) usually cannot be determined. The terminals with CAT-I (0.8 – 2.0 μm in diameter) contain numerous small, clear vesicles and 1 or 2 large dense-core vesicles.

The majority (77% of 145) of the CAT-labelled terminals form associations with unlabelled perikarya and dendrites even though TH/PNMT-immunoreactive dendrites are seen in the adjacent neuropil (Fig. 7). A small number (15% of 145) of the CAT-immunoreactive terminals form associations with CAT-labelled perikarya and dendrites; only a few (8% of 145) are with TH/PNMT-labelled perikarya and dendrites. The CAT-labelled terminals most frequently form symmetric synapses with the shaft portion of large (1.2 – 2.0 μm in diameter) TH/PNMT-labelled dendrites. In all instances, the synapses formed by the CAT-labelled terminals are symmetric while the remainder of the associations usually lack a recognizable membrane specialization but are apposed to neighboring profiles without intervening glial processes.

Associations on CAT-immunoreactive perikarya and dendrites are primarily (64% of 70) from unlabelled terminals which form both asymmetric and symmetric membrane specializations. The remaining pre-synaptic terminals are immunoreactive for CAT (30%) or TH/PNMT (6%). The CAT-labelled perikarya and dendrites form both symmetric and asymmetric synapses or lack any apparent membrane specialization in the plane of section analyzed. However, the synaptic junctions formed by TH/PNMT-containing terminals are characterized exclusively by symmetric membrane specializations.

These ultrastructural observations suggest (1) that cholinergic neurons in the RVL principally

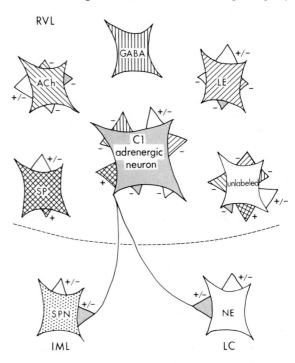

Fig. 8. Summary diagram of synaptic relations of C1 adrenergic neurons with other transmitter- or projection-identified neurons. C1 adrenergic neurons (▨) receive major (large triangles) inhibitory (symmetric synapses) inputs from neurons which contain GABA (⦀) and Leu-enkephalin (LE) (⁄⁄) as well as from neurons with unidentified (unlabelled) transmitters. The C1 neurons receive a major excitatory (asymmetric synapses) input from neurons containing substance P (SP) (✕) as well as from other unidentified neurons. Minor inputs (small triangles) to the C1 neurons are from cholinergic (ACh) (⧵), adrenergic and noradrenergic (NE) (light stippling) terminals. Whether terminals containing these transmitters arise from intrinsic or extrinsic sources is unknown. Cholinergic neurons have a major output to unidentified transmitter-containing neurons. Most of the transmitter identified neurons are innervated from similarly labelled terminals. Both cholinergic and opioid neurons are innervated by catecholaminergic (C1 adrenergic and NE) terminals. C1 adrenergic neurons project rostrally where they form inhibitory (symmetric) and excitatory (asymmetric) synapses on neurons, probably norepinephrine (NE)-containing, in the locus coeruleus (LC); they also project caudally to the IML of the spinal cord where they form direct synaptic contacts with sympathetic preganglionic neurons (SPNs) (⦂⦂).

terminate on and receive input from non-catecholaminergic neurons (see schematic Fig. 8), and (2) that the reported sympathetic activation following application of cholinergic agents to the RVL may be mediated by cholinergic inhibition of local inhibitory interneurons, possibly containing GABA or opioid peptides. The observed synapses between CAT- and TH/PNMT-containing neurons suggests that cholinergic and adrenergic neurons additionally may exert a minor reciprocal control on each other and thus may modulate their response to the more abundant input from afferents containing other transmitters.

Summary and conclusions

The first part of this chapter demonstrates that the C1 adrenergic neurons have high mitochondrial content and a close proximity to capillaries and glia suggestive of a high metabolic activity and a possible chemosensory function. Adrenergic terminals arising primarily from these neurons (1) can influence sympathetic nerve discharge through direct contacts on sympathetic preganglionic neurons in the IML of the spinal cord; and (2) are one of the more prevalent synaptic inputs to the principally noradrenergic neurons in the locus coeruleus. In both the IML and locus coeruleus, adrenergic terminals may be either excitatory (asymmetric synapses) or inhibitory (symmetric synapses) depending on their distribution on the post-synaptic target.

The second part of this chapter shows that C1 adrenergic neurons in the RVL are modulated by synaptic associations with a variety of transmitter systems (see schematic Fig. 8). Specifically, C1 adrenergic neurons receive (1) major inhibitory input (symmetric synapses) from GABA-ergic and opioid terminals as well as from unidentified (unlabelled) transmitter-containing terminals; (2) major excitatory input (asymmetric synapses) from terminals containing substance P as well as other unidentified terminals and (3) minor inputs from cholinergic, adrenergic and noradrenergic pathways. Moreover, cholinergic terminals in the RVL form symmetric synapses mainly on unidentified transmitter-containing neurons rather than the C1 neurons suggesting that the reported cardiovascular effects of cholinergic agents in the RVL are most likely mediated via inhibitory interneurons. Within the RVL, adrenergic and noradrenergic terminals innervate cholinergic and opioid neurons. Thus, these results not only provide direct evidence that a number of transmitters modulate the activity of C1 adrenergic neurons, but also suggest new directions for studies of functional interactions involving catecholaminergic regulation of other transmitter-containing neurons within the RVL.

Acknowledgements

We would like to thank Drs. C. Abate (Roche Institute of Molecular Biology), D.H. Park and T.H. Joh (Cornell University Medical College) for their generous supply of the TH and PNMT antibodies. We also would like to thank Dr. R. Giuliano for her helpful suggestions on the manuscript. Supported by NIH Grants HL 18974, MH42834 (T.A.M.) and a career development award (MH 00078) to V.M.P.

References

Andrezik, J.A., Chan-Palay, V. and Palay, S.L. (1981) The nucleus paragigantocellularis lateralis in the rat: demonstration of afferents by the retrograde transport of horseradish peroxidase. *Anat. Embryol.*, 161: 373–390.

Astier, B., Kitahama, K., Denoroy, L., Jouvet, M. and Renaud, B. (1987) Immunohistochemical evidence for the adrenergic medullary longitudinal bundle as a major ascending pathway to the locus coeruleus. *Neurosci. Lett.*, 74: 132–138.

Aston-Jones, G., Ennis, M., Pieribone, V.A., Nickell, W.T. and Shipley, M.T. (1986) The brain nucleus locus coeruleus: restricted afferent control of a broad efferent network. *Science,* 234: 734–737.

Benarroch, E.E., Granata, A.R., Ruggiero, D.A., Park, D.H. and Reis, D.J. (1986) Neurons of C1 area mediate cardiovascular responses initiated from ventral medullary surface. *Am. J. Physiol.*, 250: R932–R945.

Bousquet, P. and Schwartz, J. (1983) Alpha adrenergic drugs: pharmacological tools for the study of the central vasomotor control. *Biochem. Pharmacol.,* 32: 1459–1465.

Brown, D.L. and Guyenet, P.G. (1984) Cardiovascular neurons of the nucleus paragigantocellularis lateralis with projections to the spinal cord. *Am. J. Physiol.,* 247: R1009–1016.

Ciriello, J., Caverson, M.M. and Polosa, C. (1986) Function of the ventrolateral medulla in the control of the circulation. *Brain Res. Rev.,* 11: 359–391.

Cohen, R.S., Carlin, R.K., Grab, D.J. and Siekevitz, P. (1982) Phosphoproteins in postsynaptic densities. In W.H. Gispen and A. Routtenberg (Eds.), *Brain Phosphoproteins,* Progress in Brain Research, Vol. 56, Elsevier, Amsterdam, pp. 49–76.

Cravo, S.L., Ruggiero, D.A., Anwar, M. and Reis, D.J. (1988) Quantitative-topographic analysis of adrenergic and non-adrenergic spinal projections of cardiovascular area of RVL. *Neurosci. Abst.,* 14: 328.

Florez, J., Hurle, M.A. and Mediavilla, A. (1982) Respiratory responses to opiates applied to the medullary ventral surface. *Life Sci.,* 31: 2189–2192.

Giuliano, R., Ruggiero, D.A., Morrison, S., Ernsberger, P. and Reis, D.J. (1989) Cholinergic regulation of arterial pressure by the C1 area of the rostral ventrolateral medulla. *J. Neurosci.,* 9: 923–942.

Granata, A.R., Ruggiero, D.A., Park, D.H., Joh, T.H. and Reis, D.J. (1983) Lesions of epinephrine neurons in the rostral ventrolateral medulla abolish vasodepressor components of baroreflex and cardiopulmonary reflex. *Hypertension* 5, Suppl. V: V80–V84.

Granata, A.R., Ruggiero, D.A., Park, D.H., Joh, T.H. and Reis, D.J. (1985) Brainstem area with C1 epinephrine neurons mediates baroreflex vasodepressor responses, *Am. J. Physiol.,* 248 *(Heart Circ. Physiol.,* 17): H547–H567.

Granata, A.R., Numano, Y., Kumada, M. and Reis, D.J. (1986) A1 noradrenergic neurons tonically inhibit sympathoexcitatory neurons of the C1 area in rat brainstem. *Brain Res.,* 377: 127–146.

Guyenet, P.G. and Young, B.S. (1987) Projections of nucleus paragigantocellularis lateralis to locus coeruleus and other structures in rat. *Brain Res.,* 406: 171–184.

Helke, C.J. (1982) Neuroanatomical localization of substance P: implications for central cardiovascular control. *Peptides (Fayatteville),* X: 479–483.

Helke, C.J., Neil, J.J., Massari, V.J. and Loewy, A.D. (1982) Substance P neurons project from the ventral medulla to the interomediolateral cell column and ventral horn in the rat. *Brain Res.,* 243: 147–152.

Hökfelt, T., Fuxe, K., Goldstein, M. and Johansson, O. (1974) Immunohistochemical evidence for the existence of adrenaline neurons in the rat brain. *Brain Res.,* 66: 235–251.

Joh, T.H. and Goldstein, M. (1973) Isolation and characterization of multiple forms of phenylethanolamine *N*-methyltransferase. *Mol. Pharmacol.,* 9: 117–129.

Joh, T.H. and Ross, M.E. (1983) Preparation of catecholamine synthesizing enzymes: an immunogen for immunocytochemistry. In A.C. Cuello (Ed.), *Immunocytochemistry, Handbook Series Vol. 3,* Oxford IBRO Wiley, New York, pp. 121–138.

Jones, B.E. and Beaudet, A. (1987) Distribution of acetylcholine and catecholamine neurons in the cat brainstem: a choline acetyltransferase and tyrosine hydroxylase immunohistochemical study. *J. Comp. Neurol.,* 261: 15–32.

Kalia, M., Fuxe, K. and Goldstein, M. (1985a) Rat medulla oblongata. II. Dopaminergic, noradrenergic (A1 and A2) and adrenergic neurons, nerve fibers and presumptive terminal processes. *J. Comp. Neurol.,* 233: 308–332.

Kalia, M., Fuxe, K. and Goldstein, M. (1985b) Rat medulla oblongata. III. Adrenergic (C1 and C2) neurons, nerve fibers and presumptive terminal processes. *J. Comp. Neurol.,* 233: 333–349.

Kunos, G., Mosqueda-Garcia, R. and Mastrianni, J.A. (1987) Endorphinergic mechanism in the central cardiovascular and analgesic effects of clonidine. *Can. J. Physiol. Pharmacol.,* 65: 1624–1632.

Loewy, A.D. and Sawyer, W.B. (1982) Substance P antagonist inhibits vasomotor responses elicited from ventral medulla in rat. *Brain Res.,* 245: 279–383.

Loewy, A.D., Wallach, J.H. and McKellar, S. (1981) Efferent connections of the ventral medulla oblongata in the rat. *Brain Res. Rev.,* 3: 63–80.

Leibstein, A.G., Dermietzel, R., Willenberg, I.M. and Pauschert, R. (1985) Mapping of different neuropeptides in the lower brainstem of the rat: with special reference to the ventral surface. *J. Auton. Nerv. Syst.,* 14: 299–313.

Ljungdahl, A., Hökfelt, T., Nilsson, G. and Goldstein, M. (1978) Distribution of substance P-like immunoreactivity in the central nervous system of the rat. II. Light microscopic localization in relation to catecholaminergic containing neurons. *Neuroscience,* 3: 945–976.

Lorenz, R.G., Saper, C.B., Wong, D.L., Ciaranello, R.D. and Loewy, A.D. (1985) Co-localization of substance P- and phenylethanolamine *N*-methyltransferase-like immunoreactivity in neurons of ventrolateral medulla that project to the spinal cord: Potential role in control of vasomotor tone. *Neurosci. Lett.,* 55: 255–260.

Meeley, M.P., Ruggiero, D.A., Ishitsuka, T. and Reis, D.J. (1985) Intrinsic γ-aminobutyric acid neurons in the nucleus of the solitary tract and the rostral ventrolateral medulla of the rat: an immunocytochemical and biochemical study. *Neurosci. Lett.,* 58: 83–89.

Milner, T.A., Joh, T.H., Miller, R.J. and Pickel, V.M. (1984) Substance P, neurotensin, enkephalin, and catecholamine-synthesizing enzymes: light microscopic localizations compared with autoradiographical label in solitary efferents to the rat parabrachial region. *J. Comp. Neurol.,* 226: 434–447.

Milner, T.A., Pickel, V.M., Park, D.H., Joh, T.H. and Reis,

D.J. (1987a) Phenylethanolamine N-methyltransferase-containing neurons in the rostral ventrolateral medulla of the rat. I. Normal ultrastructure. *Brain Res.*, 411: 28 – 45.

Milner, T.A., Pickel, V.M., Chan, J., Massari, V.J., Oertel, W.H., Park, D.H., Joh, T.H. and Reis, D.J. (1987b) Phenylethanolamine N-methyltransferase-containing neurons in the rostral ventrolateral medulla. II. Synaptic relationships with GABAergic terminals. *Brain Res.*, 411: 46 – 57.

Milner, T.A., Morrison, S.F., Abate, C. and Reis, D.J. (1988a) Phenylethanolamine N-methyltransferase-containing terminals synapse directly on sympathetic preganglionic neurons in the rat. *Brain Res.*, 448: 205 – 222.

Milner, T.A., Pickel, V.M., Abate, C., Joh, T.H. and Reis, D.J. (1988b) Ultrastructural characterization of substance P-containing neurons in the rostral ventrolateral medulla in relation to neurons containing catecholamine synthesizing enzymes. *J. Comp. Neurol.*, 270: 427 – 445.

Milner, T.A., Abate, C., Reis, D.J. and Pickel, V.M. (1989a) Ultrastructural localization of phenylethanolamine N-methyltransferase-like immunoreactivity in the rat locus coeruleus. *Brain Res.*, 478: 1 – 15.

Milner, T.A., Pickel, V.M. and Reis, D.J. (1989b) Ultrastructural basis for interactions between central opioids and catecholamines. I. Rostral ventrolateral medulla. *J. Neurosci.*, 9: 2114 – 2130.

Milner, T.A., Pickel, V.M., Giuliano, R. and Reis, D.J. (1989c) Ultrastructural localization of choline acetyltransferase in the rat rostral ventrolateral medulla: evidence for major synaptic relations with non-catecholaminergic neurons. *Brain Res.* (in press).

Morrison, S.F., Milner, T.A. and Reis, D.J. (1987) Reticulospinal vasomotor neurons of the rat rostral ventrolateral medulla: relationship to sympathetic nerve activity and the C1 adrenergic cell group. *J. Neurosci.*, 8: 1286 – 1301.

Murakami, S., Okamura, H., Yanaihara, C., Yanaihara, N. and Ibata, Y. (1987) Immunocytochemical distribution of Met-enkephalin-Arg[6]-Gly[7]-Leu[8] in the lower brainstem. *J. Comp. Neurol.*, 261: 193 – 208.

Oertel, W.H., Schmechel, D.E., Tappaz, M.L. and Kopin, I.J. (1983) Production of a specific antiserum to rat brain glutamic acid decarboxylase (GAD) by injection of an antigen-antibody complex. *Neuroscience*, 6: 2689 – 2700.

Olschowka, J.A., Molliver, M.E., Grzanna, R., Rice, F.L. and Coyle, J.T. (1981) Ultrastructural demonstration of noradrenergic synapses in the rat central nervous system by dopamine-β-hydroxylase immunocytochemistry. *J. Histochem. Cytochem.*, 29: 271 – 280.

Pickel, V.M. (1981) Immunocytochemical methods. In L. Heimer and M.J. Robards (Eds.), *Neuroanatomical Tract Tracing Methods*, Plenum Press, New York, pp. 483 – 509.

Pickel, V.M. and Milner, T.A. (1987) Electron microscopy of central catecholamine systems. In: H.Y. Meltzer (Ed.), *Psychopharmacology: The Third Generation of Progress*, Raven Press, New York, pp. 49 – 59.

Pickel, V.M. and Milner, T.A. (1989) Interchangeable uses of autoradiographic and peroxidase markers for electron microscopic detection of neuronal pathways and transmitter-related antigens in single sections. In L. Heimer and M.J. Robards (Eds.), *Neuroanatomical Tract Tracing Methods, II*, Plenum Press, New York (in press).

Pickel, V.M., Chan, J. and Milner, T.A. (1986) Autoradiographic detection of ^{125}I-secondary antiserum: a sensitive light and electron microscopic labeling method compatible with peroxidase immunocytochemistry for dual localization of neuronal antigens. *J. Histochem. Cytochem.*, 34: 707 – 718.

Pieribone, V.A. and Aston-Jones, G. (1988) The iontophoretic application of Fluoro-Gold to the study of afferents to deep brain nuclei. *Brain Res.*, 475: 259 – 271.

Pilowsky, P., Minson, J., Hodgson, A., Howe, P. and Chalmers, J. (1986) Does substance P coexist with adrenaline in neurons of the rostral ventrolateral medulla in the rat? *Neurosci. Lett.*, 71: 293 – 298.

Punnen, S. and Sapru, H.N. (1986) Cardiovascular responses to medullary microinjections of opiate agonists in urethane-anesthetized rats. *J. Cardiovasc. Pharm.*, 8: 950 – 956.

Punnen, S., Willette, R.N., Krieger, A.J. and Sapru, H.N. (1986) Medullary pressor area: site of action of intravenous physostigmine. *Brain Res.*, 382: 178 – 184.

Reis, D.J., Morrison, S. and Ruggiero, D.A. (1988) The C1 area of the brainstem in tonic and reflex control of blood pressure. *Hypertension Suppl.*, 11: I8 – I13.

Ross, C.A., Armstrong, D.M., Ruggiero, D.A., Pickel, V.M., Joh, T.H. and Reis, D.J. (1981) Adrenaline neurons in the rostral ventrolateral medulla innervate thoracic spinal cord: a combined immunocytochemical and retrograde transport demonstration. *Neurosci. Lett.*, 25: 257 – 262.

Ross, C.A., Ruggiero, D.A., Joh, T.H., Park, D.H. and Reis, D.J. (1984a) Rostral ventrolateral medulla: selective projections to the thoracic autonomic cell column from the region containing C1 adrenaline neurons. *J. Comp. Neurol.*, 228: 168 – 185.

Ross, C.A., Ruggiero, D.A., Park, D.H., Joh, T.H., Sved, A.F., Fernandez-Pardal, J., Saavedra, J.M. and Reis, D.J. (1984b) Tonic vasomotor control by the rostral ventrolateral medulla: effect of electrical or chemical stimulation of the area containing C1 adrenaline neurons on arterial blood pressure, heart rate and plasma catecholamines and vasopression. *J. Neurosci.*, 4: 474 – 494.

Ruggiero, D.A., Meeley, M.P., Anwar, M. and Reis, D.J. (1985a) Newly indentified GABAergic neurons in regions of the ventrolateral medulla that regulate blood pressure. *Brain Res.*, 339: 171 – 177.

Ruggiero, D.A., Ross, C.A., Anwar, M., Park, D.H., Joh, T.H. and Reis, D.J. (1985b) Distribution of neurons containing phenylethanolamine *N*-methyltransferase in medulla and hypothalamus of rat. *J. Comp. Neurol.,* 239: 127 – 154.

Ruggiero, D.A., Giuliano, R., Anwar, M. and Reis, D.J. (1989) Anatomical substrates of cholinergic autonomic regulation. *J. Comp. Neurol.* (in press).

Saper, C.B. (1987) Function of the locus coeruleus. *Trends Neurosci.,* 10: 343 – 344.

Schramm, L.P. (1986) Spinal factors in sympathetic regulation. In A. Magro, W. Osswald, D. Reis and P. Vanhoutte (Eds.), *Central and Peripheral Mechanisms of Cardiovascular Regulation,* Plenum Press, New York, pp. 303 – 352.

Sternberger, L.A. (1979) *Immunocytochemistry,* John Wiley, New York.

Uchizono, K. (1965) Characterization of excitatory and inhibitory synapses in the CNS of the cat. *Nature,* 207: 642 – 643.

Willette, R.N., Krieger, A.J., Barcas, P.P. and Sapru, H.N. (1983) Medullary gamma-aminobutyric acid (GABA) receptors and the regulation of blood pressure in the rat. *J. Phar-macol. Exp. Ther.,* 226: 893 – 899.

Willette, R.N., Punnen, S., Krieger, A.J. and Sapru, H.N. (1984) Cardiovascular control by cholinergic mechanisms in the rostral ventrolateral medulla. *J. Pharmacol. Exp. Ther.,* 231: 457 – 463.

Willette, R.N., Morrison, S., Sapru, H.N. and Reis, D.J. (1989) Inhalation anesthetic-opioid interaction: expression of opioid actions in the medullary rostral ventrolateral reticular nucleus. *Neuropharm.* (in press).

Williams, R.G. and Dockray, G.J. (1983) Distribution of enkephalin-related peptides in rat brain: immunohistochemical studies using antisera to met-enkephalin and met-enkephalin Arg[6]Phe[7]. *Neuroscience,* 9: 563 – 586.

Yamada, K.A., Norman, W.P., Hamosh, P. and Gillis, R.A. (1982) Medullary ventral surface GABA receptors affect respiratory and cardiovascular function. *Brain Res.,* 248: 71 – 78.

Yamada, K.A., McAllen, R.M. and Loewy, A.D. (1984) GABA antagonists applied to the ventral surface of the medulla oblongata block the baroreceptor reflex. *Brain Res.,* 297: 175 – 180.

J. Ciriello, M.M. Caverson and C. Polosa (Eds.)
Progress in Brain Research, Vol. 81
© 1989 Elsevier Science Publishers B.V. (Biomedical Division)

CHAPTER 4

Central control of the circulation by the rostral ventrolateral reticular nucleus: anatomical substrates

David A. Ruggiero, Sergio L. Cravo, Victoria Arango and Donald J. Reis

Division of Neurobiology, Department of Neurology and Neuroscience, Cornell University Medical College, 411 East 69th Street, New York, NY 10021, U.S.A.

Introduction

For over a century the lower brainstem was recognized as an area of crucial importance in generating resting levels of arterial blood pressure (AP) and cardiopulmonary reflexes (Dittmar, 1873; Cushing, 1902; Ranson, 1916). Alexander's demonstration (1946) that successive rostrocaudal transections made through the medulla oblongata but not anteriorly, led to progressive blockade of the sciatic pressor reflex and eventual collapse of AP led to the theory that the vasotonic and vasoreflex centers were distributed throughout the lateral medulla; yet represented by the same cellular elements.

The subsequent failure to identify the hypothetical vasomotor center or a descending pathway from the lateral medulla to the intermediolateral cell column (IML) suggested, to the contrary, that the critical neurons were not confined to a single nucleus but rather were dispersed along the neuraxis (the multicentric concept of circulatory control; Hilton, 1975).

Recently, several findings have prompted us to re-evaluate the concept that the tonic vasomotor neurons are localized to a subregion of the lateral tegmental field in the rostral ventrolateral quadrant. The first was the localization of pressor responses to electrical or chemical stimulation of a chemosensitive area (the intermediate area) of the ventral medullary surface (Schläfke and Loeschke,

1967). The second was the fall in AP to spinal levels and blockade of the cerebral ischemic reflex provoked by bilaterally placed cold probes, pharmacologic blockade or lesions of the ventral surface (Feldberg and Guertzenstein, 1972; Guertzenstein and Silver, 1974; Feldberg, 1976) or the rostral ventrolateral tegmentum (Dampney and Moon, 1980), respectively. The third was the discovery of neurons lying near the ventral surface projecting to the IML (Amendt et al., 1978; Ross et al., 1981b; Dampney et al., 1982).

In an effort to resolve the identity of the crucial neurons, we were impressed by a striking correspondence between the sympathoexcitatory center in the rostral ventrolateral medulla and a subpopulation of catecholaminergic neurons containing the epinephrine synthesizing enzyme, phenylethanolamine *N*-methyltransferase (PNMT) — the C1 area of Hökfelt et al. (1974). Our subsequent attempts to map the microcircuitry of the functionally defined area led to the synthesis of a new anatomically discrete autonomic substructure — the rostral ventrolateral reticular nucleus or nucleus reticularis rostroventrolateralis (nucleus RVL).

Rostral ventrolateral reticular nucleus in the rat

The anatomical substrate of the functionally defined vasomotor center in the medulla oblongata is the nucleus RVL (Ross et al., 1983, 1984a,b, 1985);

and was reconstructed from its cytoarchitecture, immunocytochemistry and connectivity. In the rat, the RVL, as seen on coronal sections, is a triangular substructure in the rostral ventrolateral quadrant. The RVL (Fig. 1) is bordered dorsally by the compact and semicompact divisions of the nucleus ambiguus, medially by the rostral one-third of the inferior olive (and the nucleus gigantocellularis pars ventralis) and laterally by a ventral extension of the nucleus reticularis parvocellularis that is contiguous with the oral portion of the spinal trigeminal nucleus. The rostral pole of RVL merges medially with the lateral wings of the nucleus raphe magnus (which are interposed between the ventromedial reticular formation and the pyramids) and abuts the caudal pole of the facial nucleus, laterally. The nucleus RVL and its caudal extension, the nucleus reticularis caudoventrolateralis (nucleus CVL, which is dorsal to and partially intercalated between the two limbs of the lateral reticular "cerebellar relay" nucleus (LRN; Walberg, 1952; Fig. 2) coincide and were consequently named after the nucleus reticularis lateralis (rostroventro- and caudoventro- were prefixed) of Meessen and Olszewski (1949, Plates V – VII in rabbit). Connectivity and immunocytochemical studies revealed that the nuclei, RVL and CVL, are not equivalent to the larger nucleus paragigantocellularis lateralis (NPGCL). On the contrary, the NPGCL is a composite structure extrapolated from human (Olszewski and Baxter, 1954) to rat (Andrezik et al., 1981), and was defined arbitrarily, solely on the basis of a morphometric analysis of Nissl-stained material. In contrast to the nuclei RVL and CVL, the boundaries of NPGCL are inconsistent with connectivity data

and are, thus, more extensive medially, arbitrarily including serotonergic neurons of the lateral wings of the nucleus raphe magnus and nucleus ventralis subolivaris (NSO, the ventral subolivary nucleus). The NPGCL is also more extensive rostrocaudally and arbitrarily includes an area medially adjacent to the superior olive that is concerned with auditory feedback control (see Andrezik et al., 1981). As illustrated by Fig. 1, the cytoarchitectonic outline of nucleus RVL is relatively indistinct on Nissl-stained sections primarily because of its relatively high content of myelinated axons (Milner et al., 1987b), and secondly because of the heterogeneity of neuronal size, shape and packing density (and the proportionally greater number of small, lightly stained cell bodies).

The C1 area in the rat

As suggested by its cytoarchitecture, there is a diversity of neurochemically specific (and undefined) perikarya in the RVL. Thus far, the adrenergic perikarya of the C1 area constitute one of the largest, immunocytochemically identified "spinally-projecting" cell groups in the vasomotor area of the nucleus RVL. Figures 1 and 2 relate the cytoarchitecture of the nuclei RVL and CVL to the distributions of neurons immunocytochemically stained for the epinephrine synthesizing enzyme, PNMT at rostral versus mid-medullary levels of the ventrolateral quadrant. Adrenergic perikarya in the C1 area of RVL form a horizontally elongate cell group extending between 1.0 mm and 2.25 mm from the midline and approximately 150 – 600 μm dorsally to the rostral ventral subpial surface. On Nissl-stained tissues, perikarya of the C1 area lie

Fig. 1. Anatomy of the rostral ventrolateral reticular nucleus (nucleus RVL). Photomicrographs were taken from 40 μm coronal sections stained with thionin (a, b) or processed immunocytochemically for the adrenaline-synthesizing enzyme, PNMT (c). The C1 area (indicated by ventral arrows) is a relatively parvicellular, fibrous zone defined by a large cluster of adrenergic perikarya (Ruggiero et al., 1985c) (c). Dorsal arrows point to more intensely-stained perikarya corresponding to the respiratory (Bötzinger) complex (Ellenberger and Feldman, 1988; see their Fig. 2B). In RVL the C1-spinal neurons project exclusively to sympathetic preganglionic neurons, whereas the respiratory reticulospinal cells project to phrenic and intercostal motor nuclei. The dorsal border of the nucleus RVL is defined by motoneurons of the compact and semicompact divisions of the nucleus ambiguus. Bar = 400 μm (a); 200 μm (b); 60 μm (c).

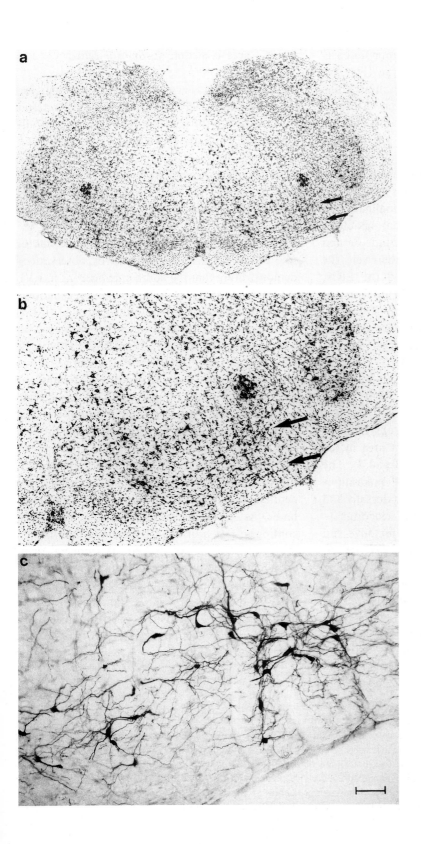

ventrally to a longitudinal column of more intensely stained spinally-projecting perikarya (Fig. 1b, dorsal arrow) equivalent to the respiratory (Bötzinger) complex of Ellenberger and Feldman (1988) and dorsally to the external arcuate and spinothalamic tracts. In the RVL, C1 neurons staining for PNMT are quantitatively equal to those containing tyrosine hydroxylase (TH, the rate limiting catecholaminergic biosynthetic enzyme) and presumably synthesize adrenaline (Armstrong et al., 1982). At mid- to caudal medullary levels, C1 immunoreactive neurons condense and form an ovoid column situated between the nucleus retroambiguus, dorsally and the LRN, ventrally, and extend from 650 to 850 μm from the ventral subpial surface and 1.8 mm from the midline. Here, adrenergic neurons are admixed with or displaced by A1 noradrenergic neurons that stain for TH but not for PNMT.

The C1 area in the human

In human postmortem material, neurons stain for TH and PNMT within an equivalent area in the rostral ventrolateral medulla (Figs. 3 and 4). The human C1 area of the ventrolateral quadrant is vertically more elongate and displaced dorsally and laterally by structures related to the neocortex — the principal subnucleus of the inferior olive and pyramids (Arango et al., 1988). As seen in the rat, the substructure of the C1 area and the original description of NPGCL as defined on Nissl-stained tissues (Olszewski and Baxter, 1954) are not equivalent. Neurons in the human RVL contain TH as well as PNMT; although whether they synthesize adrenaline remains to be established.

The C1 area is a tonic vasomotor center

This section reviews the morphophysiological evidence suggesting that neurons in the nucleus RVL (possibly those in the C1 area) are tonically active and sympathoexcitatory.

Adrenergic pathways

C1 neurons project to spinal-sympathetic preganglionic neurons

An anatomical basis for the purported vasomotor role of the C1 area is suggested by observations demonstrating that the adrenergic neurons in RVL project exclusively to sympathetic preganglionic neurons in the IML and intermediomedial (IMM) cell columns (Fig. 5). On tissues that were processed immunocytochemically for PNMT, adrenergic perikarya in the C1 area of RVL give rise to two bundles of axons: (1) one trajectory of axons arches dorsally and obliquely through the central tegmental field, coalesces in the dorsomedial medulla (underlying the rostral-subvestibular third of the nucleus tractus solitarii, NTS), and forms the principal adrenergic tegmental bundle (PT). Fibers in the PT are organized longitudinally to the neuraxis and ascend, descend or bifurcate into two limbs. At rostral medullary levels, the descending contingent (PT_d; or the C1-spinal tract) is located in the dorsal aspect of the central tegmental field; at caudal levels shifts ventromedially into the dorsomedial reticular formation and lies ventrolaterally to the hypoglossal nucleus. Commencing at the level of the area postrema to the spinomedullary junction (at the calamus scriptorius) fibers of the PT_d spray ventrally and ventrolaterally into the

Fig. 2. Anatomy of the caudal ventrolateral reticular nucleus (nucleus CVL). Photomicrographs were taken from 40 μm coronal sections stained with thionin (a, b) or immunocytochemically for PNMT (c). The A1 – C1 cell column (indicated by the ventral arrows) lies dorsal to and is partially intercalated between both limbs of the lateral reticular nucleus. Neurons in the A1 – C1 area are noradrenergic (TH-positive and PNMT-negative) and adrenergic (TH-positive and PNMT-positive). Dorsal arrows point to more intensely stained perikarya of the nucleus retroambiguus, corresponding to a portion of the rostral ventral respiratory group (Ellenberger and Feldman, 1988; see their Fig. 2A). Bar = 400 μm (a); 200 μm (b); 60 μm (c).

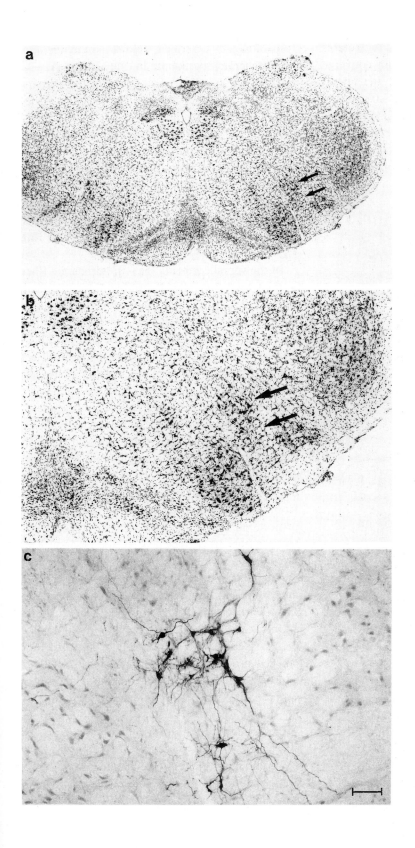

anterolateral funiculus (FAL). As the FAL rotates dorsolaterally, most fibers in PT again converge and coalesce in the dorsal aspect of the lateral funiculus. (2) A second trajectory of axons (the ventral adrenergic tegmental bundle, VT), parallels PT_d; its descending component projects directly longitudinally through the ventrolateral quadrant and primarily into the ventral aspect of the lateral

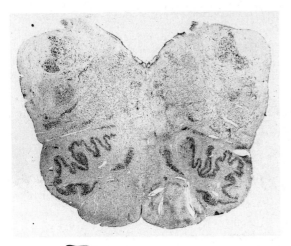

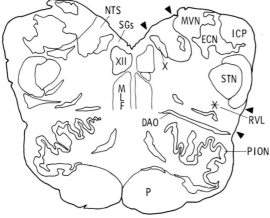

Fig. 3. Photomicrograph and drawing of a 30 μm coronal section of human rostral medulla stained with thionin. The asterisk on the schematic illustration demonstrates the location of the C1 area of nucleus RVL (see Fig. 4). Arrows on the dorsal and ventral surfaces indicate the area depicted in the darkfield photomontage of Fig. 15. Permission for the autopsies and use of the tissue samples was obtained by the responsible physicians in accordance with the requirements of the Human Rights in Research Committees.

funiculus. As described below, adrenergic (and noradrenergic) perikarya in the caudal A1 – C1 and A1 cell columns do not project to the spinal cord. Instead, these cells give rise to axons projecting in the ascending limbs of PT and VT to the A5 area, parabrachial complex, central gray, locus coeruleus, and laterodorsal tegmental nucleus, pontine raphe, nucleus raphe dorsalis, midline thalamus, hypothalamic and preoptic areas, amygdala, bed nucleus of the stria terminalis and septum (Hökfelt et al., 1974; Granata et al., 1985; Ruggiero et al., 1985a,c; Tucker et al., 1987; Ruggiero and Reis, 1988).

In the spinal cord (Fig. 5e – i), adrenergic fibers in the lateral funiculus descend as far as the sacral level. Labelled terminals were concentrated at upper thoracic spinal segments and distributed in a patchy distribution throughout the IML and IMM and in an area intercalated between both cell columns (Fig. 6). Punctate varicosities were also localized to IML and IMM in middle and lower thoracic, upper lumbar and sacral spinal segments. Lightly labelled varicosities also surrounded the central canal at upper cervical levels and represent a caudal extension of adrenergic fields in the commissural nucleus of the NTS. Terminals surrounding the spinal central canal appear to stem in part from the C2 or C3 adrenergic cell groups; the latter project via the descending limb of the periventricular fiber tract (Ruggiero et al., 1985a,c; Ruggiero and Reis, 1988).

A similar projection pattern was confirmed by anterograde transport studies (Ross et al., 1983, 1984a). Injections of anterograde tracers (tritiated amino acids or wheat-germ agglutinin-horseradish peroxidase, WGA-HRP) into the C1 area of RVL labelled processes that were restricted to the IML and IMM throughout all segments of the thoracic spinal cord.

Adrenergic-spinal neurons

By combining immunocytochemical with retrograde tracing methods in the same experiment, we have shown that adrenergic neurons in the C1 area

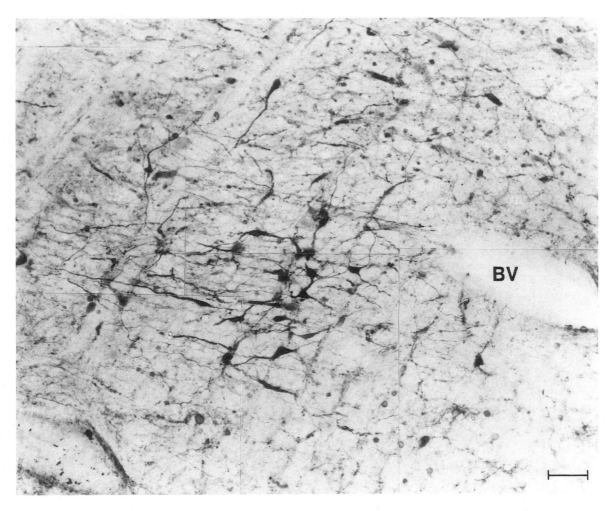

Fig. 4. Photomicrograph of adrenergic, PNMT immunoreactive, neurons of the C1 area of RVL in the human medulla oblongata (see asterisk in Fig. 3). (From Arango et al., 1988.) Bar = 60 μm.

of RVL project to the spinal cord (Ross et al., 1981a, 1983; Cravo et al., 1988). In one of these studies (Figs. 7 and 8), multiple injections of the retrograde tracer, WGA-HRP, were placed throughout the thoracic or all segments of the spinal cord, and the same sections were processed histochemically for WGA-HRP and immunocytochemically for TH or PNMT. Our most recent quantitative topographic analyses of adrenergic versus non-adrenergic spinal projections of the vasomotor area demonstrated that greater than 70% of the total number of retrogradely labelled

cells in the nucleus RVL also contained the epinephrine-synthesizing enzyme, PNMT. These data confirmed that the majority of reticulospinal neurons within the confines of the vasomotor area of RVL are adrenergic (Cravo et al., 1988).

Non-adrenergic-spinal neurons

Non-adrenergic neurons in the RVL projecting to the spinal cord form three groups: (1) longitudinal column(s) underlying (or admixed with) the compact (semicompact and external) divisions of the

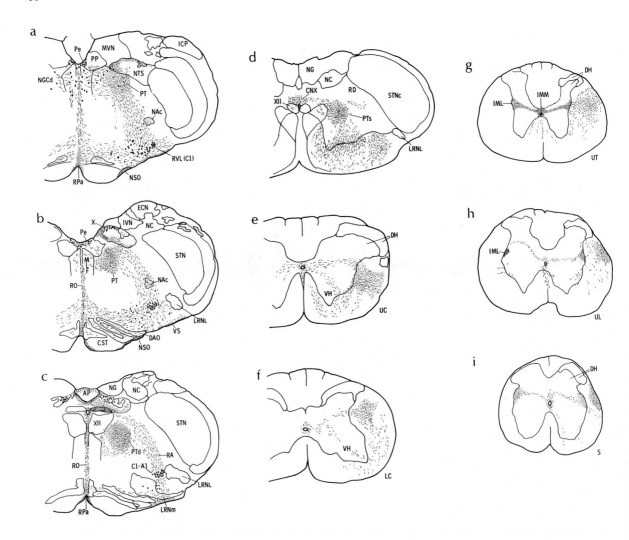

Fig. 5. Camera lucida drawings of PNMT immunoreactive cell bodies (dots), processes (axons; lines) and putative terminals (stippling) in the medulla (a – d) and spinal cord (e – i) in the rat. In the rostral medulla (a, b) axons of C1 neurons of RVL arch dorsally to form a longitudinal fiber tract – the principal adrenergic tegmental bundle. At caudal medullary levels (c, d) fibers of the descending spinal limb (PT_d) shift medially; at the spinomedullary junction they radiate ventrally and ventrolaterally into the lateral funiculus. Note that immunoreactive terminals are concentrated in the intermediolateral (IML) and intermediomedial (IMM) cell columns and that the PT_d descends as far as the sacral cord (g – i). Some fibers are also seen in the cervical central gray (e, f) particularly at upper cervical levels where they merge with a terminal field in the commissural nucleus of the NTS.

nucleus ambiguus corresponding to an area occupied by a portion of the rostral ventral respiratory group and Bötzinger complex. Non-adrenergic pre-spinal neurons in this column extend caudally into the area retroambiguus (Figs. 7b and 8c), and lie dorsally to the unlabelled catecholaminergic cell bodies of the C1 and A1 cell groups. Especially large numbers of non-adrenergic neurons were retrogradely labelled from the cervical as well as thoracic spinal segments and corroborate anterograde tracing studies which demonstrate direct projections from respiratory cell groups (including the area retroambiguus) to phrenic and intercostal motor neurons innervating the muscles of breathing (Feldman et al., 1985; Ellenberger and Feldman, 1988); (2) a ventral subpial group (Ross et al., 1981b, 1984a) underlying the C1 area and lining the ventral medullary surface (a lateral extension of the serotonergic and peptidergic cell bodies in the nucleus ventralis subolivaris and raphe pallidus); and (3) scattered immunochemically unidentified cells in the C1 area that were admixed with adrenergic perikarya.

Role of intrinsic neurons in the RVL in tonic vasomotor control

Functional evidence that the nucleus RVL harbors the hypothetical "tonic vasomotor center" in-

cludes the extraordinarily strict correspondence between the C1 area (as defined by adrenergic-spinal perikarya) and the sympathoexcitatory vasomotor neurons as defined by the following criteria: (1) Electrical stimulation of sites overlapping the C1 neurons labelled immunocytochemically for PNMT or the trajectory of the C1-spinal tract in the dorsal tegmentum (Fig. 9) provokes powerful sympathoexcitation, characterized by comparatively large increases in AP and heart rate (HR), and release of adrenal catecholamines and arginine vasopressin from the neurohypophysis (Ross et al., 1984b). (2) Chemical stimulation of the RVL by microinjecting small volumes of the perikaryal-selective excitatory amino acid L-

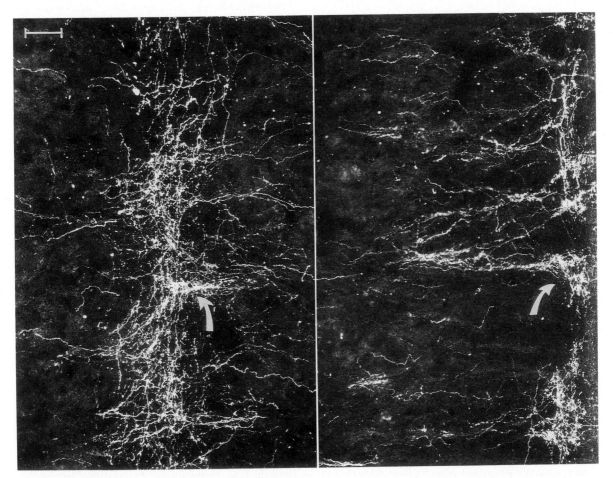

Fig. 6. Darkfield photomicrographs of a horizontal section showing a patchy distribution of PNMT-immunoreactive varicosities in the IML (right arrow) and the IMM (left arrow). Bar = 70 μm.

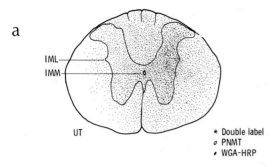

a

IML—
IMM—

UT

* Double label
o PNMT
• WGA-HRP

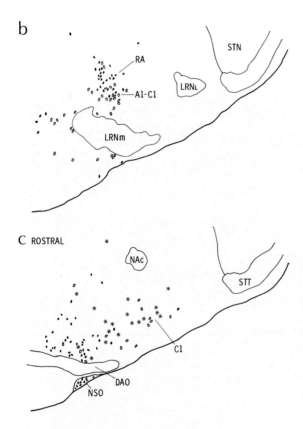

b

STN

RA

LRNl

A1-C1

LRNm

C ROSTRAL

*

NAc

*

STT

*

*

*

*

* *

* *

* * *

*

* *

* *

*

C1

*

*

DAO

NSO

glutamate (1 nmol, 15 nl, pH 7.4) in urethane-anesthetized rats (1.2 g/kg) evokes pressor responses ($\geq$ 10 mmHg) restricted to a longitudinal strip of 0.4 mm comprising the rostral one-third of the C1 area (Cravo et al., 1988) where the majority (> 70%) of thoracic-reticulospinal neurons are adrenergic. (3) Bilateral electrolytic lesions of C1 neurons or the C1-spinal tract, or chemical inactivation of C1 neurons localized by microinjection of excitotoxic agents, sodium channel blockers or inhibitory amino acids results in a collapse of AP to levels produced by spinal cord transections (Ross et al., 1983, 1984b; Granata et al., 1985). RVL-spinal sympathoexcitatory neurons recorded consistently within 100 μm of C1 (PNMT-immunoreactive) perikarya are activated antidromically by stimuli applied to the IML of the spinal cord (Morrison et al., 1988); their tonic activity is moreover synchronized to the spontaneous bursts of a sympathetic splanchnic nerve in the absence of baroreceptor input (Barman and Gebber, 1985; Morrison et al., 1988).

The RVL is an integrative reflex center

Vasomotor neurons in the nucleus RVL are critical in reflex control of the circulation and participate in the cardiopulmonary adjustments which maintain steady state conditions and reset the system preparatory or in response to movements, nocicep-

Fig. 7. Camera lucida drawings of a WGA-HRP injection site in the thoracic spinal cord (a) and coronal tissue sections (b, c) processed by a double labelling technique combining WGA-HRP histochemistry with an immunocytochemical method (PAP) for demonstrating PNMT. Note that the majority of double-labelled perikarya (asterisks) were restricted to the C1 area of the nucleus RVL (c). These compose a longitudinal strip of approximately 0.4 mm overlapping the functionally defined vasomotor area. Adrenergic cells in the C1 area receive direct projections from the caudal NTS (see Fig. 13) and may mediate

baroreceptor and other cardiopulmonary reflexes. In contrast, perikarya in the nucleus CVL were retrogradely labelled in the nucleus retroambiguus (RA) and were clearly a separate population from the PNMT-immunoreactive cell bodies in the A1 – C1 area. Reticulospinal neurons in RA also receive afferents from cardiopulmonary divisions of NTS and demonstrate striking overlap with cells projecting to RVL (see Fig. 10b), vasodepressor sites (Day and Renaud, 1983) and respiratory premotor neurons (Ellenberger and Feldman, 1988). Cells in the RVL and CVL, including the C1 and A1 columns project to the forebrain (e.g. paraventricular hypothalamic and preoptic nuclei, Tucker et al., 1987) and may integrate neuroendocrine and cardiopulmonary reflexes.

tive stimulation and behaviors such as the defense alerting-response. The evidence that primary baroreceptor afferents signal adrenergic neurons in RVL is strong; yet equally compelling are data suggesting that the nucleus is an integrative reflex center, subserving somatosympathetic, chemoreceptor and neuroendocrine reflexes, and conceivably, the autonomic adjustments to emotionally arousing stimulation by virtue of descending afferents from the forebrain. That such pathways exist is supported by the following evidence: (1) the dependence of these reflexes on the integrity of RVL; (2) the wealth of pharmacologically and functionally characterized receptors in the area; and (3) stimulation of rostral brain areas projecting directly (or indirectly) to RVL (including the amygdala and cerebral cortex) elicits changes in AP and baroreceptor reflex excitability.

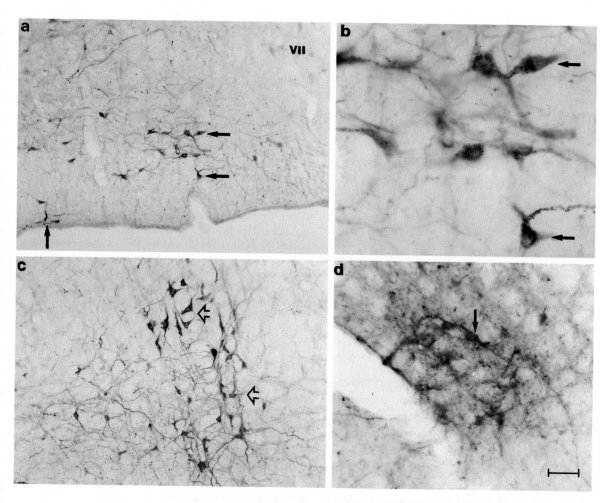

Fig. 8. Photomicrographs demonstrating PNMT-immunoreactive perikarya in the C1 area of the RVL (brown diffuse reaction product) also containing WGA-HRP (black granular reaction product) transported from the thoracic spinal cord (a). (b) Some double-labelled cells are indicated by arrows. (c) PNMT-immunoreactive cells in the A1 – C1 area (ventral arrow) are clearly a separate population from those that are retrogradely labelled in the nucleus retroambiguus (dorsal arrow). (d) Photomicrograph showing the close apposition of fibers anterogradely labelled with WGA-HRP transported from an injection into the caudal NTS, to PNMT-immunoreactive cell bodies in the A1 – C1 area (see Fig. 13). Bar = 72 μm (a, c); 22 μm (b); 36 μm (d).

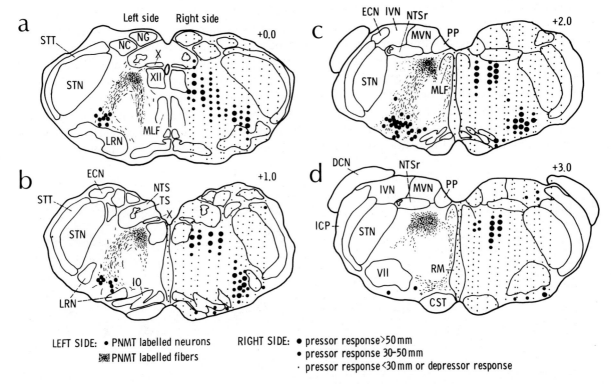

LEFT SIDE: ● PNMT labelled neurons
               ▧ PNMT labelled fibers

RIGHT SIDE: ● pressor response >50 mm
              ● pressor response 30-50 mm
              · pressor response <30 mm or depressor response

Fig. 9. Locations of the medullary pressor sites most responsive to constant current electrical stimulation compared to the locations of C1 cells and fibers immunocytochemically labelled for PNMT. Left side of each section: PNMT-labelled C1 neurons and PNMT-labelled fibers. Right side of each section: pressor responses to electrical stimulation with 25 μA (100 Hz, 0.5 msec, 10-sec train). Responses between 30 and 50 mmHg are indicated by *small solid circles,* whereas those greater than 50 mmHg are indicated by *larger solid circles.* Responses less than 30 mmHg or depressor responses are indicated by *small dots.* The location of the pressor region in the ventrolateral medulla corresponds to the location of the C1 neurons, and the location of the pressor region in the dorsomedial medulla corresponds to the location of the PNMT-labelled descending fiber bundle (From Ross et al., 1984b).

Afferents to the nucleus RVL

Afferents to the nucleus RVL were therefore studied systematically by microinjecting retrograde tracers into the functionally-defined vasomotor area — a longitudinal strip of approximately 0.4 mm including the rostral one-third of the C1 area. Cases were analyzed with injection deposits that consistently involved the pyramidal-shaped nucleus RVL, which included the C1 subnucleus, the ventromedullary surface and the reticular area intercalated between C1 and the compact/semi-compact divisions of the nucleus ambiguus. Those cases with injection sites that spread into the medial reticular formation, raphe magnus or

nucleus reticularis parvocellularis were discarded. Small injection sites that were restricted to individual loci of RVL yielded variable patterns of transport. The data plotted in Fig. 10 are therefore based on a large injection encompassing the whole nucleus and are representative of several cases. Photomicrographs of retrogradely labelled neurons are provided in Figs. 11 and 12.

Afferents to the RVL were widespread albeit limited to nuclei relaying primary (NTS) and higher order visceral afferents (parabrachial complex), somatic including nociceptive signals (spinal cord and central gray) and afferents from forebrain centers such as those involved in the hypothalamic defense-alerting reflex. Confirming

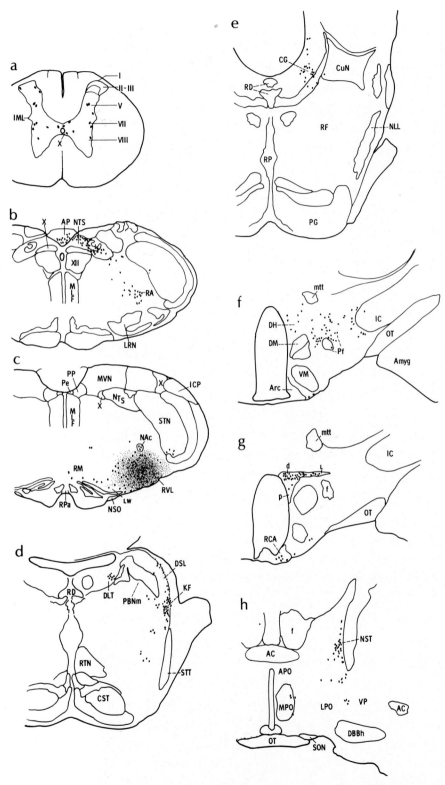

Fig. 10. Camera lucida drawings of coronal tissue sections through spinal cord (a), hindbrain (b – d), midbrain (e), and forebrain (f – h) demonstrating the distribution of retrogradely-labelled perikarya from a representative WGA-HRP injection restricted to the nucleus RVL (c) (see text for details).

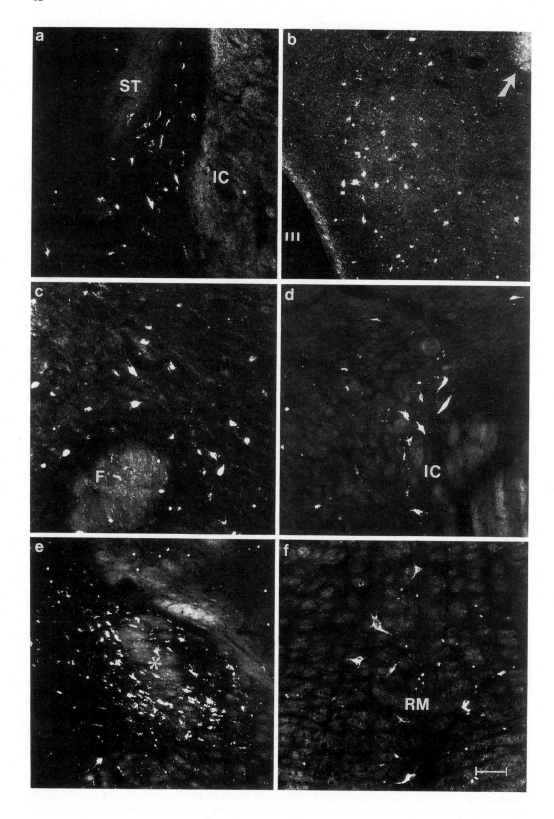

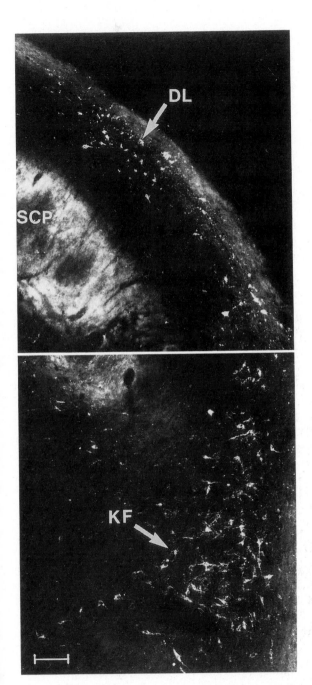

Fig. 12. Darkfield photomontage of retrograde transport of WGA-HRP from RVL to neurons in the nucleus of Koelliker-Fuse (KF), and the dorsal-lateral subdivision (DL) of the lateral parabrachial nucleus. SCP (superior cerebellar peduncle). Bar = 60 μm.

Fig. 11. Darkfield photomicrographs of neurons backfilled from an injection of WGA-HRP restricted to the rostral ventrolateral reticular nucleus (RVL). (a) Bed nucleus of the stria terminalis (ST) adjacent to the internal capsule (IC); (b) dorsal hypothalamic nucleus adjacent to third ventricle (III), arrow indicates the mammillothalamic tract; (c) perifornical nucleus surrounding the fornix (F); (d) lateral hypothalamic nucleus (adjacent to internal capsule); (e) nucleus tractus solitarii surrounding the solitary tract; and (f) nucleus raphe magnus (RM). Bar = 60 μm.

our previous observations (Ruggiero et al., 1984; Ross et al., 1985), afferents to the vasomotor area showed some similarities although marked differences with those innervating the NPGCL (Andrezik et al., 1981). Whereas inputs to nucleus RVL appear to be functionally specific, those to NPGCL were not, and also derived from secondary auditory nuclei, vestibular complex, and somatic "premotor" areas of the medial and pontine reticular formation. In the medulla, most afferents to the RVL were labelled in the NTS and area postrema (see below). Other cells were backfilled in the nucleus CVL, overlapping vasodepressor (Day and Renaud, 1983) and respiratory-premotor neurons (Ellenberger and Feldman, 1988); nucleus raphe magnus (thought to modulate spinal afferent neurotransmission and opiate-induced analgesia; see Basbaum et al., 1978); and the lateral tegmental field (where neurons with sympathetic nerve-related activity discharge prior to sympathoexcitatory neurons in RVL; Gebber and Barman, 1985). In the pons, afferents were labelled in the parabrachial complex (where cardiopulmonary units coexist) and the laterodorsal tegmental nucleus [the "micturition center" where neurons, along with cells in nucleus RVL (this report), project to the sacral IML (Loewy et al., 1979)]. Projections to RVL from the central gray and hypothalamus provide anatomical substrates for (a) the sympathoexcitation and increased discharge rates of RVL neurons triggered by stimulating equivalent sites (Ciriello et al., 1985; Sun and Guyenet, 1986), and (b) the hypothalamic-mesencephalic defense responses mediated by excitatory relays from nucleus RVL to the IML (Hilton et al., 1983; Hilton and Smith, 1984). In contrast to Chan et al. (1986), injections of retrograde tracers (including fluorescent dyes) into the RVL did not transport to the nucleus ambiguus. Projection cells in the area postrema (as reported by Ross et al., 1985) were found to be the sole source of hindbrain catecholaminergic afferents according to Blessing et al. (1987). A noradrenergic innervation of RVL in contrast was reported previously to arise from the A5 area (Sun and Guyenet, 1986). Whether a dopaminergic input arises from the hypothalamus is unknown. Neither the insular cortex nor central nucleus of the amygdala (regions innervating the NTS) provide direct projections to the RVL.

Major discrepancies with data from other species (rabbit or cat) are as follows: (1) the predominantly unilateral projection from NTS to RVL as revealed in the rat is in sharp contrast with the bilateral distribution reported in rabbits and cats, and (2) there is a more limited distribution of afferents from the hypothalamus and hindbrain in the cat and rabbit (Dampney et al., 1982, 1987). Whether these differences reflect interspecific variations or are related to technical parameters is unresolved. As described below, some of the afferents and local receptors in nucleus RVL have been characterized functionally. In general, electrical or chemical stimulation of most afferents to RVL have marked effects on AP and HR, respiration and baroreflex excitability; others, in particular the higher order afferents may serve as components of appetitive or emotional behaviors that occur during the sleep – wake cycle or in conditioned learning.

Baroreceptor reflex

That neurons in the RVL mediate baroreceptor reflexes was initially predicted by its afferent projections from an area of cardiopulmonary representation in the NTS. The origins of afferents from the NTS were first revealed by injecting retrograde tracers into the RVL (Ross et al., 1985). Projections to the RVL were traced primarily ipsilaterally to cells in caudal subdivisions of NTS receiving primary cardiopulmonary afferents including the dorsal, intermediate and ventral subnuclei and the commissural nucleus of the vagus (Ciriello, 1983; Kalia and Richter, 1985).

In order to characterize the projection field in RVL, injections of anterograde tracers were made into the caudal NTS. Labelled axons traversed the lateral tegmental field (LTF) and entered the ventrolateral medulla (Fig. 13). Punctate varicosities resembling terminal boutons were lightly distributed over three areas: (1) the LTF, (2) a previously unidentified pyramidal-shaped substructure in the ventrolateral medulla (defining the nucleus RVL and differentiating it from the NPGCL), and (3) a patchy strip lining the ventral subpial surface. In the RVL, putative terminals were concentrated over the C1 area and dorsally along the longitudinal cell columns subjacent to and including the nucleus ambiguus. These fields were contiguous caudally with varicosities in the A1 – C1 and A1 noradrenergic areas and the more dorsal nucleus retroambiguus (defining the nucleus CVL). Photomicrographs of anterogradely labelled fields in the RVL and CVL are provided in Fig. 14.

Anatomical evidence that C1 adrenergic neurons are involved in the baroreflex arc was obtained by a novel procedure combining anterograde tracers with an immunocytochemical method localizing catecholaminergic enzymes on the same tissue (Figs. 8 and 13) (see Ruggiero and Reis, 1988). With this technique, microinjections of WGA-HRP or tritiated amino acids into the caudal NTS anterogradely labelled processes surrounding PNMT (or TH) immunoreactive perikarya that were concentrated in lateral aspects of the C1 area of RVL. The projection fields also coincided with the A1 – C1 and A1 columnar organization of the nucleus CVL. Such data provide strong suggestive

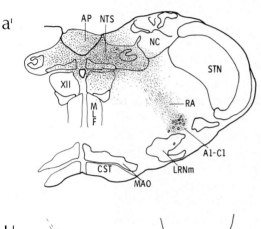

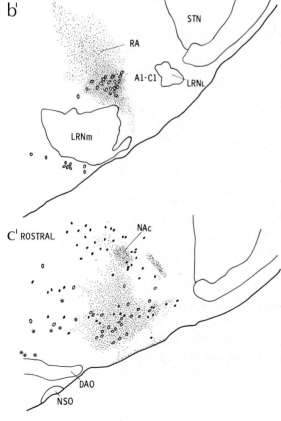

Fig. 13. Camera lucida drawing of a WGA-HRP injection site in the nucleus tractus solitarii (NTS) and area postrema (AP) (a′) and coronal tissue sections (b′, c′) processed by a combined labelling technique. Tissues were processed immunocytochemically for PNMT and histochemically for WGA-HRP reaction product. Note that the cell bodies immunoreactive for PNMT (open circles) in the C1 area of RVL (c′) and the A1 – C1 area of CVL (b′) are surrounded by fields of punctate varicosities resembling terminal boutons (fine stippling) that were anterogradely labelled from the NTS and AP. Putative terminals also overlap non-adrenergic reticular neurons in dorsal parts of the RVL and CVL, as well as the compact, semicompact and loose formations of the nucleus ambiguus. Comparing these data with the distributions of reticulospinal neurons, as depicted in Fig. 7, suggests that C1 and non-adrenergic-premotor neurons in the ventrolateral medulla relay cardiopulmonary signals to the IML. Asterisks denote adrenergic PNMT-positive perikarya in the medial aspect of the C1 area of RVL that were retrogradely labelled from the NTS; these data suggest that C1 neurons projecting to the NTS might modulate incoming signals of primary cardiopulmonary afferents or preganglionic output neurons of the dorsal motor nucleus where adrenergic processes are also concentrated (see Fig. 28-2 of Ruggiero and Reis, 1988). Bidirectional cardiovascular feedback loops between NTS and RVL also have been demonstrated electrophysiologically (Ciriello and Caverson, 1986).

66

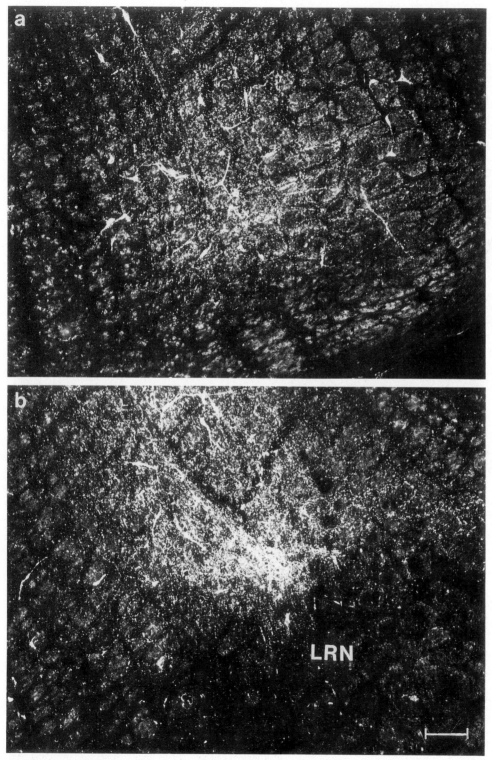

Fig. 14. Darkfield photomicrographs showing anterogradely labelled processes in the nucleus RVL (a) and nucleus CVL (b) from an injection of WGA-HRP into the caudal two-thirds of the NTS. In panel (a), the terminal field at this level of nucleus RVL is separated from the ventral medullary surface by large myelinated fiber tracts. Some labelled processes run perpendicularly to and perforate the fiber tracts forming a patchy distribution on the ventral subpial surface (not visible on this micrograph). Bar = 70 μm.

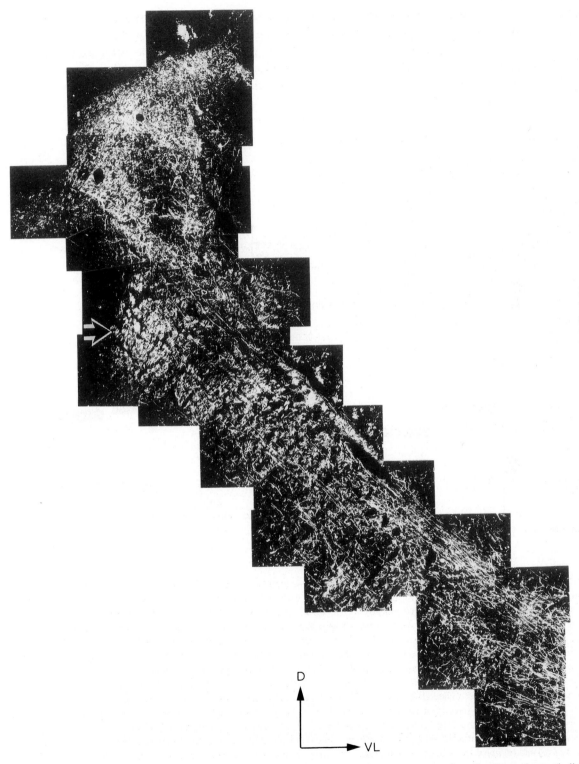

Fig. 15. A montage of darkfield photomicrographs of the human medulla oblongata corresponds to the diagonal area (indicated by arrows on Fig. 3) that extends from the NTS (dorsomedially) to the RVL (ventrolaterally). Tissues were treated by using antibodies to tyrosine hydroxylase. Note that immunoreactive processes extend between the NTS and the RVL. The pathway appears to be reciprocating: (1) on immunocytochemically processed tissues axons of adrenergic cells in RVL extend into the NTS, and (2) WGA-HRP injected into the NTS (on tissue blocks of human postmortem material) transports towards the RVL (Arango and Ruggiero, in progress). Arrows indicate dorsal (D) and ventrolateral (VL) directions. (Modified after Arango et al., 1988.)

evidence for synaptic relays from the NTS to both adrenergic and noradrenergic neurons in the RVL and CVL. In other "dual transport" experiments (Ross et al., 1985), NTS efferents were found to surround premotor neurons in the C1-vasomotor area of RVL projecting to the IML and IMM in the thoracic spinal cord. Since a large percentage of adrenergic neurons in the NTS-projection field project to the IML (compare Figs. 7 and 13), it is conceivable that the C1 neurons represent an

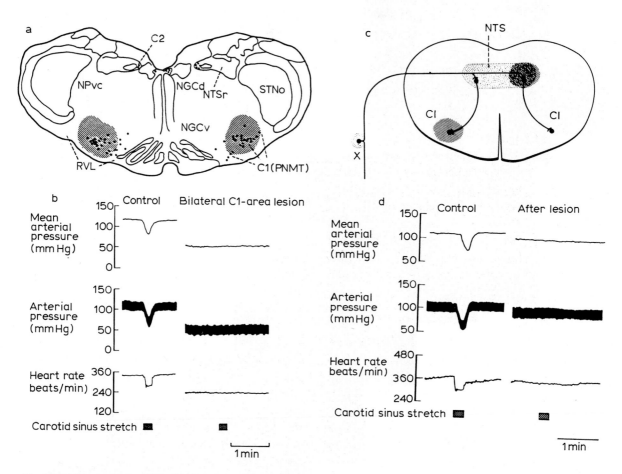

Fig. 16. (a) Representative bilateral lesions in rostral ventrolateral medulla as compared to the distributions of phenylethanolamine N-methyltransferase (PNMT)-labelled cells in the C1 area. After each experiment, animals were perfused with paraformaldehyde and sections were processed immunocytochemically for PNMT. In animals with C1 lesions, PNMT-stained cells on the side contralateral to a unilateral C1 lesion were plotted from the same experiments. Note that the lesions destroyed the bulk of neurons in the region. (b) Effect of bilateral lesions of C1 area on resting mean AP, HR, and responses to carotid sinus stretch in anesthetized and paralyzed rat. Note that after bilateral lesions, AP falls to approximately 55 mmHg, i.e. lower than the maximal vasodepression produced by sinus stretch and reflex responses disappear. (c) Model used to test a proposed baroreceptor reflex pathway, based on the anatomical findings that vagal afferents bilaterally innervate nucleus tractus solitarii (NTS, *light shading*), whereas NTS projections to C1 area are primarily unilateral. A lesion of NTS on right side (*hatched area*) isolates the reflex arc on the left side. A subsequent lesion of left C1 area (area identified by PNMT-labelled cell bodies represented by *hatched lines*) should abolish reflexes yet preserve resting arterial pressure. (d) Combined ipsilateral (left) C1 area and contralateral (right) NTS lesions abolish responses to carotid sinus stretch in an anesthetized and paralyzed rat. Note that while AP is maintained, reflex responses to sinus stretch disappear. For (b) and (d) *upper trace*, mean arterial pressure (mmHg); *middle trace*, arterial blood pressure (mmHg); *lower trace*, heart rate (beats/min). (Modified from Granata et al., 1985.)

anatomical substrate of the baroreceptor reflex.

Similar pathways from the NTS to the ventrolateral medulla may exist in humans (Fig. 15): (a) axons of catecholaminergic neurons (labelled for TH and PNMT) course between the NTS and RVL; (b) injections of WGA-HRP into the NTS of the human postmortem brainstem consistently label an arc of fibers issuing from ventrolateral aspects of the NTS that course towards the C1 area of RVL; and (c) fibers of C1 neurons in the human RVL contribute to a homologous adrenergic tegmental bundle located in an identical region of the dorsal-medial medulla (Arango et al., 1988; Arango and Ruggiero, in preparation).

The functional importance of the pathway from the NTS to RVL is implied by two findings. First, are the electrophysiological data demonstrating that the spontaneous firing of neurons of RVL, antidromically activated from the IML is coupled with sympathetic discharge locked to the cardiac cycle and inhibited by stimulation of arterial baroreceptors (Brown and Guyenet, 1984; Barman and Gebber, 1985; Morrison et al., 1988). Second, are the observations that the vasodepressor responses to electrical stimulation of the cervical vagus or stretch of the carotid sinus were effectively abolished by electrolytic lesions or pharmacologic blockade of C1 neurons in the RVL; yet were unaltered by destroying the nucleus CVL or other NTS projection sites (Granata et al., 1985). The C1 area of RVL, thus, may mediate baroreceptor and possibly other cardiopulmonary reflexes relayed by the NTS (see Fig. 16 for details).

Somatosympathetic reflexes

Spinal afferents to the RVL also may mediate the somatosympathetic reflex elevations in AP and HR to stimuli normally provoked by exercise, postures and nociception. Our work (Ruggiero et al., 1986b; Stornetta et al., 1988) has demonstrated that lumbosacral dorsal horn cells relaying primary and most likely, higher order somatic afferents, project bilaterally although predominantly contralaterally to the RVL and variably to other autonomic relay stations including the hypothalamus, central gray, locus coeruleus, parabrachial complex, A5 area, NTS and the nucleus CVL. Yet the pressor responses to sciatic or sural nerve stimulation were blocked by lesions (or chemical blockade) restricted to the contralateral RVL but unaltered by mid-collicular transections interrupting spinal afferents to the forebrain or by lesions of all other afferent fields including the LRN, A5 area and parabrachial complex. These data demonstrate that the spinoreticular limb of the somatosympathetic reflex is coupled to the RVL and not to the LRN of Walberg (1952) as proposed by earlier studies (e.g. Iwamoto et al., 1982).

Ventral surface chemosensitivity and cerebrovascular reflexes

Neurons in the C1 area of the RVL are morphologically specialized for their roles in chemoreceptor reflexes associated with the ventral medullary surface and in the cerebrovasodilation accompanying reductions in cerebral blood flow or oxygen perfusion. They possess abundant mitochondria and are in close proximity to the ventral subpial surface and intraparenchymal microvessels (Milner et al., 1987b; Ruggiero et al., 1985c). That the RVL mediates ventral surface reflexes is suggested by the extremely tight correspondence between C1 neurons and chemosensitive sites along the ventral surface where neurotransmitters stimulate changes in AP and HR, and by the fact that the cardiovascular responses are blocked by selective inactivation of C1 neurons or destruction of the C1-spinal tract (Benarroch et al., 1986). Lesions of an electrophysiologically identified vasomotor center in RVL also block the sympathoexcitatory reflex to cerebral ischemia (Dampney and Moon, 1980; Guyenet and Brown, 1986) and profoundly impair the diffuse cerebrovascular vasodilation generated by hypoxia but not by hypercarbia (Underwood et al., 1986).

What is the neurotransmitter of tonic sympatho-spinal neurons in RVL?

C1 adrenergic neurons likely play an integral role in the cardiovascular integrative functions of RVL as corroborated by their connectivity and tight correspondence with a functionally defined tonic vasomotor center. Still unresolved, however, is the identity of the neurotransmitter(s) responsible for

the tonic background excitation of spinal preganglionic neurons. Whether the sympathoexcitatory drive from the RVL is mediated by adrenaline coreleased with another neurotransmitter or by an independent pool of neurons perforce having similar projection pathways has yet to be determined (Figs. 17 and 18). Whereas adrenergic perikarya presently constitute one of the largest neurochemically identified prespinal cell groups in

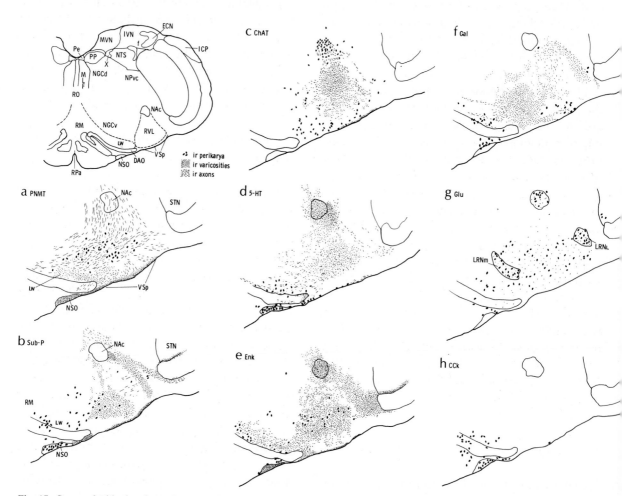

Fig. 17. Camera lucida drawings of a coronal section of the rostral medulla (top) illustrating the nucleus RVL. Drawings illustrate the distributions of identified neurons (closed circles), axons (lines) and fine punctate varicosities (stippling) labelled immunocytochemically for PNMT (a); substance P (b); choline acetyltransferase (c); 5-hydroxytryptamine (d); leu-enkephalin (e); galanin (f); glutaminase (g) and cholecystokinin (h). Not illustrated are perikarya and processes in RVL immunostaining for neuropeptide Y (NPY), glutamic acid decarboxylase (GAD, the enzyme synthesizing GABA), tyrosine hydroxylase (TH), atrial natriuretic factor and corticotropin releasing hormone. The tight correspondence of adrenergic perikarya with terminal fields staining for substance P, acetylcholine, serotonin, enkephalins, TH and galanin suggest multiple putative neurotransmitter interactions involved in the tonic and reflex control of AP.

the vasomotor area of RVL (greater than 70% of the cells projecting from RVL to IML are adrenergic; a conservative estimate given the

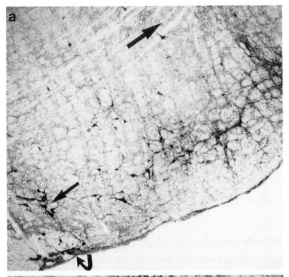

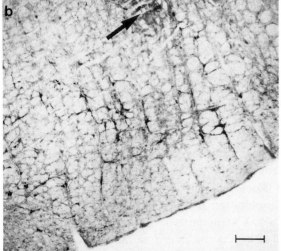

Fig. 18. Photomicrographs of perikarya and processes in the RVL demonstrating: (a) substance P-immunoreactivity (straight and curved arrows on lower left depict substance P immunoreactive cells in the lateral wings of the nucleus raphe magnus and subolivary nucleus, respectively); and (b) leu-enkephalin immunoreactivity. Dorsal arrows point to the compact division of the nucleus ambiguus. Our mapping studies of the ventral medulla suggest that most peptidergic cells (including substance P- and enkephalin-immunoreactive neurons) lie medially to the C1 area and predominantly in nuclei of the medullary raphe and pararaphe. Bar = 60 μm.

limitations of the double-label methodology), other candidates include neuropeptide Y (cosynthesized in C1 neurons, Hökfelt et al., 1983), substance P (Lorenz et al., 1985), enkephalin (Hökfelt et al., 1979), galanin (a 29-amino acid peptide isolated from porcine intestine, and present in noradrenergic cells projecting to the hypothalamus; see Levin et al., 1987), atrial natriuretic peptide (Skofitsch et al., 1985) and choline acetyltransferase (ChAT, the enzyme synthesizing acetylcholine (Ruggiero et al., 1986a; Giuliano et al., 1988b). Our recent findings suggest that a few neurons in RVL synthesize corticotropin-releasing factor (Giuliano et al., 1988a).

Perikarya containing glutamic acid decarboxylase (GAD), the enzyme synthesizing GABA (Meeley et al., 1985; Ruggiero et al., 1985b) and glutaminase (present in glutamate-neurons; antisera were generously provided by Dr. T. Kaneko, Kyoto University; Ruggiero and Kaneko, in preparation) while abundant in the RVL are scattered without organization. They immunostain extremely weakly and inconsistently (requiring prior intracerebral injections of colchicine for their expression) and while overlapping the C1 area do not resemble the morphology of premotor neurons projecting to the IML.

Neuropharmacology of the RVL

The RVL is the site of action for a broad spectrum of pharmacologic agents involved in cardiopulmonary control and derives its afferents from a variety of monoaminergic and peptidergic cell groups. The neurotransmitters of these afferent neurons and whether they derive locally or via distal sources are unresolved questions, yet their diversity is exemplified by a wealth of pharmacologically defined receptors in the RVL including: (1) *amino acids* such as GABA (the benzodiazepine complex, Ernsberger et al., 1988a), and glycine (^{3}H-strychnine, Zarbin et al., 1981); (2) *neuropeptides* (neuropeptide Y, Martel et al., 1986; neurotensin, Kessler et al., 1987, and corticotropin-releasing factor, De Souza et al.,

1985); (3) *acetylcholine* [(M2 muscarinic "cardiac" receptors labelled by ^{3}H-QNB (Giuliano et al., 1987; Ernsberger et al., 1988b,c)]; and (4) *catecholamines*: α_1-adrenergic (Young and Kuhar, 1980), and α_2-adrenergic (Unnerstall et al., 1984; Ernsberger et al., 1986) receptors; and lastly (5) *imidazole* receptors (Ernsberger et al., 1986, 1988d).

The wealth of receptor types in RVL is supported by the immunocytochemical localization of fine punctate varicosities (resembling terminal boutons) staining for the above neurotransmitters or their synthetic enzymes. Particularly high densities of processes staining for ChAT, substance P, enkephalins and 5-hydroxytryptamine overlapped adrenergic and non-adrenergic cells in the C1 area, and the area containing the respiratory cell columns (Ellenberger and Feldman, 1988); others lined the ventral medullary surface. Scattered processes in RVL were also labelled for glutaminase, GAD (Milner et al., 1987a; Ruggiero et al., 1985b), TH (Ruggiero et al., 1985c; see Milner et al., this volume) and corticotropin-releasing factor (Giuliano et al., 1988a). Extensive peptidergic, cholinergic and GABAergic plexi overlapping the vasomotor area are consistent with ultrastructural data demonstrating synapses with C1 neurons (Milner 1987a, 1988, 1989), and with the effects these agents have on AP and HR when microinjected into RVL.

Excitatory mechanisms in RVL appear to involve the neurotransmitter, acetylcholine and amino acids such as L-glutamate. That cholinergic mechanisms in the C1 area regulate AP is suggested by the following evidence: (1) local cholinergic cells and terminals in RVL labelled for ChAT synapse on both adrenergic and unidentified neurons in the RVL (Ruggiero et al., 1986a; Giuliano et al., 1988b; Milner et al., in preparation); and (2) systemically administered cholinergic agonists provoke 3-fold increases in the spontaneous activity of RVL neurons in the C1 area and increases in AP and HR mediated by the M2-cardiac receptor. The pressor response is blocked by RVL lesions or by microinjections of the M2

antagonist, AF-DX 116 that are confined to the C1 area but is unaffected by the M1 antagonist, pirenzepine, or the antinicotinic agent, hexamethonium (Giuliano et al., 1988b).

Glutamate, another excitatory neurotransmitter in RVL (Sun and Guyenet, 1986) elevates AP when injected into the C1 area (Ross et al., 1984b) and conceivably may arise, in part, from local neurons, as demonstrated by the immunocytochemical localization of glutaminase (see Fig. 17g). Bulbospinal neurons, possibly those in RVL, may employ glutamate as an excitatory neurotransmitter as suggested by two findings: (1) asymmetric putative glutamatergic synapses in IML, and (2) the observation that a glutamate receptor antagonist blocks RVL-evoked discharge of sympathetic preganglionic neurons (see Morrison et al., this volume).

GABAergic mechanisms in RVL appear to be tonically active and interact with a myriad of afferents converging there, mediating the baroreceptor and, perhaps, other cardiopulmonary reflexes. In support are pools of GABAergic (GAD-immunopositive) perikarya and punctate varicosities in RVL (Meeley et al., 1985; Ruggiero et al., 1985b), including symmetric (presumably inhibitory) synapses on C1 adrenergic and neurochemically unidentified neurons (Milner et al., 1987a); biochemical evidence for synthesis, content and Ca^{2+}-dependent release of GABA from terminals in the C1 area (Meeley et al., 1983, 1985), and functional data demonstrating that disinhibition of RVL neurons by microinjecting GABA antagonists (e.g. bicuculline) into the C1 area evokes prolonged elevations in AP and HR, simulating baroreceptor withdrawal (Feldberg, 1976; Ross et al., 1984b; Benarroch et al., 1986).

Enkephalinergic elements surrounding both adrenergic and neurochemically unidentified cells in the ventral medulla may explain the dose-related (naloxone-sensitive) changes in AP and HR and attenuation of the carotid occlusion reflex elicited by stimulating opiate-receptors in RVL (e.g. Punnen et al., 1984). Interactions between opiate peptides and catecholamines in the central regulation of AP are suggested by comparable cardiovascular actions of adrenergic agonists (see below) and ultrastructural evidence for synapses between chemically identified neurons in the RVL (Milner et al., 1989).

Adrenergic, α_2 and β, receptors in the RVL have been implicated as sites of action of the antihypertensive agents, clonidine (Bousquet and Schwartz, 1983; Bousquet et al., 1984; Ernsberger et al., 1987a,b) and propranolol, respectively (Privitera et al., 1988). Recent studies have suggested that the potent vasodepressor response to clonidine is mediated not by α_2-receptors but rather by a new class of imidazole receptors in RVL; presumably via a biologically active non-catecholaminergic ligand, clonidine-displacing factor (CDS) (Meeley et al., 1986; Ernsberger et al., 1987a,b, 1988d).

Conclusions

In conclusion, neurons in the RVL, perhaps the hypothetical tonic vasomotor center, generate basal levels of sympathetic tone and AP and integrate cardiopulmonary and cerebrovascular reflexes. The critical zone precisely coincides a chemosensory area of the rostral ventrolateral quadrant (the C1 area) where most reticulospinal neurons projecting to the IML cosynthesize the putative neurotransmitters, adrenaline and neuropeptide Y. Receptors in the RVL are responsive to a broad spectrum of cardioactive pharmacologic agents and the RVL is a major site of action of the imidazole, clonidine — a clinically effective antihypertensive drug (Bousquet and Schwartz, 1983; Granata et al., 1986). Nonetheless, still elusive is the identity of the neurotrans-

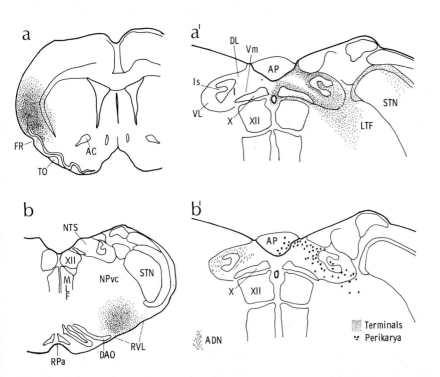

Fig. 19. An anatomical substrate for forebrain control of cardiopulmonary function. Camera lucida drawings of WGA-HRP injection sites in (a) the insular pressor area (IPA) and (b) the nucleus RVL. Anterograde transport from the IPA (a') labels terminals in cardiopulmonary subdivisions of the NTS (including an area receiving primary afferents of the aortic depressor nerve (ADN; Ciriello, 1983). The distribution of the cortical projections to the NTS (a') shows an extraordinarily tight correspondence with neurons that are retrogradely labelled from the RVL (b').

mitter in RVL generating sympathetic tone and whether it is, in fact, the C1 neurons of RVL which contribute to exaggerated sympathetic tone and, in turn, the circulatory changes involved in the initiation, expression or maintenance of neurogenic hypertension.

Stress, one of several acquired factors believed to be involved in the genesis of hypertension, may be related to the observation that the sympathetic component of the alerting response is coupled by an excitatory pathway to the RVL (Hilton et al., 1983; Hilton and Smith, 1984). The potential importance of the forebrain in the circulatory responses to stress is suggested by our anatomical observations of extensive relays from substructures coinciding the defense areas to the vasomotor

region of RVL and, also, by the striking correlation between the insular pressor area [where electrical or chemical (L-glutamate or kainate) excitation of perikarya elevates AP and HR], and cells in the insular cortex which project to subdivisions of NTS relaying cardiopulmonary afferents to the RVL (see Figs. 19 and 20). Most intriguing are the recent findings that neurochemically unidentified neurons residing in RVL and NTS have direct projections to the thalamus and areas of the frontal and cingulate cortices, bypassing the thalamus (Ruggiero et al., 1985a, 1987; Meyer et al., 1986), where frontal ablations have provoked components of sham rage and focal autonomic response (Kennard, 1945). Conceivably, sites in the RVL where signals from the forebrain converge

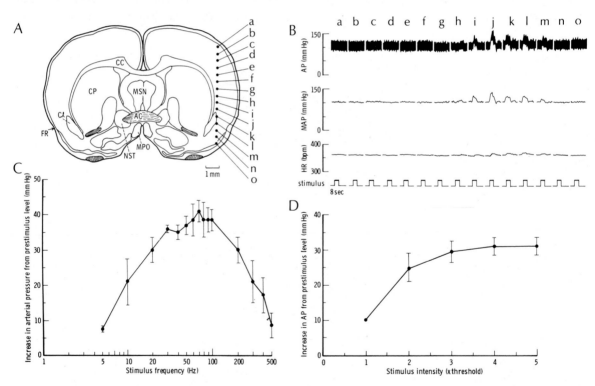

Fig. 20. Changes in arterial pressure (AP) and heart rate (HR) elicited by electrical stimulation of the insular cortex of an anesthetized rat. (A) Drawing of a coronal section of the forebrain at the level of the decussation of the anterior commissure. An electrode track that penetrates the cortex is shown with stimulus sites (a – o) illustrated by *filled circles* 500 μm apart. At each site the cortex was stimulated with an 8-sec stimulus train of square-wave pulses (0.5 msec pulse duration, 50 Hz at 100 μA). (B) AP, mean arterial pressure (MAP), and HR responses elicited from the stimulus sites. Effects of stimulus frequency (C) and intensity (D) on pressor response elicited from the insular cortex expressed as a change in AP (mmHg) from the prestimulus level (mean ± S.E.M., n = 4). The stimulus parameters are the same as in (A) and (B). (From Ruggiero et al., 1987.)

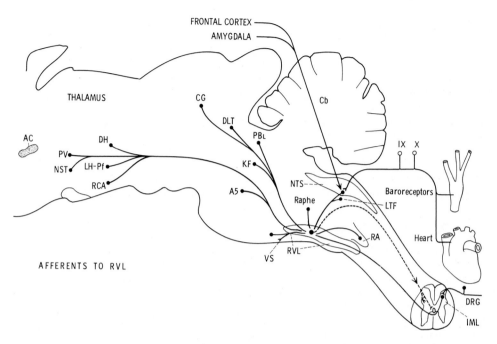

FRONTAL CORTEX
AMYGDALA

THALAMUS
CG
Cb
AC
DLT
PV
DH
PBL
IX X
NST
LH-Pf
KF
Baroreceptors
RCA
NTS
LTF
A5
Raphe
RA
Heart
VS
RVL
DRG
IML

AFFERENTS TO RVL

Fig. 21. Summary schematic drawing demonstrating that afferents to the nucleus RVL, unlike those to NPGCL derive from a discrete and functionally specific set of autonomic/limbic substructures distributed throughout the neuraxis. Afferents to RVL may play a role in somatosympathetic reflexes (via the spinal cord and raphe magnus), baroreceptor and other cardiopulmonary reflexes (via the NTS or RA), chemoreceptor and ventral surface reflexes (via the NTS or specialized processes of RVL neurons contacting the ventral subpial surface or intraparenchymal microvessels) and the defense-alerting and other conditioned autonomic responses to stress (via the central gray and forebrain). A potential-indirect route from the insular cortex and amygdala to nucleus RVL may occur by their projections to the subcortical forebrain (e.g. bed nucleus of stria terminalis and hypothalamus) or to neurons in the lower brainstem (e.g. NTS) (see text). The precise organization of the terminal fields and receptors in RVL and CVL and their relationships to vasomotor versus respiratory premotor neurons projecting respectively to the IML or phrenic and intercostal spinal motor nuclei has yet to be established.

with and in part reciprocate afferents from visceral, nociceptive and other sensory nuclei (Fig. 21) (Ruggiero et al., 1985a, 1986b, 1987; Stornetta et al., 1988) provide substrates whereby baroreceptor excitation lowers AP and depresses central afferent neurotransmission and electrocortical activity (Dworkin, 1988). The anatomical pathways, as described here, suggest that neurons in nucleus RVL may integrate the tonic and reflex control of AP and, perhaps, the autonomic adjustments to aversive and behaviorally-provoked stimulation.

References

Alexander, R.S. (1946) Tonic and reflex functions of medullary sympathetic cardiovascular centers. *J. Neurophysiol.,* 9: 205 – 217.

Amendt, K., Czachurski, J., Dembowsky, K. and Seller, H. (1978) Neurons within the "chemosensitive area" on the ventral surface of the brainstem which project to the intermediolateral column. *Pfluegers Arch.,* 375: 289 – 292.

Andrezik, J.A., Chan-Palay, V. and Palay, S.L. (1981) The nucleus paragigantocellularis lateralis in the rat. Conformation and cytology. *Anat. Embryol.,* 161: 355 – 371.

Arango, V., Ruggiero, D.A., Callaway, J.L., Anwar, M., Mann, J.J. and Reis, D.J. (1988) Catecholaminergic neurons in the ventrolateral medulla and nucleus of the solitary tract in the human. *J. Comp. Neurol.,* 273: 224 – 240.

Armstrong, D.M., Ross, C.A., Pickel, V.M., Joh, T.H. and Reis, D.J. (1982) Distribution of dopamine-, noradrenaline- and adrenaline-containing cell bodies in the rat medulla oblongata demonstrated by the immunocytochemical localization of catecholamine biosynthetic enzymes. *J. Comp. Neurol.,* 212: 173 – 187.

Barman, S.M. and Gebber, G.L. (1985) Axonal projection patterns of ventrolateral medullospinal sympathoexcitatory

76

neurons. *J. Neurophysiol.,* 53: 1551 – 1566.

Basbaum, A.I., Clanton, C.H. and Fields, H.L. (1978) Three bulbospinal pathways from the rostral medulla of the cat: an autoradiographic study of pain modulating systems. *J. Comp. Neurol.,* 178: 209 – 224.

Benarroch, E.E., Granata, A.R., Ruggiero, D.A., Park, D.H. and Reis, D.J. (1986) Neurons of the C1 area mediate cardiovascular responses initiated from the ventral medullary surface. *Am. J. Physiol. (Regulatory),* 250: R932 – R945.

Blessing, W.W., Hedger, S.C., Joh, T.H. and Willoughby, J.O. (1987) Neurons in the area postrema are the only catecholamine-synthesizing cells in the medulla or pons with projections to the rostral ventrolateral medulla (C$_1$-area) in the rabbit. *Brain Res.,* 419: 336 – 340.

Bousquet, P. and Schwartz, J. (1983) α-Adrenergic drugs: pharmacological tools for the study of the central vasomotor control. *Biochem. Pharmacol.,* 32: 1459 – 1465.

Bousquet, P., Feldman, J., Bloch, R. and Schwartz, J. (1984) Central cardiovascular effects of α-adrenergic drugs: differences between catecholamines and imidazolines. *J. Pharmacol. Exp. Ther.,* 230: 232 – 236.

Brown, D.L. and Guyenet, P.G. (1984) Cardiovascular neurons of brain stem with projection to spinal cord. *Am. J. Physiol.,* 247: R1009 – R1016.

Chan, S.H.H., Chan, J.Y.H. and Ong, B.T. (1986) Anatomic connections between nucleus reticularis rostroventrolateralis and some medullary cardiovascular sites in the rat. *Neurosci. Lett.,* 71: 277 – 282.

Ciriello, J. (1983) Brainstem projections of aortic baroreceptor afferent fibers in the rat. *Neurosci. Lett.,* 36: 37 – 42.

Ciriello, J. and Caverson, M.M. (1986) Bidirectional cardiovascular connections between ventrolateral medulla and nucleus of the solitary tract. *Brain Res.,* 367: 273 – 281.

Ciriello, J., Caverson, M.M. and Calaresu, F.F. (1985) Lateral hypothalamic and peripheral cardiovascular input to ventrolateral medullary neurons. *Brain Res.,* 347: 173 – 176.

Cravo, S.L., Ruggiero, D.A., Anwar, M. and Reis, D.J. (1988) Quantitative-topographic analysis of adrenergic and non-adrenergic spinal projections of cardiovascular area of RVL. *Soc. Neurosci. Abstr.,* 14: 328.

Cushing, H. (1902) Some experimental and clinical observations concerning states of increased intracranial tension. *Am. J. Med. Sci.,* 124: 375 – 400.

Dampney, R.A.L. and Moon, E.A. (1980) Role of ventrolateral medulla in vasomotor response to cerebral ischemia. *Am. J. Physiol.,* 239: H349 – H358.

Dampney, R.A.L., Czachurski, J., Dembowsky, K., Goodchild, A.K. and Seller, H. (1987) Afferent connections and spinal projections of the pressor region in the rostral ventrolateral medulla of the cat. *J. Auton. Nerv. Syst.,* 20: 73 – 86.

Dampney, R.A.L., Goodchild, A.K., Robertson, L.G. and Montgomery, W. (1982) Role of ventrolateral medulla in vasomotor regulation: a correlative anatomical and physiological study. *Brain Res.,* 249: 223 – 235.

Day, T.A. and Renaud, L.P. (1983) Depressor area within caudal ventrolateral medulla of the rat does not correspond to the A1 catecholamine cell group. *Brain Res.,* 279: 299 – 302.

DeSouza, E.B., Insel, T.R., Perrin, M.H., Rivier, J., Vale, W.W. and Kuhar, M.J. (1985) Corticotropin-releasing factor receptors are widely distributed within the rat central nervous system: an autoradiographic study. *J. Neurosci.,* 5: 3189 – 3203.

Dittmar, C. (1873) Ein neuer Beweis für die Reizbarkeit der centripetalen Endfasern des Ruckenmarks. *Akad. Wissenschaften, Leipzig. Mathematisch-physische Klasse.* Berichte 22: 18 – 45.

Dworkin, B. (1988) Hypertension as a learned response: the baroreceptor reinforcement hypothesis. In T. Elbert, W. Langosch, A. Steptoe and D. Vaitl (Eds.), *Behavioral Mechanisms in Cardiovascular Disorders,* pp. 17 – 47.

Ellenberger, H.H. and Feldman, J.L. (1988) Monosynaptic transmission of respiratory drive to phrenic motoneurons from brainstem bulbospinal neurons in rats. *J. Comp. Neurol.,* 269: 47 – 57.

Ernsberger, P., Arango, V., Meeley, M.P. and Reis, D.J. (1986) Selective binding of an endogenous clonidine-like substance to imidazole binding sites and distribution of these sites in the medulla oblongata of the rat. *Soc. Neurosci. Abstr.,* 12: 1334.

Ernsberger, P., Meeley, M.P., Mann, J.J. and Reis, D.J. (1987a) Clonidine binds to imidazole binding sites as well as α_2-adrenoceptors in the ventrolateral medulla. *Eur. J. Pharmacol.,* 134: 1 – 13.

Ernsberger, P., Meeley, M.P. and Reis, D.J. (1987b) Imidazole binding sites in the ventrolateral medulla (VLM) labeled with ^{3}H-cimetidine are modulated by a clonidine-displacing substance. *Fed. Proc.,* 46: 1460.

Ernsberger, P., Arango, V., Iacovitti, L. and Reis, D.J. (1988a) Photoaffinity labeling of benzodiazepine receptors in slide-mounted sections and β-adrenergic receptors in intact cells. *Soc. Neurosci. Abstr.,* 14: 170.

Ernsberger, P., Arango, V. and Reis, D.J. (1988b) A high density of muscarinic receptors in the rostral ventrolateral medulla of the rat is revealed by correction for autoradiographic efficiency. *Neurosci. Lett.,* 85: 179 – 186.

Ernsberger, P., Arneric, S.P., Arango, V. and Reis, D.J. (1988c) Quantitative distribution of muscarinic receptors and choline acetyltransferase in rat medulla: examination of transmitter-receptor mismatch. *Brain Res.,* 452: 336 – 344.

Ernsberger, P., Meeley, M.P. and Reis, D.J. (1988d) An endogenous substance with clonidine-like properties: selective binding to imidazole sites in the ventrolateral medulla. *Brain Res.,* 441: 309 – 318.

Feldberg, W. (1976) The ventral surface of the brain stem: a scarcely explored region of pharmacological sensitivity.

Neuroscience, 1: 427 – 441.

Feldberg, W. and Guertzenstein, P.G. (1972) A vasodepressor effect of pentobarbitone sodium. *J. Physiol. (Lond.),* 224: 83 – 103.

Feldberg, W. and Guertzenstein, P.G. (1976) Vasodepressor effects obtained by drugs acting on the ventral surface of the brain stem. *J. Physiol. (Lond.),* 229: 395 – 408.

Feldman, J.L., Loewy, A.D. and Speck, D.F. (1985) Projections from the ventral respiratory group to phrenic and intercostal motoneurons in the cat: an autoradiographic study. *J. Neurosci.,* 5: 1993 – 2000.

Gebber, G.L. and Barman, S.M. (1985) Lateral tegmental field neurons of cat medulla: a potential source of basal sympathetic nerve discharge. *J. Neurophysiol.,* 54: 1498 – 1512.

Giuliano, R., Ernsberger, P. and Reis, D.J. (1987) Cholinergic vasopressor mechanism in rostral ventrolateral medulla is mediated by the M2 muscarinic receptor. *Soc. Neurosci. Abstr.,* 13: 808.

Giuliano, R., Ruggiero, D.A., Milner, T.A., Anwar, M. and Reis, D.J. (1988a) Corticotropin-releasing factor: anatomical substrates of autonomic regulation. *Soc. Neurosci. Abstr.,* 14: 23.

Giuliano, R., Ruggiero, D.A., Morrison, S., Ernsberger, P. and Reis, D.J. (1988b) Cholinergic regulation of arterial blood pressure by the C1 area of the rostral ventrolateral medulla. *J. Neurosci.,* 9: 923 – 942.

Granata, A.R., Ruggiero, D.A., Park, D.H., Joh, T.H. and Reis, D.J. (1985) Brain stem area with C1 epinephrine neurons mediates baroreflex vasodepressor responses. *Am. J. Physiol.,* 248 (*Heart Circ. Physiol.,* 17): H547 – H567.

Granata, A.R., Numao, Y., Kumada, M. and Reis, D.J. (1986) A1 noradrenergic neurons tonically inhibit sympathoexcitatory neurons of the C1 area in rat brainstem. *Brain Res.,* 377: 127 – 146.

Guertzenstein, P.G. and Silver, A. (1974) Fall in blood pressure produced from discrete regions of the ventral surface of the medulla by glycine and lesions. *J. Physiol. (Lond.),* 242: 489 – 503.

Guyenet, P.G. and Brown, D.L. (1986) Unit activity in nucleus paragigantocellularis lateralis during cerebral ischemia in the rat. *Brain Res.,* 364: 301 – 314.

Hilton, S.M. (1975) Ways of viewing the central nervous control of the circulation-old and new. *Brain Res.,* 87: 213 – 219.

Hilton, S.M. and Smith, P.R. (1984) Ventral medullary neurons excited from the hypothalamic and mid-brain defence areas. *J. Auton. Nerv. Syst.,* 11: 35 – 42.

Hilton, S.M., Marshall, J.M. and Timms, R.J. (1983) Ventral medullary relay neurons in the pathway from the defence areas of the cat and their effect on blood pressure. *J. Physiol. (Lond.),* 345: 149 – 166.

Hökfelt, T., Fuxe, K., Goldstein, M. and Johansson, O. (1974) Immunohistochemical evidence for the existence of adrenaline neurons in rat brain. *Brain Res.,* 66: 235 – 251.

Hökfelt, T., Terenius, L., Kuypers, H.G.J.M. and Dann, O.

(1979) Evidence for enkephalin immunoreactive neurons in the medulla oblongata projecting to the spinal cord. *Neurosci. Lett.,* 14: 55 – 60.

Hökfelt, T., Lundberg, J.M., Tatemoto, K., Mutt, V., Terenius, L., Polak, J., Bloom, S., Sasek, C., Elde, R. and Goldstein, M. (1983) Neuropeptide Y (NPY) and FMRF amide neuropeptide-like immunoreactivities in catecholamine neurons of the rat medulla oblongata. *Acta Physiol. Scand.,* 117: 315 – 318.

Iwamoto, G.A., Kaufman, M.P., Botterman, B.R. and Mitchell, J.H. (1982) Effects of lateral reticular nucleus lesions on the exercise pressor reflex in cats. *Circ. Res.,* 51: 400 – 403.

Kalia, M. and Richter, D. (1985) Morphology of physiologically identified slowly adapting lung stretch receptor afferents stained with intra-axonal horseradish peroxidase in the nucleus of the tractus solitarius of the cat. I. A light microscopic analysis. *J. Comp. Neurol.,* 241: 503 – 520.

Kennard, M.A. (1945) Focal-autonomic representation in the cortex and the relation to sham rage. *J. Neuropathol. Exp. Neurol.,* 4: 296 – 304.

Kessler, J.P., Moyse, E., Kitabgi, P., Vincent, J.P. and Beaudet, A. (1987) Distribution of neurotensin binding sites in the caudal brainstem of the rat: a light microscopic radioautographic study. *Neuroscience,* 23: 189 – 198.

Levin, M.C., Sawchenko, P.E., Howe, P.R.C., Bloom, S.R. and Polak, J.M. (1987) Organization of galanin-immunoreactive inputs to the paraventricular nucleus with special reference to their relationships to catecholaminergic afferents. *J. Comp. Neurol.,* 261: 562 – 582.

Loewy, A.D., Saper, C.B. and Baker, R.P. (1979) Descending projections from the pontine micturition center. *Brain Res.,* 172: 533 – 538.

Lorenz, R.G., Saper, C.B., Wong, D.L., Ciaranello, R.D. and Loewy, A.D. (1985) Colocalization of substance P and phenylethanolamine *N*-methyltransferase-like immunoreactivity in neurons of the ventrolateral medulla that project to the spinal cord: potential role in control of vasomotor tone. *Neurosci. Lett.,* 55: 255 – 260.

Martel, J.-C., St. Pierre, S. and Quiron, R. (1986) Neuropeptide Y receptors in rat brain: autoradiographic localization. *Peptides,* 7: 55 – 60.

Meeley, M.P., Underwood, M.D., Talman, W.T. and Reis, D.J. (1983) Content and in vitro release of endogenous amino acids in the area of the nucleus tractus solitarius (NTS). *Soc. Neurosci. Abstr.,* 9: 262.

Meeley, M.P., Ruggiero, D.A., Ishitsuka, T. and Reis, D.J. (1985) Intrinsic GABA neurons in the nucleus of the tractus solitarius and the rostral ventrolateral medulla in the rat: an immunocytochemical and biochemical study. *Neurosci. Lett.,* 58: 83 – 89.

Meeley, M.P., Ernsberger, P.R., Granata, A.R. and Reis, D.J. (1986) An endogenous clonidine-displacing substance from bovine brain: receptor binding and hypotensive actions in the ventrolateral medulla. *Life Sci.*, 38: 1119–1126.

Meessen, H. and Olszewski, J. (1949) A *Cytoarchitectonic Atlas of the Rhombdencephalon of the Rabbit*, Karger, Basel.

Meyer, G., Galindo-Mireles, D., Gonzalez-Hernandez, T., Castañeyra-Perdomo, A. and Ferres-Torres, R. (1986) Direct projections from the reticular formation of the medulla oblongata to the anterior cingulate cortex in the mouse and the rat. *Brain Res.*, 398: 207–211.

Milner, T.A., Pickel, V.M., Chan, J., Massari, V.J., Oertel, W.H., Park, D.H., Joh, T.H. and Reis, D.J. (1987a) Adrenergic neurons in the rostral ventrolateral medulla. II. Synaptic interactions with GABA-ergic terminals. *Brain Res.*, 411: 46–57.

Milner, T.A., Pickel, V.M., Park, D.H., Joh, T.H. and Reis, D.J. (1987b) Phenylethanolamine *N*-methyltransferase-containing neurons in the rostral ventrolateral medulla of the rat. I. Normal ultrastructure. *Brain Res.*, 411: 28–45.

Milner, T.A., Pickel, V.M., Abate, C., Joh, T.H. and Reis, D.J. (1988) Ultrastructural characterization of substance P-like immunoreactive neurons in the rostral ventrolateral medulla in relation to neurons containing catecholamine-synthesizing enzymes. *J. Comp. Neurol.*, 270: 427–445.

Milner, T.A., Pickel, V.M. and Reis, D.J. (1989) Ultrastructural basis for interactions between central opioids and catecholamines. I. Rostral ventrolateral medulla. *J. Neurosci.*, 9: 2114–2130.

Morrison, S.F., Milner, T.A. and Reis, D.J. (1985) Reticulospinal vasomotor neurons of the rat rostral ventrolateral medulla: relationship to sympathetic nerve activity and the C1 adrenergic cell group. *J. Neurosci.*, 8: 1286–1301.

Olszewski, J. and Baxter, D. (1954) *Cytoarchitecture of the Human Brainstem*, Karger, Basel.

Privitera, P.J., Granata, A.R., Underwood, M.D., Gaffney, T.E. and Reis, D.J. (1989) C1 area of the rostral ventrolateral medulla as a site for the central hypotensive action of propranolol. *J. Pharmacol. Exp. Ther.*, 246: 529–535.

Punnen, S., Willette, R., Krieger, A.J. and Sapru, H.N. (1984) Cardiovascular response to injections of enkephalin in the pressor area of the ventrolateral medulla. *Neuropharmacology*, 23: 939–946.

Ranson, S.W. (1916) New evidence in favor of a vasoconstrictor center in the brain. *Am. J. Physiol.*, 42: 1–8.

Ross, C.A., Armstrong, D.M., Ruggiero, D.A., Pickel, V.M., Joh, T.H. and Reis, D.J. (1981a) Adrenaline neurons in the rostral ventrolateral medulla innervate thoracic spinal cord: combined immunocytochemical and retrograde transport demonstration. *Neurosci. Lett.*, 25: 257–262.

Ross, C.A., Ruggiero, D.A. and Reis, D.J. (1981b) Projections to the spinal cord from neurons close to the ventral surface of the hindbrain of the rat. *Neurosci. Lett.*, 21: 143–148.

Ross, C.A., Ruggiero, D.A., Joh, T.H. Park, D.H. and Reis, D.J. (1983) Adrenaline synthesizing neurons in the rostral

ventrolateral medulla: a possible role in the tonic vasomotor control. *Brain Res.*, 273: 356–361.

Ross, C.A., Ruggiero, D.A., Joh, T.H., Park, D.H. and Reis, D.J. (1984a) Rostral ventrolateral medulla: selective projections to the thoracic autonomic cell column from the region containing C1 adrenaline neurons. *J. Comp. Neurol.*, 228: 168–184.

Ross, C.A., Ruggiero, D.A., Park, T.H., Sved, A.F., Fernandez-Pardal, J., Saavedra, J.M. and Reis, D.J. (1984b) Tonic vasomotor control by the rostral ventrolateral medulla: effect of electrical or chemical stimulation of the area containing C1 adrenaline neurons on arterial pressure, heart rate and plasma catecholamines and vasopressin. *J. Neurosci.*, 4: 479–494.

Ross, C.A., Ruggiero, D.A. and Reis, D.J. (1985) Projections from the nucleus tractus solitarii to the rostral ventrolateral medulla. *J. Comp. Neurol.*, 242: 511–534.

Ruggiero, D.A. and Reis, D.J. (1988) Neurons containing phenylethanolamine *N*-methyltransferase: a component of the baroreceptor reflex? In J.M. Stolk, D.C. U'Prichard, and K. Fuxe (Eds.), *Epinephrine in the Central Nervous System*, Oxford University Press, New York, pp. 291–307.

Ruggiero, D.A., Ross, C.A., Anwar, M. and Reis, D.J. (1984) The rostral ventrolateral medulla: immunocytochemistry of intrinsic neurons and afferent connections. *Soc. Neurosci. Abstr.*, 10: 229.

Ruggiero, D.A., Anwar, M., Park, D.H. and Reis, D.J. (1985a) Autonomic projections of medullary adrenaline-synthesizing neurons. *Soc. Neurosci. Abstr.*, 11: 491.

Ruggiero, D.A., Meeley, M.P., Anwar, M. and Reis, D.J. (1985b) Newly identified GABAergic neurons in regions of the ventrolateral medulla which regulate blood pressure. *Brain Res.*, 339: 171–177.

Ruggiero, D.A., Ross, C.A., Anwar, M., Park, D.H., Joh, T.H. and Reis, D.J. (1985c) Distribution of neurons containing phenylethanolamine *N*-methyltransferase in medulla and hypothalamus of rat. *J. Comp. Neurol.*, 239: 127–154.

Ruggiero, D.A., Giuliano, R. and Reis, D.J. (1986a) Cholinergic neurons in autonomic brainstem nuclei. *Fed. Proc.*, 46: 493.

Ruggiero, D.A., Stornetta, R.L., Morrison, S.F. and Reis, D.J. (1986b) Spinal projections to brainstem autonomic centers. *Soc. Neurosci. Abstr.*, 12: 1156.

Ruggiero, D.A., Mraovitch, S., Granata, A.R., Anwar, M. and Reis, D.J. (1987) A role of insular cortex in cardiovascular function. *J. Comp. Neurol.*, 257: 189–207.

Schläfke, M. and Löschke, H.H. (1967) Lokalisation eines an der Regulation von Atmung und Kreislauf beteiligten Gebiets an der ventralen Oberflaeche der Medulla oblongata durch Kalteblockade. *Pfluegers Arch.*, 297: 201–220.

Skofitsch, G., Jacobowitz, D.M., Eskay, R.L. and Zamir, N. (1985) Distribution of atrial naturetic factor-like immunoreactive neurons in the rat brain. *Neuroscience*, 16: 917–948.

Stometta, R., Morrison, S.L., Ruggiero, D.A. and Reis, D.J. (1989) Neurons in the rostral ventrolateral medulla mediate the somatic pressor reflex. *Am. J. Physiol.,* 25: R448 – 462.

Sun, M.K. and Guyenet, P.G. (1986) Hypothalamic glutamatergic input to medullary sympathoexcitatory neurons in rats. *Am. J. Physiol.,* 251: R798 – R810.

Sun, M.-K., Filtz, T. and Guyenet, P.G. (1986) Role of glutamate in baroreflexes. *Soc. Neurosci. Abstr.,* 12: 580.

Tucker, D.C., Saper, C.B., Ruggiero, D.A. and Reis, D.J. (1987) Organization of central adrenergic pathways. I. Relationships of ventrolateral medullary projections to the hypothalamus and spinal cord. *J. Comp. Neurol.,* 259: 591 – 603.

Underwood, M.D., Iadecola, C. and Reis, D.J. (1986) Bilateral lesion of the C1 area of the rostral ventrolateral medulla globally impairs the cerebrovascular response to hypoxia.

Soc. Neurosci. Abstr., 12: 1320.

Unnerstall, J.R., Kopaitic, T.A. and Kuhar, M.J. (1984) Distribution of α_2-agonist binding sites in the rat and human central nervous system: analysis of some functional, anatomic correlates of the pharmacological effects of clonidine and related adrenergic agents. *Brain Res. Rev.,* 7: 69 – 101.

Walberg, F. (1952) Lateral reticular nucleus in medulla oblongata in mammals; comparative anatomical study. *J. Comp. Neurol.,* 96: 283 – 343.

Young, W.S., III and Kuhar, M.J. (1980) Noradrenergic α_1- and α_2-receptors: light microscopic autoradiographic localization. *Proc. Natl. Acad. Sci. U.S.A.,* 77: 1696 – 1700.

Zarbin, M.A., Wamsley, J.K. and Kuhar, M.J. (1981) Glycine receptor: light microscopic autoradiographic localization with ^{3}H-strychnine. *J. Neurosci.,* 1: 532 – 547.

Contribution of Ventrolateral Medullary Neurons to Vasomotor Tone

J. Ciriello, M.M. Caverson and C. Polosa (Eds.)
Progress in Brain Research, Vol. 81
© 1989 Elsevier Science Publishers B.V. (Biomedical Division)

CHAPTER 5

Inhibitory vasomotor neurons in the caudal ventrolateral region of the medulla oblongata

W.W. Blessing and Yu-Wen Li

Centre for Neuroscience, Departments of Medicine and Physiology, Flinders University of South Australia, Bedford Park, 5042 S.A., Australia

Introduction

In this chapter we give a brief history of the discovery of sympathoinhibitory vasomotor neurons in the caudal ventrolateral medulla and then we address particular aspects of their function, drawing on published work and presenting new experimental evidence.

Definition of inhibitory vasomotor neuronal groups within the medulla oblongata is a relatively recent achievement, facilitated by advances in neuroanatomical methodology. In retrospect it is easy to see that the interpretation of traditional electrical stimulation, recording and lesion studies (e.g. Alexander, 1946; Chai and Wang, 1962) should have been more circumspect because the problem of fibres of passage is particularly relevant to studies within the medulla oblongata. The first hints of the existence of vasodepressor neurons outside of the nucleus tractus solitarius (NTS) came from "ventral surface" pharmacological studies of Feldberg and his colleagues (Feldberg 1976; Feldberg and Guertzenstein, 1976). These authors defined a nicotine sensitive vasodepressor area on the ventral surface of the cat medulla, near the exiting rootlets of the hypoglossal nerve. Emphasis was placed on the concept of the "surface" of the medulla and no attempt was made to interpret this finding in terms of the known neuroanatomy of the region. Presumably the vasodepressor response depends on the action of nicotine diffusing to particular neuronal cell bodies or dendritic processes located within the ventrolateral medulla. Studies in other species have shown that a vasodepressor response can be elicited by stimulation of neurons in the caudal ventrolateral medulla and evidence (see below) suggests that the vasodepressor cells are located between the nucleus ambiguus and lateral reticular nucleus, a region of the reticular formation in which neurons are poorly demonstrated with Nissl stains (Fig. 1).

Neuroanatomical interest in the caudal ventrolateral region of the medulla followed the studies of Dahlstrom and Fuxe (1964, 1965), Ungerstedt (1971) and Swanson and Hartman (1975) who defined the A1 group of noradrenaline-containing neurons, some years before the C1 adrenaline containing-cells were located in the rostral ventrolateral medulla (Hökfelt et al., 1974). Although Ungerstedt emphasized the rostral projections of the A1 cells it was generally assumed that these neurons projected to the spinal cord, probably to the sympathetic preganglionic cells. Functional studies followed this line of thinking. Coote and his colleagues used electrical stimulation and extracellular recording techniques to suggest that the A1 cells have a sympathoinhibitory function in the cat (Coote and McLeod, 1974a,b), a possibility also considered by Dembowsky et al.

(1981). Support for this conclusion came from studies in the rabbit where it was shown that electrolytic lesions in the region of the caudal ventrolateral medulla containing the A1 cells caused acute hypertension, manifested after recovery from anaesthesia (Blessing et al., 1981b). Surviving animals had increased peripheral vascular resistance. However, interpretion of findings from all these studies was complicated by the finding that

A1 cells probably do not project to the spinal cord (see below).

A new generation of functional studies utilized focal intramedullary injections of pharmacological agents known to excite or inhibit nerve cell bodies, thereby reducing problems of interpretation due to effects on fibres of passage (Goodchild et al., 1982). Injection of L-glutamate into the caudal ventrolateral medulla in anaesthetized rabbits (Fig.

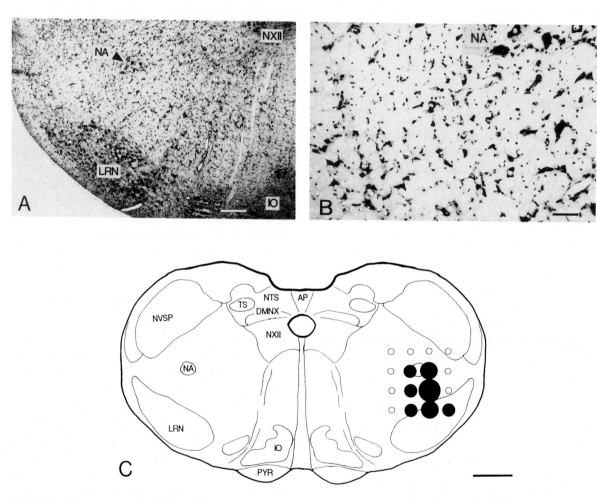

Fig. 1. (A) Photomicrograph of a Nissl stained transverse section of rabbit medulla oblongata at the rostrocaudal level of the mid inferior olive (IO), the hypoglossal nucleus (NXII) and the exiting rootlets of the hypoglossal nerve (bar = 400 μm). (B) Higher power photomicrograph of the region between the nucleus ambiguus (NA) and the lateral reticular nucleus (LRN) showing that the neurons in this region stain poorly for Nissl substance (bar = 100 μm). (C) Location of vasodepressor neurons in the caudal ventrolateral medulla of the rabbit between the nucleus ambiguus and the lateral reticular nucleus. The closed circles indicate sites from which vasodepressor responses were elicited by small injections of L-glutamate (see text). No significant change in arterial pressure was elicited from regions marked with an open circle (bar = 1 mm).

2), rats and cats caused a dramatic fall in arterial pressure, accompanied by inhibition of peripheral sympathetic vasomotor tone (Blessing and Reis, 1982; Willette et al., 1983a; McAllen and Woollard, 1984; Pilowsky et al., 1985). The possible physiological importance of this observation was emphasized by the ability of neuroinhibitory agents to increase arterial pressure when injected into the same region of the caudal ventrolateral medulla (Blessing and Reis, 1983; Willette et al., 1983b). In particular muscimol, a long acting GABA receptor stimulating agent, caused a major increase in arterial pressure (Fig. 3A), sometimes associated with cardiac arrhythmias and pulmonary congestion. These observations suggested that the vasodepressor neurons are tonically active, at least in the anaesthetized animal.

Pharmacological studies using receptor antagonists suggested the existence of tonically active inputs to the vasodepressor neurons. Inhibitory GABA (Fig. 3B) and glycine-like inputs were demonstrated (Blessing and Reis, 1983; Willette et

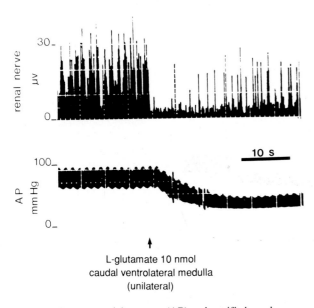

Fig. 2. Effect on arterial pressure (AP) and rectified renal sympathetic nerve activity of a unilateral injection of L-glutamate into the caudal ventrolateral medullary area containing the vasodepressor neurons in the urethane-anaesthetized, paralyzed and mechanically ventilated rabbit.

al., 1984c). In addition, the depressor neurons apparently possess inhibitory receptors for opiates (Willette et al., 1984a). Interestingly, although a nicotine-sensitive depressor response was originally described (Feldberg and Guertzenstein, 1976) the presence of a nicotinic receptor on the vasodepressor neurons has not yet been demonstrated by focal intramedullary injections of the appropriate pharmacological agents.

Vasodepressor neurons; their output pathway and the neurotransmitters involved

The early identification of the vasodepressor neurons as A1 noradrenaline-synthesizing neurons, inhibiting sympathetic preganglionic neurons by a direct spinal projection, has been complicated by the findings of intra-axonal transport studies in the rat (Loewy et al., 1981; Westlund et al., 1983) and the rabbit (Blessing et al., 1981) showing that the A1 cells do not project to the spinal cord. Lesion studies coupled with biochemical assay of catecholamine levels in the spinal cord suggested that A1 cells might have descending projections in the cat (Fleetwood-Walker et al., 1983) but this finding has not been confirmed. Retrograde transport studies in the cat (Amendt et al., 1979), rabbit (Blessing et al., 1981a) and rat (Ross et al., 1985a) show that the majority of neurons projecting to the spinal cord from the ventrolateral medulla originate in the rostral region, similar to the situation in other species. This finding has been confirmed by anterograde tracing procedures in the cat (Caverson et al., 1983; Dampney et al., 1987) and in the rat (Ross et al., 1985b). Anterograde studies in the rabbit (Li and Blessing, 1989) have confirmed the projection from the rostral ventrolateral medulla to the intermediolateral column and we have not yet been able to demonstrate a similar projection from the caudal ventrolateral medulla.

Blessing and Reis (1982) hypothesized that the A1 noradrenaline-containing neurons might mediate the depressor response by means of a short inhibitory projection to sympathoexcitatory neurons present in the rostral ventrolateral medulla (Dampney et al., 1982; Ross et al., 1984). Willette et al. reported the first evidence that vasomotor responses elicited by chemical stimulation of the caudal ventrolateral medulla are indeed mediated by an action on neurons in the rostral ventrolateral medulla (Willette et al., 1984b). Their evidence did not bear directly on the question of the neurotransmitter in the vasodepressor neurons. Granata and colleagues (Granata et al., 1985a, 1986) provided pharmacological evidence in support of the hypothesis that the vasodepressor cells belong to the A1 group of neurons. Day and colleagues used focal electrical stimulation in the rat

caudal ventrolateral medulla to suggest that the depressor response depends on neurons situated in the nucleus ambiguus and in the region slightly dorsomedial to these cells (Day et al., 1983), implying that the depressor neurons could not be A1 cells. However, chemical stimulation and inhibition studies show the location of vasodepressor neurons in the rat as being ventral to the nucleus ambiguus, in a region which does include A1 neurons (e.g. Willette et al., 1983b; Gordon, 1987; Guyenet, 1987; Kubo and Kihara, 1988). What is required is evidence from very small injections of excitatory or inhibitory pharmacological agents. We have completed such experiments in the rabbit

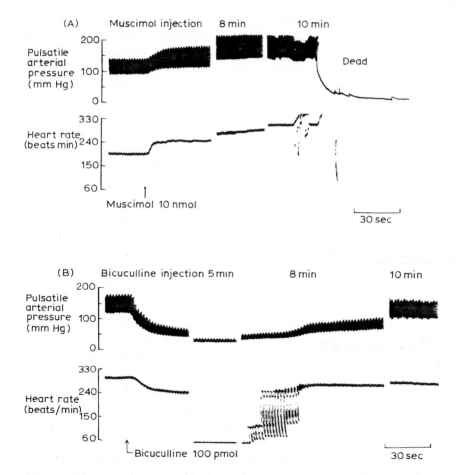

Fig. 3. Effect on arterial pressure and heart rate of bilateral injections of either muscimol (A) or bicuculline (B) into the caudal ventrolateral medullary area containing the vasodepressor neurons in the urethane-anaesthetized, paralyzed and mechanically ventilated rabbit. (Modified from Blessing and Reis, 1983.)

using either 25 or 10 nl of 0.5 or 0.1 nmol L-glutamate (Li and Blessing, 1988). These studies have confirmed that the depressor neurons in this species are concentrated in the region of the reticular formation which lies between the nucleus ambiguus and the lateral reticular nucleus (Fig. 1), on the medial aspect of the A1 neurons, overlapping with the medial half of this group. The size of the vasodepressor area is not greatly reduced by the use of the smaller amounts of L-glutamate and it seems that the depressor neurons are distributed within a small region of the reticular formation just ventral to the nucleus ambiguus at a rostrocaudal level corresponding with the caudal two thirds of the area postrema. There are A1 neurons in the vasodepressor region in the rabbit and it is not possible to exclude their participation in the depressor response by more selective intra-medullary injections.

However, evidence from other sources weighs strongly against the role of the A1 cells as mediators of the vasodepressor response. Sun and Guyenet (1986) provided neuroanatomical evidence from double labelling studies that no A1 cells project to the rostral ventrolateral medulla. This double labelling work in the rat is consistent with the available evidence from other retrograde intra-axonal transport studies in this species (Chan et al., 1986) and in the cat (Dampney et al., 1987). These studies show that the majority of neurons projecting from caudal to the rostral ventrolateral medulla are situated just medial and dorsal to the A1 group. The situation is similar in the rabbit. Figure 4 (A – D) shows the distribution of retrogradely labelled medullary neurons in this species after injection of Fluorogold or rhodamine-labelled latex beads into the rostral ventrolateral medulla. By combining retrograde transport of

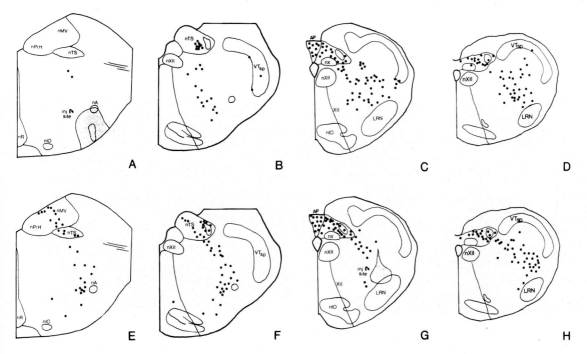

Fig. 4. Distribution of retrogradely labelled neurons after injection of either Fluorogold or rhodamine-labelled latex beads into the rostral (A – D) or the caudal (E – H) ventrolateral medulla in the rabbit. Abbreviations: AP = area postrema; LRN = lateral reticular nucleus; nA = nucleus ambiguus; nIO = inferior olive; nMv = medial vestibular nucleus; nPrH = nucleus prepositus hypoglossae; DMNX = dorsal motor nucleus of the vagus; nXII = hypoglossal nucleus; VTsp = spinal tract of the trigeminal nerve; XII = hypoglossal nerve.

88

Fluorogold with tyrosine hydroxylase immunohistochemistry (Blessing et al., 1987a) and by combining either Fluorogold or rhodamine-labelled beads with FAGLU catecholamine histofluorescence (unpublished data) we have consistently shown that no A1 neurons project to the rostral ventrolateral medulla in the rabbit although in this species there are some non-catecholamine containing retrogradely-labelled neurons scattered amongst the A1 cells. These anatomical results make it extremely unlikely that the vasodepressor neurons belong to the A1 group.

There is a growing body of evidence which suggests that GABA may function as a neurotransmitter in the caudal vasodepressor neurons, a suggestion first made by Willette and colleagues (Willette et al., 1983b). Although the availability of antibodies against GABA conjugates has facilitated neuroanatomical studies of GABA-containing cell bodies in the neocortex similar neurons in the

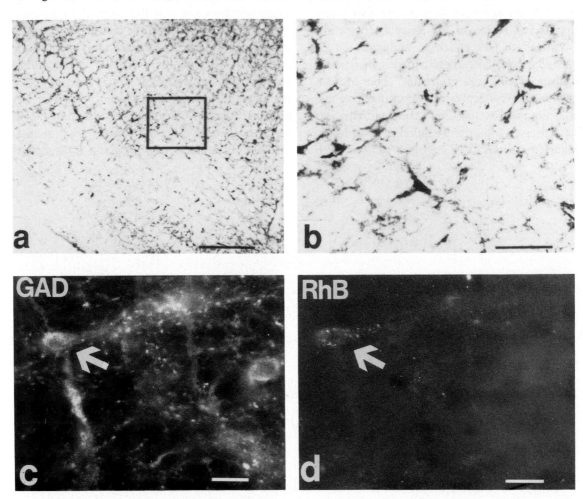

Fig. 5. (A, B) Photomicrographs of rabbit caudal ventrolateral medulla after pre-treatment with colchicine and immunohistochemical processing for glutamic acid decarboxylase (GAD) using the avidin-biotin-peroxidase system, primary antiserum diluted 1/10 000. Immuno-positive neurons are scattered throughout the lateral reticular formation. Bar = 500 μm (A) and 100 μm (B). (C, D) Fluorescence immunohistochemistry for GAD (using FITC labelled second antibody and primary antibody diluted 1 in 1000) and retrograde transport of rhodamine-labelled latex beads (RhB) to the caudal ventrolateral medulla after injection of tracing agent into the rostral ventrolateral medulla. The neuron indicated by the arrow contains both GAD and rhodamine beads. Bar = 20 μm (C) and (D).

medulla oblongata have been surprisingly difficult to detect. Even with colchicine pre-treatment it is difficult to detect any GABA-containing neurons in the NTS or in the ventrolateral medulla using the avidin-biotin-peroxidase technique and a specific (Somogyi et al., 1985) GABA-detecting antibody (unpublished observations). Neurons containing glutamic acid decarboxylase (GAD) have been demonstrated in the rat medulla after appropriate pre-treatment with colchicine (Blessing et al., 1984; Meeley et al., 1985; Mugnaini and Oertel, 1985). Similar studies using the same antibody in the rabbit have shown that GAD-containing neurons are distributed widely throughout the medulla oblongata, at least some neurons being present in all nuclei except the somatic motor nuclei of the cranial nerves and the lateral reticular nucleus (unpublished observations). There are GAD-containing neurons in the caudal ventrolateral medulla (Fig. 5) but there is no obvious, isolated group of cells forming a "vasodepressor nucleus". We have been in-

vestigating whether any of the GAD-positive neurons contain retrogradely transported tracing agents after injection of these substances into the rostral ventrolateral medulla. We have injected Fluorogold or rhodamine-labelled beads into the rostral or the caudal ventrolateral medulla then, after 3 – 5 days, injected colchicine into appropriate sites. After the rabbit survived for a further day the medulla oblongata was processed for GAD immunohistochemistry using the immuno-fluorescence procedure. In most transverse sections through the caudal ventrolateral medullary region there were one or two doubly labelled neurons after injection of tracer agent into the rostral ventrolateral medulla (Fig. 5C,D). We have not been able to demonstrate a GAD-positive projection from the NTS at the level of the area postrema to the rostral ventrolateral medulla and, at present, we agree with Ruggiero et al. (1985) that this projection probably does not exist. In contrast, when the tracing agent is injected into the caudal ventrolateral medulla it is retrogradely

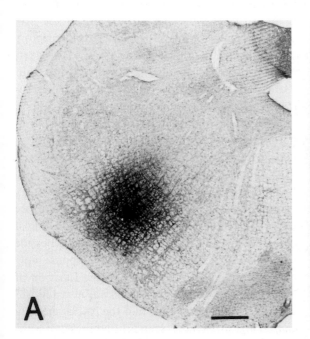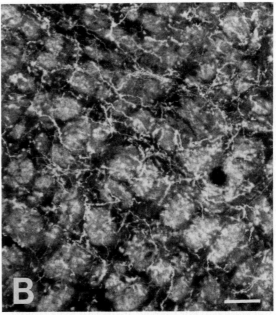

Fig. 6. Photomicrographs showing injection site for Phaseolus Vulgaris Leucoagglutinin in the caudal ventrolateral medulla (A) and anterogradely labelled nerve terminals in the rostral ventrolateral medulla (B). Bar = 660 µm (A) and 60 µm (B).

transported into GAD-positive neurons in the NTS at the level of the area postrema (unpublished data).

The introduction of Phaseolus Vulgaris Leuco-agglutinin (PHA-L) as an anterograde intra-axonal tracing agent (Gerfen and Sawchenko, 1984) with iontophoretic deposition of the tracer, has facilitated the study of intramedullary neuronal connections. We have commenced a series of such studies in the rabbit. Early results (Li and Blessing, 1989) have confirmed the existence of a dense projection from the NTS, at the level of the area postrema, to both the caudal and the rostral ventrolateral medulla. This is consistent with the retrograde studies in the rabbit (Fig. 4), rat (Ross et al., 1985b) and cat (Dampney et al., 1987) and with the early anterograde autoradiographic study of Loewy and Burton (1978). The PHA-L studies in the rabbit reveal a dense and remarkably localized projection from the caudal ventrolateral medulla to the portion of the rostral ventrolateral medulla which contains the spinally projecting sympathoexcitatory neurons (Fig. 6). Ultrastructural studies after appropriate retrograde labelling of the rostral sympathoexcitatory neurons are necessary to confirm a synaptic relationship between caudal and rostral cells but light microscopic examination of varicosities anterogradely labelled with PHA-L-strongly suggests that these terminals innervate rostral neurons.

An indirect confirmation of the hypothesis that the vasodepressor neurons exert their effect by a tonic inhibitory action on sympathoexcitatory neurons in the rostral ventrolateral medulla has been provided by Pilowsky et al. (1987) who showed that inhibiting the vasodepressor neurons with local injections of muscimol results in release of neuropeptide Y-like immunoreactivity into the spinal CSF. The source of this neuropeptide Y is likely to be perikarya in the rostral ventrolateral medulla (Blessing et al., 1986, 1987b) and the data are consistent with the idea that removal of the inhibitory input from the vasodepressor cells results in an increase in the discharge rate of the rostral neurons.

Pharmacological evidence supporting the hypothesis that GABA is the neurotransmitter in the vasodepressor neurons has been obtained in the rabbit (Blessing, 1988). Bilateral injection of bicuculline, a GABA-receptor antagonist, into the rostral ventrolateral medulla caused a dose-dependent reduction in the magnitude of the sympathoinhibitory and vasodepressor response elicited by injection of L-glutamate into the caudal ventrolateral medulla. However, injection of bicuculline into the rostral ventrolateral medulla caused a major rise in arterial pressure associated with an increase in peripheral sympathetic vasomotor tone. Although this observation is consistent with the idea that the caudal tonically active depressor neurons are GABAergic the change in baseline values weakens the interpretation of the experiment. A more convincing demonstration that the depressor response depends on activation of GABAergic receptors in the rostral ventrolateral medulla was provided by experiments in which both muscimol and bicuculline were injected into the rostral ventrolateral medulla, simultaneously. By adjusting the dose of each agent it was possible to keep the baseline arterial pressure at the pre-injection value. In this situation, GABA receptors are presumably made inaccessible to GABA released from nerve terminals but activity of the sympathoexcitatory neurons can be altered by neurotransmitters acting at non-GABAergic receptors. In agreement with this idea, the pressor sympathoexcitatory response elicited by injecting L-glutamate into the rostral medulla was preserved after muscimol-bicuculline GABAergic blockade. In contrast, the depressor sympathoinhibitory response normally elicited by injecting L-glutamate into the caudal ventrolateral medulla was almost completely abolished by the combined blockade (Fig. 7). Furthermore, the pressor response normally observed with inhibition of the function of the caudal vasodepressor neurons was also abolished. Injection of strychnine into the rostral medulla caused a gradual increase in arterial pressure without significant effect on either the depressor or the pressor response elicited by stimulation or inhibition of the caudal sympathoinhibitory cells (Blessing, 1988). Thus, the combined anatomical and pharmacological data suggest that the vasodepressor neurons, utilizing GABA as a transmitter, exert their action by a short inhibitory projection to the sympathoexcitatory neurons in the rostral ventrolateral medulla.

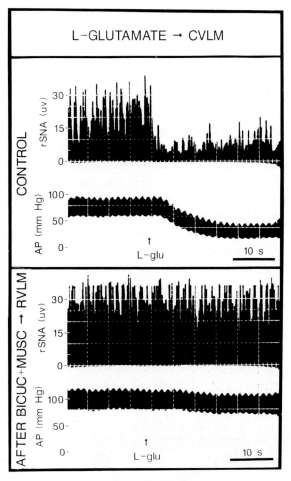

Fig. 7. Oscilloscope records of rectified spinal sympathetic nerve activity (SNA) and arterial pressure (AP) showing the effect of unilateral injection of L-glutamate (10 nmol) into the caudal ventrolateral medulla (CVLM) before and after bilateral combined injection of muscimol (0.5 nmol) and bicuculline (0.5 nmol) into the rostral ventrolateral medulla (RVLM). (From Blessing, 1988.)

Role of vasodepressor neurons in baroreceptor-vasomotor reflex

Coote and McLeod (1974a,b) first suggested that neurons in the caudal ventrolateral medulla participate in the baroreceptor-vasomotor reflex. West et al. (1981) made electrolytic lesions in the caudal ventrolateral medulla of rabbits. In surviving unanaesthetized animals it was possible to demonstrate that constriction of the inferior vena cava did not reduce aortic blood flow as much as would be expected if the baroreceptor-vasomotor reflex was functioning normally. This evidence is consistent with the view that neurons in the caudal ventrolateral medulla are somehow involved in the central processing of this reflex. However, interpretation of the experiments is complicated by the high mortality rate associated with anodal stainless steel electrolytic lesions in the caudal ventrolateral medulla. Badoer et al. (1987) and Head et al. (1987) showed that cathodal lesions produced much less dramatic cardiovascular sequelae, although they did not assess the baroreceptor-vasomotor reflex in their rabbits.

When studies in anaesthetized animals confirmed the presence of tonically active vasodepressor neurons in the caudal ventrolateral medulla there was a renewed interest in the possibility that these neurons might constitute the inhibitory link in the central processing of the baroreceptor-vasomotor reflex. Willette et al. (1983b) showed that the rise in arterial pressure seen after bilateral injection of muscimol into the caudal ventrolateral medulla was associated with blockade and reversal of the depressor response normally elicited by stimulation of the central end of the cut aortic depressor nerve. A similar phenomenon occurs in the rabbit (Fig. 8 and Blessing and Willoughby, 1987) and this finding strongly suggests that the depressor neurons play an important part in the central processing of the baroreceptor-vasomotor reflex. However, when more physiological methods are used to alter peripheral baroreceptor function, a more complicated result is obtained. Blessing and Willoughby (1987) made recordings of sympathetic

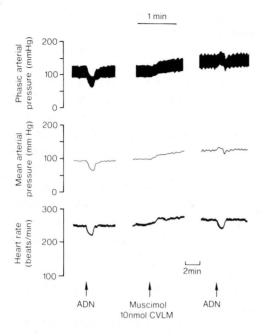

Fig. 8. Polygraph tracing the depressor response elicited by electrical stimulation of the aortic nerve depressor (ADN) before and after bilateral injections of muscimol into the caudal ventrolateral medulla (CVLM).

vasomotor activity from the cut renal nerve and altered baroreceptor activity by temporary occlusion of either the inferior vena cava or the descending aorta using cuff occluders. After bilateral caudal ventrolateral injections of muscimol, in doses which completely abolish the vasodepressor response to local injection of L-glutamate, the normal changes in renal nerve activity were still observed when the vascular occluders were inflated. The inhibitory response was diminished or abolished when muscimol increased resting arterial pressure to such an extent that occlusion of the aorta failed to further increase arterial pressure. However, when the elevated arterial pressure was lowered by occlusion of the inferior vena cava activity in the renal nerve was observed to increase. Furthermore, renal nerve activity acutely decreased when arterial pressure was suddenly restored to the high value when the inferior vena cava cuff was deflated (Blessing and Willoughby, 1987). In recent experiments we have obtained the same result with the venous cuff after bilateral injection of muscimol into the caudal ventrolateral medulla at two rostrocaudal levels (Fig. 9).

The failure of muscimol to abolish baroreceptor-initiated changes in sympathetic nerve activity contrasts with the complete blockade of

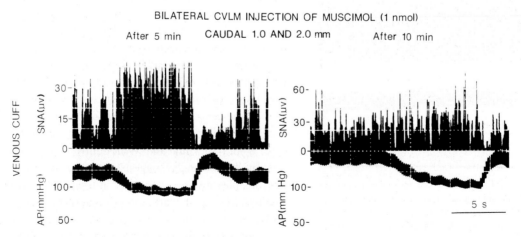

Fig. 9. Oscilloscope records of rectified renal sympathetic nerve activity (SNA) and arterial pressure (AP) 5 and 10 min after bilateral injection of muscimol into the caudal ventrolateral medulla at 1 and 2 mm caudal to the rostral border of the area postrema. The increase in nerve activity observed in response to occlusion of the inferior vena cava is preserved.

vasopressin secretion observed after similar injections of muscimol into the caudal ventrolateral medulla (Blessing and Willoughby, 1985) and the result suggests that the depressor neurons are not integral links in the central pathway mediating the baroreceptor-vasomotor reflex. This result is in agreement with the findings from electrolytic lesion experiments. When bilateral electrolytic lesions (either cathodal or anodal) are made in the caudal ventrolateral medulla in the anaesthetized rabbit there is no acute increase in arterial pressure. In these rabbits the renal nerve response to vascular occlusion and the vasodepressor response to electrical stimulation of the aortic depressor nerve are preserved (Blessing and Willoughby, 1987). Granata et al. (1985b) made a similar observation concerning the depressor response elicited by stimulating the central end of the cut vagus nerve in the rat.

There are other observations at variance with the idea that the vasodepressor neurons are directly

linked into central pathways mediating the baroreceptor-vasomotor reflex. In baroreceptor-denervated rabbits, muscimol injections into the caudal ventrolateral medulla increase arterial pressure more rapidly and to higher levels than occurs after similar injections in baroreceptor-intact animals (Fig. 10). This suggests that the tonic activity of at least some of the vasodepressor neurons in not entirely dependent on baroreceptor-derived excitatory input. The rise in arterial pressure which occurs after inhibition of the vasodepressor neurons may well take place despite the buffering action of baroreceptors, acting via some central pathway which does not directly involve neurons in the caudal ventrolateral medulla. More information is required concerning this question especially since the depressor response elicited by chemical stimulation of the NTS in the rat does seem to be dependent on the integrity of neuronal responses in the caudal ventrolateral medulla (Urbanski and Sapru, 1988). It may be that there are species differences. In the rabbit we have found that injection of L-glutamate into the NTS elicits little or no vasodepressor response (unpublished observations). We agree that the sensitivity of the baroreceptor-sympathoinhibitory reflex is decreased by procedures which elevate arterial pressure by inhibiting neuronal function in the caudal ventrolateral medulla. The question is whether or not this sensitivity is due to direct interruption of the central baroreceptor-vasomotor pathway or whether it is a secondary effect of reduction of output from the vasodepressor neurons to some other region, possibly the rostral ventrolateral medulla.

Recent papers based on the assumption that the vasodepressor neurons constitute the central inhibitory link in the baroreceptor-vasomotor reflex have suggested the presence of an excitatory amino acid-mediated link between the NTS and the vasodepressor neurons. Injection of DL-amino-5-phosphonovaleric acid (APV) (Gordon, 1987; Kubo and Kihara, 1988) or kynurenic acid (Guyenet et al., 1987) into the caudal ventrolateral medulla causes a rise in arterial pressure associated with blockade or reversal of the aortic nerve-depressor

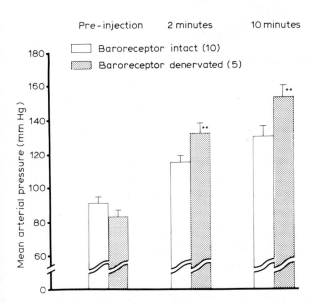

Fig. 10. Arterial blood pressure before and 2 and 10 min after bilateral injection of muscimol (1 nmol) into the caudal ventrolateral medulla in anaesthetized rabbits with either intact (open bars) or denervated baroreceptors. ** Significantly different from values in intact animals; $p < 0.01$. (Data from Blessing and Willoughby, 1987.)

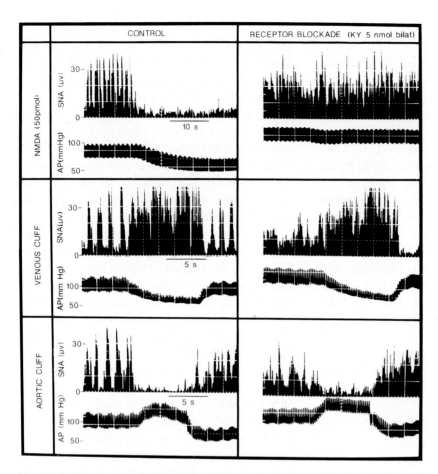

Fig. 11. Oscilloscope records of rectified renal sympathetic nerve activity (SNA) and arterial pressure (AP) before and after bilateral injection of kynurenic acid into the caudal ventrolateral medulla. The sympathoinhibitory effect of local injection of *N*-methyl-D-aspartate is blocked but the reflex changes in sympathetic nerve activity induced by vascular occlusion are preserved. (From Blessing, 1989.)

response. This effect is also observed in the rabbit (Blessing, 1989). However, sympathetic vasomotor activity in the renal nerve still responds appropriately to changes in arterial pressure after injection of either APV or kynurenic acid into the caudal ventrolateral medulla (Fig. 11). It is interesting to note that sympathetic activity in the renal nerve does not increase in parallel to the increase in arterial pressure which occurs after injection of kynurenic acid or APV. The nerve activity actually decreases in some rabbits (Blessing, 1989) and this suggests that baroreceptor-mediated inhibition still reaches the sympathoexcitatory neurons even though the caudal depressor cells are

functionally isolated from their excitatory amino acid input. In both rabbits (Blessing, 1989) and rats (Gordon, 1987) amino acid antagonists do not prevent the neuroexcitatory action of locally applied L-glutamate (as judged by the preservation of the vasodepressor response) even though these agents do interfere with the aortic nerve-depressor response when they are injected into the caudal ventrolateral medulla. This suggests that the endogenous excitatory amino acid neurotransmitter impinging on the vasodepressor neurons is not L-glutamate itself.

It should be stressed that there are many neurotransmitter systems impinging on the depressor neurons. In addition, further work may demonstrate subgroups of these cells, with outputs affecting different vascular beds, as has been suggested for the rostral sympathoexcitatory neurons (Dampney and McAllen, 1988). At present, we believe that the vasodepressor neurons in the caudal ventrolateral medulla are not directly linked into the baroreceptor-vasomotor reflex but it is clear that more experimental evidence is necessary before the presumably complex functions of the vasodepressor cells can be demonstrated.

Acknowledgements

Our experimental work was supported by the National Health and Medical Research Council, The National Heart Foundation of Australia and The Neurosurgical Research Foundation of South Australia. Mr. Paul Cranwell and Mr. Roger McCart provided excellent technical assistance. Dr. Wolfgang Oertel kindly provided the antiserum to glutamic acid decarboxylase.

References

Alexander, R.S. (1946) Tonic and reflex functions of medullary sympathetic cardiovascular centers. *J. Neurophysiol.,* 9: 205 – 217.

Amendt, K., Czachurski, J., Dembowsky, K. and Seller, H. (1979) Bulbospinal projections to the intermediolateral cell column: a neuroanatomical study. *J. Auton. Nerv. Syst.,* 1: 103 – 117.

Badoer, E., Head, G.A., Aberdeen, J.A. and Korner, P.I. (1987) Localization of the main noradrenergic neuron groups in the pons and medulla of the rabbit and the importance of cathodal lesions for prolonged survival. *J. Neurosci. Methods,* 19: 11 – 27.

Blessing, W.W. (1988) Depressor neurons in rabbit caudal medulla act via GABA receptors in rostral medulla. *Am. J. Physiol.,* 254: H686 – H692.

Blessing, W.W. (1989) Baro-vasomotor reflex is preserved after N-methyl-D-aspartate receptor blockade in rabbit caudal ventrolateral medulla. *J. Physiol. Sept.* (in press).

Blessing, W.W. and Reis, D.J. (1982) Inhibitory cardiovascular function of neurons in the caudal ventrolateral medulla of the rabbit: relationship to the area containing A_1 noradrenergic cells. *Brain Res.,* 253: 161 – 171.

Blessing, W.W. and Reis, D.J. (1983) Evidence that GABA and glycine-like inputs inhibit vasodepressor neurons in the caudal ventrolateral medulla of the rabbit. *Neurosci. Lett.,* 37: 57 – 62.

Blessing, W.W. and Willoughby J.O. (1985) Inhibiting the rabbit caudal ventrolateral medulla prevents baroreceptor-initiated secretion of vasopressin. *J. Physiol. (Lond.),* 367: 253 – 265.

Blessing, W.W. and Willoughby, J.O. (1987) Depressor neurons in rabbit caudal medulla do not transmit the baroreceptor-vasomotor reflex. *Am. J. Physiol.,* H777 – H786.

Blessing, W.W., Goodchild, A.K., Dampney, R.A.L. and Chalmers, J.P. (1981a) Cell groups in the lower brainstem of the rabbit projecting to the spinal cord, with special reference to catecholamine-containing neurons. *Brain Res.,* 221: 35 – 55.

Blessing, W.W., West, M.J. and Chalmers, J. (1981b) Hypertension, bradycardia, and pulmonary edema in the conscious rabbit after brainstem lesions coinciding with the A1 group of catecholamine neurons. *Circ. Res.,* 49: 949 – 958.

Blessing, W.W., Oertel, W.H. and Willoughby, J.O. (1984) Glutamic acid decarboxylase immunoreactivity is present in perikarya of neurons in nucleus tractus solitarius of rat. *Brain Res.,* 322: 346 – 350.

Blessing, W.W., Howe, P.R.C., Joh, T.H., Oliver, J.R. and Willoughby, J.O. (1986) Distribution of tyrosine hydroxylase and neuropeptide Y-like immunoreactive neurons in rabbit medulla oblongata, with attention to colocalization studies, presumptive adrenaline-synthesizing perikarya, and vagal pre-ganglionic neurons. *J. Comp. Neurol.,* 248: 285 – 300.

Blessing, W.W., Hedger S.C., Joh, T.H. and Willoughby, J.O. (1987a) Neurons in the area postrema are the only catecholamine-synthesizing cells in the medulla or pons with projections to the rostral ventrolateral medulla (C_1-area) in the rabbit. *Brain Res.,* 419: 336 – 340.

Blessing, W.W., Oliver, J.R., Hodgson, A.H., Joh, T.H. and Willoughby, J.O. (1987b) Neuropeptide Y-like immunoreactive C_1 neurons in the rostral ventrolateral medulla of the rabbit project to sympathetic preganglionic neurons in the spinal cord. *J. Auton. Nerv. Syst.,* 18: 121 – 129.

Caverson, M.M., Ciriello, J. and Calaresu, F.R. (1983) Direct pathway from cardiovascular neurons in the ventrolateral medulla to the region of the intermediolateral nucleus of the upper thoracic cord: an anatomical and electrophysiological investigation in the cat. *J. Auton. Nerv. Syst.,* 9: 451 – 475.

Chai, C.Y. and Wang, S.C. (1962) Localization of central cardiovascular mechanisms in lower brain stem of the cat. *Am. J. Physiol.,* 202: 25 – 30.

Chan, S.H.H., Chan, J.Y.H. and Ong, B.T. (1986) Anatomic connections between nucleus reticularis rostroventrolateralis and some medullary cardiovascular sites in the rat. *Neurosci. Lett.,* 71: 277 – 282.

Coote, J.H. and McLeod, V.H. (1974a) Evidence for the involvement in the baroreceptor reflex of a descending inhibitory pathway. *J. Physiol. (Lond.)*, 241: 477–496.

Coote, J.H. and McLeod, V.H. (1974b) The influence of bulbospinal monoaminergic pathways on sympathetic nerve activity. *J. Physiol. (Lond.)*, 241: 453–475.

Dahlstrom, A. and Fuxe, K. (1964) Evidence for the existence of monoamine containing neurons in the central nervous system. I. Demonstration of monoamines in the cell bodies of brain stem neurons. *Acta Physiol. Scand.*, 62 Suppl. 232: 1–55.

Dahlstrom, A. and Fuxe, K. (1965) Evidence for the existence of monoamine containing neurons in the central nervous system. II. Experimentally induced changes in the intraneuronal amine levels of bulbospinal nervous systems. *Acta Physiol. Scand.*, 64: 7–85.

Dampney, R.A.L. and McAllen, R.M. (1988) Differential control of sympathetic fibres supplying hindlimb skin and muscle by subretrofacial neurones in the cat. *J. Physiol. (Lond.)*, 395: 41–56.

Dampney, R.A.L., Goodchild, A.K., Robertson, L.G. and Montgomery, W. (1982) Role of ventrolateral medulla in vasomotor regulation: a correlative anatomical and physiological study. *Brain Res.*, 249: 223–235.

Dampney, R.A.L., Czachurski, J., Dembowsky, K., Goodchild, A.K. and Seller, H. (1987) Afferent connections and spinal projections of the pressor region in the rostral ventrolateral medulla of the cat. *J. Auton. Nerv. Syst.*, 20: 73–86.

Day, T.A., Ro, A. and Renaud, L.P. (1983) Depressor area within caudal ventrolateral medulla of the rat does not correspond to the A_1-catecholamine cell group. *Brain Res.*, 279: 299–302.

Dembowsky, K, Lackner, K., Czachurski, J. and Seller, H. (1981) Tonic catecholaminergic inhibition of the spinal somatosympathetic reflexes originating in the ventrolateral medulla oblongata. *J. Auton. Nerv. Syst.*, 3: 277–290.

Feldberg, W. (1976) The ventral surface of the brain stem: a scarcely explored region of pharmacological sensitivity. *Neuroscience*, 1: 427–441.

Feldberg, W. and Guertzenstein, P.G. (1976) Vasodepressor effects obtained by drugs acting on the ventral surface of the brainstem. *J. Physiol. (Lond.)*, 258: 337–355.

Fleetwood-Walker, S.M., Coote, J.H. and Gilbey, M.P. (1983) Identification of spinally projecting neurons in the A_1 catecholamine cell group of the ventrolateral medulla. *Brain Res.*, 273: 25–33.

Gerfen, C.R. and Sawchenko, P.E. (1984) An anterograde neuroanatomical tracing method that shows the detailed morphology of neurons, their axons and terminals: immunohistochemical localization of an axonally transported plant lectin, Phaseolous Vulgaris Leucoagglutinin (PHA-L). *Brain Res.*, 290: 219–238.

Goodchild, A.K., Dampney, R.A.L. and Bandler, R. (1982) A method of evoking physiological responses by stimulation of cell bodies, but not axons of passage, within localized regions of the central nervous system. *J. Neurosci. Methods*, 6: 351–363.

Gordon, F.J. (1987) Aortic baroreceptor reflexes are mediated by NMDA receptors in caudal ventrolateral medulla. *Am. J. Physiol.*, 252: R628–R633.

Granata, A.R., Kumada, M. and Reis, D.J. (1985a) Sympathoinhibition by A1-noradrenergic neurons is mediated by neurons in the C1 area of the rostral medulla. *J. Auton. Nerv. Syst.*, 14: 387–395.

Granata, A.R., Ruggiero, D.A., Park, D.H. Joh, T.H. and Reis, D.J. (1985b) Brainstem area with C_1 epinephrine neurons mediates baroreceptor vasodepressor responses. *Am. J. Physiol.*, 248: H547–567.

Granata, A.R., Numao, Y., Kumada, M. and Reis, D.J. (1986) A1 noradrenergic neurons tonically inhibit sympathoexcitatory neurons of C1 area in rat brainstem. *Brain Res.*, 377: 127–146.

Guyenet, P.G., Filtz, T.M. and Donaldson, S.R. (1987) Role of excitatory amino acids in rat vagal and sympathetic baroreflexes. *Brain Res.*, 407: 272–284.

Head, G.A., Badoer, E. and Korner, P.I. (1987) Cardiovascular role of A_1 catecholaminergic neurons in the rabbit. Effect of chronic lesions on responses to methyldopa, clonidine and 6-OHDA induced transmitter release. *Brain Res.*, 412: 18–28.

Hökfelt, T., Fuxe, K., Goldstein, M. and Johansson, O. (1974) Immunohistochemical evidence for the existence of adrenaline neurons in the rat brain. *Brain Res.*, 66: 235–251.

Kubo, T. and Kihara, M. (1988) *N*-Methyl-D-aspartate receptors mediate tonic vasodepressor control in the caudal ventrolateral medulla of the rat. *Brain Res.*, 451: 366–370.

Li, Y.-W. and Blessing, W.W. (1988) Precise localization of vasodepressor neurons in the caudal ventrolateral medulla of the rabbit. *Proc. Aust. Physiol. Pharmacol. Soc.*, 19: 198P.

Li, Y.-W. and Blessing, W.W. (1989) Neuronal connections between the nucleus tractus solitarius and the caudal and rostral ventrolateral medulla in the rabbit. *Proc. Aust. Neurosci. Soc.*, Feb.

Loewy, A.D. and Burton, H. (1978) Nuclei of the solitary tract: efferent projections to the lower brainstem and spinal cord of the cat. *J. Comp. Neurol.*, 181: 421–450.

Loewy, A.D., Wallach, J.H. and McKellar, S. (1981) Efferent connections of the ventral medulla oblongata in the rat. *Brain Res. Rev.*, 3: 63–80.

McAllen, R.M. and Woollard, S. (1984) Exploration of the cat's ventral medullary surface by microinjections of excitant amino acid. *J. Physiol. (Lond.)*, 346: 35.

Meeley, M.P. Ruggiero, D.A., Ishitauka, T. and Reis, D.J. (1985) Intrinsic gamma-aminobutyric acid neurons in the nucleus of the solitary tract and the rostral ventrolateral medulla of the rat: an immunocytochemical and biochemical study. *Neurosci. Lett.*, 58: 83–89.

Mugnaini, E. and Oertel, W.H. (1985) An atlas of the distribution of GABAergic neurons and terminals in the rat CNS as revealed by GAD immunohistochemistry. In A. Bjorklund and T. Hökfelt (Eds.), *Handbook of Chemical Neuroanatomy, Vol. 4, GABA and Neuropeptides in the CNS, Part 1,* Elsevier, Amsterdam, pp. 436 – 608.

Pilowsky, P., West, M. and Chalmers, J. (1985) Renal sympathetic nerve responses to stimulation, inhibition and destruction of the ventrolateral medulla in the rabbit. *Neurosci. Lett.,* 60: 51 – 55.

Pilowsky, P., Morris, M.J., Minson, J.B., West, M.J., Chalmers, J.P., Willoughby, J.O. and Blessing, W.W. (1987) Inhibition of vasodepressor neurons in the caudal ventrolateral medulla of the rabbit increases both arterial pressure and the release of neuropeptide Y-like immunoreactivity from the spinal cord. *Brain Res.,* 420: 380 – 384.

Ross, C.A., Ruggiero, D.A., Park, D.H., Joh, T.H., Sved, A.F., Fernandez-Pardal, J. Saavedra, J.M. and Reis, D.J. (1984) Tonic vasomotor control by the rostral ventrolateral medulla: effect of electrical or chemical stimulation of the area containing C1 adrenaline neurons on arterial pressure, heart rate and plasma catecholamines and vasopressin. *J. Neurosci.,* 4: 474 – 494.

Ross, C.A., Ruggiero, D.A., Joh, T.H., Park, D.H. and Reis, D.J. (1985a) Rostral ventrolateral medulla: selective projections to the thoracic autonomic cell column from the region containing C1 adrenaline neurons. *J. Comp. Neurol.,* 228: 168 – 185.

Ross, C.A., Ruggiero, D.A. and Reis, D.J. (1985b) Projections from the nucleus tractus solitarii to the rostral ventrolateral medulla. *J. Comp. Neurol.,* 242: 511 – 534.

Ruggiero, D.A., Meeley, M.P., Anwar, M. and Reis, D.J. (1985) Newly identified GABAergic neurons in regions of the ventrolateral medulla which regulate blood pressure. *Brain Res.,* 339: 171 – 177.

Somogyi, P., Hodgson, A.J., Chubb, I.W., Penke, B. and Erdei, A. (1985) Antisera to gamma-aminobutyric acid. II. Immunocytochemical application to the central nervous system. *J. Histochem. Cytochem.,* 33: 240 – 248.

Sun, M.-K. and Guyenet, P.G. (1986) Effect of clonidine and gamma-aminobutyric acid on the discharges of medullospinal sympathoexcitatory neurons in the rat. *Brain Res.,* 368: 1 – 17.

Swanson, L.W. and Hartman, B.K. (1975) The central adrenergic system: an immunofluorescence study of the location of cell bodies and their efferent connections in the rat utilizing dopamine-beta-hydroxylase as a marker. *J. Comp. Neurol.,* 163: 467 – 506.

Ungerstedt, U. (1971) Stereotaxic mapping of the monoamine pathways in the rat brain. *Acta Physiol.,* 367: 1 – 48.

Urbanski, R.W. and Sapru, H.N. (1988) Evidence for a sympathoexcitatory pathway from the nucleus tractus solitarii to the ventrolateral medullary pressor area. *J. Auton. Nerv. Syst.,* 23: 161 – 174.

West, M.W., Blessing, W.W. and Chalmers, J. (1981) Arterial baroreceptor reflex function in the conscious rabbit after brainstem lesions coinciding with the A1 group of catecholamine neurons. *Circ. Res.,* 49: 959 – 970.

Westlund, K.N., Bowker, R.M., Ziegler, M.G. and Coulter, J.D. (1983) Noradrenergic projections to the spinal cord of the rat. *Brain Res.,* 263: 15 – 31.

Willette, R.N., Barcas, P.P., Krieger, A.J. and Sapru, H.N. (1983a) Vasopressor and depressor areas in the rat medulla: identification by microinjection of L-glutamate. *Neuropharmacology,* 22: 1071 – 1079.

Willette, R.N., Krieger, A.J., Barcas P.P. and Sapru, H.N. (1983b) Medullary gamma aminobutyric acid (GABA) receptors and the regulation of blood pressure in the rat. *J. Pharmacol. Exp. Ther.,* 226: 893 – 899.

Willette, R.N., Punnen, S., Krieger, A.J. and Sapru, H.N. (1984a) Hypertensive response following stimulation of opiate receptors in the caudal ventrolateral medulla. *Neuropharmacology,* 23: 401 – 406.

Willette, R.N., Punnen, S., Krieger, A.J. and Sapru, H.N. (1984b) Interdependence of rostral and caudal ventrolateral medullary areas in the control of blood pressure. *Brain Res.,* 321: 169 – 174.

Willette, R.N., Barcas, P.P., Krieger, A.J. and Sapru, H.N. (1984c) Endogenous GABAergic mechanisms in the medulla and the regulation of blood pressure. *J. Pharmacol. Exp. Ther.,* 230: 34 – 39.

J. Ciriello, M.M. Caverson and C. Polosa (Eds.)
Progress in Brain Research, Vol. 81
© 1989 Elsevier Science Publishers B.V. (Biomedical Division)

CHAPTER 6

Differential regulation of sympathetic nerve activity by lateral and medial subregions of the rostral ventral medulla

Kurt J. Varner, Cynthia L. Grosskreutz, Bryan F. Cox and Michael J. Brody

Department of Pharmacology and Cardiovascular Center, University of Iowa, Iowa City, IA 52242, U.S.A.

Introduction

Numerous studies have demonstrated that neural networks within the rostral ventral medulla (RVM) play a critical role in maintaining the level of arterial pressure (AP) (see Guertzenstein, 1973; Feldberg, 1976; Granata et al., 1985). More recent studies examining the role of RVM in the control of AP have focused on the rostral ventrolateral medulla (RVLM). This subregion of the RVM in the rat centered 2 mm lateral to midline, 1 mm dorsal to the ventral surface of the brainstem, is bounded rostrally by the caudal pole of the facial nucleus and includes part of the nucleus paragigantocellularis (Ross et al., 1984a). Activation of RVLM by electrical stimulation or the microinjection of excitatory amino acids increases AP (Dampney and Moon, 1980; Dampney et al., 1982; Ross et al., 1983, 1984b). In contrast, bilateral electrolytic lesions or the microinjection of agents such as gamma-aminobutyric acid (GABA) or tetrodotoxin into RVLM reduces AP to levels resembling those produced by spinal cord transection (Guertzenstein and Silver, 1974; Feldberg, 1976; Dampney and Moon, 1980; Ross et al., 1983, 1984b; Granata et al., 1985). Anatomical (Ross et al., 1983, 1984a; Minson et al., 1987) and electrophysiological (Barman and Gebber, 1985; Morrison et al., 1988) evidence indicates that control of

tonic sympathetic outflow and AP by RVLM is mediated over direct bulbo-spinal projections to the interomediolateral (IML) autonomic nucleus in the spinal cord. Many, but not all, of these bulbospinal neurons contain the epinephrine synthesizing enzyme phenylethanolamine *N*-methyltransferase (Ross et al., 1983; Minson et al., 1987). Some of these same neurons may colocalize neuropeptide Y (Everitt et al., 1984; Blessing et al., 1986).

Recently, a second more medial subregion of the RVM (rostral ventromedial medulla, RVMM) that is also involved in the control of AP has been identified. The RVMM is located 1 mm lateral to the midline, in the same dorso-ventral and rostrocaudal plane as the RVLM and contains part of the nucleus gigantocellularis. Activation or inactivation of RVMM, using methods similar to those described above, elicits changes in AP comparable to those from RVLM (Cox and Brody, 1987a; Grosskreutz and Brody, 1987; Minson et al., 1987). Like RVLM, the region containing RVMM also contains bulbo-spinal neurons. Many of these neurons, in particular those located in ventral RVMM and below contain serotonin or substance P (Bowker et al., 1981; Loewy and McKellar, 1981; Helke et al., 1982). In addition, a significant number of bulbo-spinal neurons whose transmitter has not yet been determined, are intermingled with, and dorsal to, the serotonergic and substance P-containing cells.

Although RVMM and RVLM appear to be equally important in the control of sympathetic outflow and AP, recent studies from our laboratory suggest that RVLM and RVMM differ in terms of their afferent input and control of vasomotor function. Cox and Brody (1988a,b, 1989a,b) demonstrated using lidocaine microinjection and electrical stimulation that RVLM and RVMM differentially control regional vascular resistances in urethane-anesthetized rats. Although anesthetization of RVMM and RVLM produced similar falls in renal and mesenteric vascular resistances and AP, the fall in hindquarter vascular resistance produced by blocking RVMM was significantly larger than that seen with block of RVLM. Electrical stimulation of RVLM and RVMM elicited equivalent graded increases in AP, however, the increase in renal vascular resistance was much greater with stimulation of RVLM, whereas stimulation of RVMM elicited a much greater increase in hindquarter vascular resistance. The hemodynamic responses elicited by electrical stimulation of RVLM were partially attenuated by the microinjection of lidocaine into the RVMM (Cox and Brody, 1988a,b 1989a,b). In contrast, the responses evoked by stimulation of RVMM were not affected by inactivation of RVLM. These data indicated that the integrity of RVMM is required for the full expression of the cardiovascular responses elicited by stimulation of the RVLM. A similar conclusion was reached by Minson and coworkers (1987) who demonstrated that electrolytic lesions of a site corresponding closely to the RVLM failed to attenuate the pressor response elicited by the microinjection of glutamate into a more medial site (1.3 mm lateral to midline).

Cox and Brody (1987a, 1988a,b 1989a,b) also demonstrated that the vasomotor activity of RVLM and RVMM are differentially influenced by changes in respiratory tidal volume. In urethane-anesthetized rats under conditions of normal tidal volume (2.5 ml), bilateral microinjec-

tion of lidocaine (200 nl, 4%) into either RVLM or RVMM produced marked falls in AP, renal sympathetic nerve activity (RSNA) and regional vascular resistances. However, under conditions of reduced tidal volume (1.5 ml), the decreases in AP, RSNA and regional vascular resistances elicited by inactivation of RVLM were attenuated. The vasomotor responses elicited by inactivation of the RVMM were unaffected by a reduction in tidal volume. The differential RVLM responses apparently reflected state-dependent changes in afferent input from mechanoreceptors in the lungs and chest wall, since removal of vagal afferents and prevention of chest wall movement prevented attenuation of lidocaine-induced responses from RVLM under conditions of reduced tidal volume.

Further evidence of differences in afferent input to RVLM and RVMM was provided by the finding that the pressor and vasoconstrictor responses in the renal, mesenteric and hindquarter vasculature elicited by electrical stimulation of the lateral hypothalamus were blocked by the microinjection of lidocaine into RVMM, but not RVLM (Cox and Brody, 1987a). This result was consistent with the findings of a preliminary study using retrogradely transported rhodamine latex microspheres, which demonstrated direct hypothalamic projections to RVMM, but not to RVLM.

It is apparent that RVLM and RVMM differentially control vasomotor function. It may be presumed that this control is exerted via differential control of sympathetic outflow, however, this has not been directly tested. In fact, only a few studies have attempted to determine directly the contribution of the RVM to tonic sympathetic nerve activity (SNA) (McAllen et al., 1982; Pilowsky et al., 1985; Dean and Coote, 1986; Cox and Brody, 1988a, 1989a). The studies to be reviewed attempted to determine (1) whether the RVLM and RVMM control the sympathetic outflow to individual sympathetic nerves differentially and (2) whether the RVLM and/or RVMM is the sole source of sympathetic outflow in the anesthetized rat.

Methods

Studies were performed on male Sprague-Dawley rats (300–400 g) anesthetized with urethane. Catheters were placed into the femoral artery and vein for the recording of AP and the administration of drugs, respectively. The trachea was cannulated and the animals artificially ventilated using a rate (75 strokes/min) and stroke volume (2.5 ml) which mimic natural respiration. The neuromuscular blocking agent pancuronium (0.48 mg/kg, i.v. initial dose) was administered to prevent spontaneous respiration.

After placing the animal in a stereotaxic head holder, either the lumbar chain, renal or splanchnic sympathetic nerves were isolated retroperitoneally through an incision in the left flank and placed on bipolar platinum electrodes. The electrode and nerve were then covered with Wacker Sil-Gel. The sympathetic nerve signal recorded using a bandpass of 30–1000 Hz, was quantified using a window discriminator and spike counter and displayed as a continuous time-frequency histogram on a polygraph along with AP. The level of background noise in the neural recordings was estimated after sacrificing the animal.

Microinjections of lidocaine (200 nl, 4%) were used to reversibly interrupt neuronal transmission in RVLM and/or RVMM. The injections were made stereotaxically by placing an array of microinjectors bilaterally into the RVLM (−11.8 mm caudal to bregma, 1 mm dorsal to the ventral surface of the medulla and 2 mm lateral to midline) and into the RVMM (same coronal plane 1 mm lateral to midline) (Paxinos and Watson, 1986). Residual neurogenic cardiovascular tone after lidocaine injection into RVM was estimated by i.v. administration of the ganglionic blocking agent trimethaphan (3.3 mg/kg).

Results and discussion

The microinjection of lidocaine into either RVLM or RVMM reduced the level of mean arterial pressure (MAP) to approximately 55 mmHg. An additional fall in MAP of approximately 10 mmHg was elicited by the combined anesthetization of RVMM and RVLM or the administration of the ganglionic blocking agent trimethaphan. These results are consistent with previous reports from this laboratory (Cox and Brody, 1987a; Grosskreutz and Brody, 1988) and indicate that under conditions of normal tidal volume, neural systems in the RVMM and RVLM contribute equally to the neurogenic maintenance of AP. In addition, the combined inactivation of both regions effectively eliminates the neurogenic contribution to the maintenance of AP.

Although the microinjection of lidocaine into RVMM or RVLM elicited similar reductions in AP, inactivation of these regions elicited a differential pattern of sympathetic nerve responses. Renal sympathetic nerve activity (RSNA) was reduced by approximately 50% after anesthetization of either RVLM or RVMM. In contrast, the reduction in lumbar chain sympathetic nerve activity (LSNA) was greater after inactivation of RVLM than after inactivation of RVMM (approximately 70 and 55%, respectively). Similarly, inactivation of RVLM elicited greater reductions in splanchnic sympathetic nerve activity (SSNA) (approximately 50%) than did inactivation of RVMM (approximately 30%). Combined inactivation of RVLM and RVMM eliminated LSNA, while RSNA and SSNA were only reduced by approximately 60%. The administration of trimethaphan virtually abolished the residual 40% of RSNA and all but 15% of SSNA which is presumed to reflect the activity of preganglionic fibers unaffected by ganglionic blockade.

These data suggest that the subregions of the RVM exert differential control over the activities of the lumbar chain and splanchnic sympathetic nerves in the anesthetized rat. The RVMM and RVLM appear to contribute equally to RSNA. These results also point out a dissociation between the control of arterial pressure and activity of the renal and splanchnic sympathetic nerves. Although combined inactivation of RVMM and RVLM essentially eliminated the neurogenic component of AP, a considerable portion of SNA, apparently not involved in vasomotor control, remained on these two nerves.

There are several possible explanations for the source and function of the residual component of SNA, all of which await future investigation. First, the residual activity may represent a component of SNA involved in the tonic control of non-vasomotor systems such as the juxtaglomerular apparatus or the renal tubules. Second, this activity may arise from spinal sympathetic generators (Ardell et al., 1982; Taylor and Schramm, 1987) which are unmasked by the inactivation of supraspinal sites. As a final alternative to be suggested, this activity may originate from supramedullary sites such as Kolliker-Fuse nucleus (Cox and Brody, 1987b), medial thalamus, lateral hypothalamus, and/or posterior medial hypothalamus (Huang et al., 1988; Varner et al., 1988).

In summary, the studies reviewed in this paper provide several novel observations concerning the control of sympathetic outflow by the RVLM and RVMM. First, there is differential control of SNA by these two regions with the RVLM exerting greater control over SSNA and LSNA than does the RVMM. Renal sympathetic nerve activity appears to be controlled equally by both regions. Secondly, a substantial component of RSNA and SSNA appears to be non-vasomotor in function and may originate from spinal and/or other supraspinal generators of SNA. Taken together, these studies provide direct evidence that the medial and lateral subregions of the RVM differentially control sympathetic outflow.

Summary

Microinjections of lidocaine were used to examine the contributions of two subregions of the RVM, RVLM (2 mm lateral to midline) and RVMM (1 mm lateral to midline) to the maintenance of AP and SNA in urethane-anesthetized rats. Lidocaine microinjected into either site reduced AP to similar levels. Blockade of RVLM and RVMM produced a small further reduction in AP and essentially abolished neurogenic maintenance of AP. Blockade of either RVLM or RVMM elicited similar falls in RSNA. In contrast, inactivation of RVLM elicited larger falls in lumbar chain (LSNA) and splanchnic (SSNA) SNA than did inactivation of the RVMM. Combined blockade of RVLM and RVMM essentially eliminated LSNA, while RSNA and SSNA were reduced only 60%. From these data we conclude that (1) RVLM and RVMM contribute equally to the neurogenic maintenance of AP; (2) RVLM and RVMM differentially control the activity of individual sympathetic nerves; and (3) a substantial portion of RSNA and SSNA originates outside the RVM and may not be involved in vasomotor control.

Acknowledgements

The authors wish to thank Lynn Apel for secretarial assistance in the preparation of this manuscript. This work was supported in part by grants HLB-14388, HL-07121-13 and a gift from the Searle Family Trust.

References

Ardell, J.L., Barman, S.M. and Gebber, G.L. (1982) Sympathetic nerve discharge in chronic spinal cat. *Am. J. Physiol. (Heart Circ. Physiol.* 12), 243: H426–H470.

Barman, S.M. and Gebber, G.L. (1985) Axonal projection pattern of ventrolateral medullospinal sympathoexcitatory neurons. *J. Neurophysiol.*, 53: 1567–1582.

Blessing, W.W., Howe, P.R.C., Joh, T.J., Oliver, J.R. and Willoughby, J.O. (1986) Distribution of tyrosine hydroxylase and neuropeptide Y-like immunoreactive neurons in the rabbit medulla oblongata, with attention to colocalization studies, presumptive adrenaline-synthesizing perikarya, and vagal preganglionic cells. *J. Comp. Neurol.*, 248: 285–300.

Bowker, R.M., Steinbusch, H.W.M. and Coulter, J.D. (1981) Serotonergic and peptidergic projections to the spinal cord demonstrated by a combined retrograde HRP histochemical and immunocytochemical staining method. *Brain Res.*, 211: 412–417.

Cox, B.F. and Brody, M.J. (1987a) Decreased tidal volume (TV) alters arterial pressure (AP) control by rostral ventrolateral medulla (RVLM) – peripheral hemodynamic mechanisms and central sites. *Fed. Proc.*, 46: 744.

Cox, B.F. and Brody, M.J. (1987b) Tonic control of arterial

pressure and regional hemodynamics by pontine regions. *Soc. Neurosci. Abst.,* 13: 1246.

Cox, B.F. and Brody, M.J. (1988a) Tidal volume affects the response to inactivation of the rostral ventrolateral medulla. *Hypertension,* 11: I-186–I-189.

Cox, B.F. and Brody, M.J. (1988b) Evidence for two functionally distinct vasomotor subregions of rostral ventral medulla. *Clin. Exp. Hyper.* A10 (Suppl. 1): 11–18.

Cox, B.F. and Brody, M.J. (1989a) Mechanisms of respiration-induced changes in vasomotor control exerted by RVLM. *Am. J. Physiol. (Regulatory Integrative Comp. Physiol.)* (in press).

Cox, B.F. and Brody, M.J. (1989b) Subregions of rostral ventral medulla differentially control arterial pressure and regional hemodynamics. *Am. J. Physiol. (Regulatory Integrative Comp. Physiol.)* (in press).

Dean, C. and Coote, J.H. (1986) A ventromedullary relay involved in the hypothalamic and chemoreceptor activation of sympathetic postganglionic neurons to skeletal muscle, kidney, and splanchnic area. *Brain Res.,* 377: 279–295.

Dampney, R.A.L. and Moon, E.A. (1980) Role of ventrolateral medulla in vasomotor response to cerebral ischemia. *Am. J. Physiol. (Heart Circ. Physiol.* 8), 239: H349–H358.

Dampney, R.A.L., Goodchild, A.K., Robertson, L.G. and Montgomery, W. (1982) Role of ventrolateral medulla in vasomotor regulation: a correlative anatomical and physiological study. *Brain Res.,* 249: 223–235.

Everitt, B.J. Hökfelt, T., Terenius, L., Tatemoto, K., Mutt, V. and Goldstein, M. (1984) Differential co-existence of neuropeptide Y (NPY)-like immunoreactivity with catecholamines in the central nervous system of the rat. *Neuroscience,* 11: 443–462.

Feldberg, W. (1976) The ventral surface of the brain stem: a scarcely explored region of pharmacological sensitivity. *Neuroscience,* 1: 427–441.

Granata, A.R., Ruggiero, D.A., Park, D.H., Joh, T.H. and Reis, D.J. (1985) Brain stem area with C1 epinephrine neurons mediates baroreflex vasodepressor responses. *Am. J. Physiol. (Heart Circ. Physiol.* 17), 248: H547–H567.

Grosskreutz, C.L. and Brody, M.J. (1988) Role of the rostral ventrolateral medulla (RVLM) in neural control of arterial pressure (AP). *FASEB J.,* 2: A1487.

Guertzenstein, P.A. (1973) Blood pressure effects obtained by drugs applied to the ventral surface of the brain stem. *J. Physiol. (Lond.),* 229: 395–408.

Guertzenstein, P.A. and Silver, A. (1974) Fall in blood pressure from discrete regions of the ventral surface of the medulla by glycine and lesions. *J. Physiol. (Lond.),* 242: 489–503.

Helke, C.J., Neil, J.J., Massari, V.J. and Loewy, A.D. (1982) Substance P neurons project from the ventral medulla to the intermediolateral cell column and ventral horn in the rat. *Brain Res.,* 243: 147–152.

Huang, Z.S., Varner, K.J., Barman, S.M. and Gebber, G.L. (1988) Diencephalic regions contributing to sympathetic nerve discharge in anesthetized cats. *Am. J. Physiol. (Regulatory Integrative Comp. Physiol.* 23), 254: R249–R256.

Loewy, A.D. and McKellar, S. (1981) Serotonergic projections from the ventral medulla to the intermediolateral cell column in the rat. *Brain Res.,* 211: 146–152.

McAllen, R.M., Neil, J.J. and Loewy, A.D. (1982) Effects of kainic acid applied to the ventral surface of the medulla oblongata on vasomotor tone, the baroreceptor reflex and hypothalamic autonomic responses. *Brain Res.,* 238: 65–76.

Minson, J.B., Chalmers, J.P., Caon, A.C. and Renaud, B. (1987) Separate areas of rat medulla oblongata with populations of serotonin- and adrenalin-containing neurons alter blood pressure after L-glutamate stimulation. *J. Auton. Nerv. Syst.,* 19: 39–50.

Morrison, S.F., Milner, T.A. and Reis, D.J. (1988) Reticulospinal vasomotor neurons of the rat rostral ventrolateral medulla: relationship to sympathetic nerve activity and the C1 adrenergic cell group. *J. Neurosci.,* 8: 1286–1301.

Paxinos, G. and Watson, C. (1986) *The Rat Brain in Stereotaxic Coordinates, 2nd edn.,* Academic Press, New York.

Pilowsky, P., West, M. and Chalmers, J. (1985) Renal sympathetic nerve responses to stimulation, inhibition and destruction of rostral ventrolateral medulla in the rabbit. *Neurosci. Lett.,* 60: 51–55.

Ross, C.A., Ruggiero, D.A., Joh, T.H., Park, D.H. and Reis, D.J. (1983) Adrenaline synthesizing neurons in the rostral ventrolateral medulla: a possible role in tonic vasomotor control. *Brain Res.,* 273: 356–361.

Ross, C.A., Ruggiero, D.A., Joh, T.H., Park, D.H. and Reis, D.J. (1984a) Rostral ventrolateral medulla: selective projections to the thoracic autonomic cell column from the region containing C1 adrenaline neurons. *J. Comp. Neurol.,* 228: 168–185.

Ross, C.A., Ruggiero, D.A., Park, D.H., Joh, T.J., Sved, A.F., Fernandez-Pardal, J., Saavedra, J.M. and Reis, D.J. (1984b) Tonic vasomotor control by the rostral ventrolateral medulla: effect of electrical or chemical stimulation of the area containing C1 adrenaline neurons on arterial pressure, heart rate, and plasma catecholamines and vasopressin. *J. Neurosci.,* 4: 474–494.

Taylor, R.F. and Schramm, L.P. (1987) Differential effects of spinal transection on sympathetic nerve activities in rats. *Am. J. Physiol. (Regulatory Integrative Comp. Physiol.* 22), 253: R611–R618.

Varner, K.J., Barman, S.M. and Gebber, G.L. (1988) Cat diencephalic neurons with sympathetic nerve-related activity. *Am. J. Physiol. (Regulatory Integrative Comp. Physiol.* 23), 254: R257–R262.

J. Ciriello, M.M. Caverson and C. Polosa (Eds.)
Progress in Brain Research, Vol. 81
© 1989 Elsevier Science Publishers B.V. (Biomedical Division)

CHAPTER 7

Sympathoexcitatory neurons of the rostroventrolateral medulla and the origin of the sympathetic vasomotor tone

Patrice G. Guyenet, James R. Haselton and Miao-Kun Sun

Department of Pharmacology, University of Virginia School of Medicine, Charlottesville, VA 22908, U.S.A.

Introduction

The rostral ventrolateral medulla (RVLM) represents the area of the medulla limited medially by the gigantocellular field, the inferior olive and the nucleus interfascicularis hypoglossi (an outlying collection of serotonergic cells, definition after Loewy and McKellar, 1981). Ventrally, the RVLM extends to the ventral medullary surface, laterally to the trigeminal tract (or subtrigeminal portion of lateral reticular nucleus in cats), and caudally to the rostral tip of the lateral reticular nucleus. The dorsal aspect of the RVLM includes the rostral compact and subcompact subdivisions of nucleus ambiguus (for a definition of these terms, see Bieger and Hopkins, 1987). The medial two thirds of RVLM project massively to the intermediolateral cell column (Guyenet and Young, 1987 for references). A large component of this pathway consists of neurons immunoreactive for phenylethanolamine N-methyltransferase (PNMT; C_1 neurons), which project monosynaptically onto sympathetic preganglionic neurons (Milner et al., 1988). Depending on the study, between 25 and 50% of the reticulospinal projection of RVLM is found to be devoid of PNMT immunoreactivity (e.g. Tucker et al., 1987). The RVLM has reciprocal connections with the nucleus tractus solitarius, the area postrema, more caudal aspects of the ventrolateral medulla (region of the A_1 NE neurons), the parabrachial nuclei, and various hypothalamic structures (Andrezik et al., 1981; Ross et al., 1985). The RVLM also receives inputs from various hypothalamic structures, the central gray matter and the cord.

The pivotal role of the RVLM in vasomotor control is now well established (e.g. Ross et al., 1984b). Acute lesions of this structure or inhibition of neuronal activity by local microinjections of substances which inhibit neuronal activity (muscimol, GABA) result in the virtual elimination of the sympathetic vasomotor tone of anesthetized animals. Conversely the microinjection of substances which depolarize neurons such as glutamate or kainic acid produce massive sympathoexcitation (Willette et al., 1983 and for refs. see Ross et al., 1984b). However, the neuronal circuitry responsible for the vasomotor function of the RVLM is just beginning to be unraveled. One of several key issues is whether the RVLM simply contains a major collection of efferent bulbospinal cells whose tonic activity is driven synaptically by neurons located elsewhere in the brain. In other words, the question is to determine whether the reticulospinal projections of RVLM are simply the equivalent for sympathetic vasomotor control of the bulbospinal premotoneurons of the respiratory system (for review see Feldman, 1986) or whether

RVLM contains its own intrinsic tone-generating mechanism. If this latter proposition is correct, the question becomes to determine the neuronal basis of this tone-generating mechanism. This short chapter will largely focus on this particular issue.

RVLM neurons with intrinsic pacemaker activity "in vitro"

In coronal slices incubated in oxygenated saline, neurons with a regular, non-bursting rate of discharge are frequently encountered in the RVLM (mean firing rate at 30°C: 9 spikes/sec, range 4 – 13; mean rate at 37°C: 22 spikes/sec). Intracellular recordings (Fig. 1) reveal that their action potentials arise from a gradual interspike depolarization and not from EPSPs. Hyperpolarization to − 75 mV by intracellular current injection eliminates all pacemaking activity but does not reveal the presence of EPSPs (Fig. 1E). In addition, resetting of the pacemaking activity is produced by brief intracellular current pulses designed

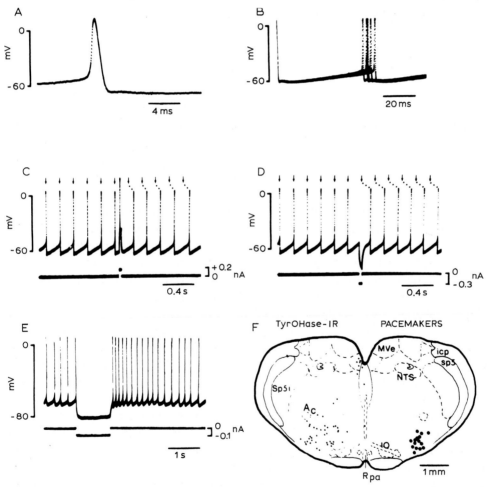

Fig. 1. Pacemaker neurons of rostral ventrolateral medulla. These neurons were recorded in tissue slices (rat) at 30°C. (A) Typical action potential; (B) five superimposed oscilloscope sweeps triggered on the upswing of individual spikes to demonstrate regularity of discharge; (C, D) resetting of pacemaking activity by intracellular depolarization (C) or hyperpolarization (D); (E) interruption of pacemaker activity by hyperpolarizing current (note lack of EPSP); (F) location of C_1 adrenergic neurons (left, tyrosine-hydroxylase immunostaining of 40 μm coronal section) and pacemaker neurons (right, intracellular staining with Lucifer Yellow). (Reprinted from Sun and Guyenet, 1988 a, b, c with permission from Brain Res.)

either to trigger a premature action potential (depolarizing pulse; Fig. 1C) or to delay the occurrence of a spike (hyperpolarizing pulse, Fig. 1D). These properties suggest strongly that the tonic activity of these cells is due to intrinsic pacemaking activity although it cannot yet be excluded that the spontaneous interspike depolarization might depend on or be facilitated by the presence in the tissue of some neuromodulator. The action potential of RVLM pacemaker neurons is largely sodium-dependent as it is blocked by tetrodotoxin. This agent suppresses all pacemaking activity (unpublished results of Sun and Guyenet). Contrary to the noradrenergic cells of the locus coeruleus (Williams et al., 1984) RVLM pacemakers do not seem able to produce spontaneous regenerative calcium spikes.

Modulators of RVLM pacemaker activity

The firing rate of these pacemaker cells is increased 30 – 80% by manipulations likely to produce enhancement of the intracellular cAMP concentration (Sun and Guyenet, unpublished data). Such treatments include incubation in presence of 8-brcAMP (0.5 – 1 mM), forskolin (10 μM) or β-adrenergic agonists (isoproterenol, epinephrine 1 – 10 μM). Substances such as dideoxy forskolin (10 μM), phenylephrine (up to 10 μM), and clonidine (up to 1 μM) produce no effect while adenosine (10 – 100 μM) produces inhibition (antagonized by theophylline 10 μM). Both isoproterenol and the cAMP analog increase the rate of depolarization of the membrane during the interspike interval without affecting either threshold and duration of the action potential or the early afterhyperpolarization. After TTX blockade, β-adrenergic agonists produce a depolarization associated with a decreased membrane resistance suggesting that cAMP activates an inward sodium or calcium current (unpublished results of Sun and Guyenet). The α_2-adrenergic agonist clonidine (up to 1 μM) produces no effect by itself nor does it antagonize the excitation caused by β-adrenergic receptor stimulation. Thus,

RVLM pacemakers do not possess α_2-adrenoceptors. Neither β- nor α-adrenergic receptor antagonists, administered alone or in combination, reduce the pacemaking activity indicating

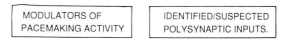

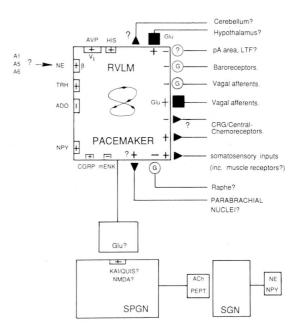

Fig. 2. Inputs of RVLM pacemakers. Summary diagram representing on left a list of substance which up or down regulate the intrinsic pacemaker activity of RVLM pacemakers (based on unpublished "in vitro" experiments of Sun and Guyenet). The right side summarizes the list of probable inputs to these cells and is a composite of results obtained by numerous investigators (see text for details). These inputs represent polysynaptic pathways in most cases (e.g. vagal afferents, baroreceptors, somatosensory inputs, etc.). Question marks are indicated where no single-unit evidence is available yet, but input is highly probable. Abbreviations: A_1, A_5, A_6 = brainstem noradrenergic cell groups; ADO = adenosine; AVP = vasopressin; CGRP = calcitonin gene-related peptide; CRG = central respiratory generator; G = GABA; Glu = glutamate-receptor agonist; HIS = histamine; LTF = lateral tegmental field; mENK = methionin enkaphalin; NE = noradrenaline: NPY = neuropeptide Y; pA = periambigual area (area of the A_1 cells or ventrolateral medullary depressor area); TRH = thyrotropin-releasing hormone; SPGN = sympathetic preganglionic neuron; SGN = sympathetic ganglionic neuron.

that the basal discharge of these neurons "in vitro" is not dependent on the presence of catecholamines.

The pacemaker activity of these RVLM neurons is also enhanced by V_1 vasopressin-receptor agonists, histamine, thyrotropin-releasing hormone, substance P, calcitonin gene-related peptide, neuropeptide Y and histamine. It is slowed by metenkephalin (1 μM) and adenosine but it is unaffected by angiotensin II and CRF (unpublished results of Sun and Guyenet, summarized in Fig. 2).

RVLM pacemaker neurons are reticulospinal neurons and do not belong to the C_1 adrenergic cell group

The intraspinal microinjection of rhodamine-tagged microbeads ($T_2 - T_3$) results in the retrograde labelling of many neurons in the rat RVLM. Lucifer Yellow was injected into RVLM pacemaker neurons in slices prepared from rats subjected one week before to intraspinal microbead injections. The majority of Lucifer Yellow-stained neurons was found to contain rhodamine beads demonstrating that RVLM pacemaker neurons have a spinal axonal projection (Sun et al., 1988b). Since these cells are recorded in the portion of the RVLM whose spinal projections terminate exclusively in the intermediolateral cell column and central autonomic areas of the spinal gray matter (see Guyenet and Young, 1987 for references), it follows that the pacemaker neurons innervate this structure and must play a role in sympathetic control.

In order to determine if RVLM pacemaker neurons are phenotypically adrenergic, they were stained intracellularly with Lucifer Yellow "in vitro" and the tissue was subsequently processed for the detection of either tyrosine-hydroxylase or phenylethanolamine N-methyltransferase with an indirect immunofluorescence technique (Texas red labelled secondary antibody). Neither enzyme could be detected in a total sample of 24 intracellularly stained RVLM pacemakers (Sun et al., 1988 b,c). On the other hand, 9 of 21 randomly sampled silent neurons also located in the RVLM were found to be strongly immunoreactive for tyrosine-hydroxylase (Sun et al., 1988c). From these experiments, it appears that RVLM pacemaker neurons project to the intermediolateral cell column and do not belong to the C_1 group of PNMT-immunoreactive neurons. Furthermore, the C_1 adrenergic cells do not display intrinsic pacemaker activity under similar "in vitro" conditions.

The RVLM reticulospinal neurons with intrinsic pacemaker activity therefore have characteristics which are ideally suited to fulfill a tone-generator role with regard to the sympathetic vasomotor output. However, because these neurons represent at best 50% of the projection of RVLM to the intermediolateral cell column, the balance consisting of C_1 adrenergic cells, a thorough understanding of the role of the RVLM in vasomotor control must at the very least incorporate some reasonable concept regarding the specific role played by these two main cell types. The following sections will attempt to address this question in part by describing the properties of reticulospinal sympathoexcitatory neurons "in vivo".

General properties of reticulospinal RVLM sympathoexcitatory cells recorded "in vivo" and major synaptic inputs

A very well documented body of evidence acquired in three different species (rat, cat and rabbit, Brown and Guyenet, 1985; Terui et al., 1986; Barman and Gebber, 1985) indicates that the RVLM contains a large concentration of barosensitive reticulospinal neurons with projections specifically targeted to the intermediolateral cell column and many of which have spontaneous activity under anesthesia. Cross-species experimentation also indicates that the bulk of these cells have a median conduction velocity close to 3 m/sec indicative of lightly myelinated projection. A representative example of the properties of these cells in the rat is shown in Fig. 3. As a group, these cells also receive a number of synaptic inputs in addition to that which conveys the inhibitory baroreceptor feedback. Inputs from spinal somatic sensory afferent pathways (excitatory, Morrison et al., 1986), vagal visceral afferent pathways (excitation and inhibition, Sun and Guyenet, 1987) renal visceral afferents (Saeki et al., 1988), the central respiratory generator (Terui et al., 1986; McAllen, 1987; Haselton and Guyenet, unpublished, see Fig. 4),

the hypothalamus (Brown and Guyenet, 1985; Terui et al., 1986), the midline raphe (inhibition, McCall, in press), the lateral tegmental field (mostly excitation, Barman and Gebber, 1987) have been particularly well documented with single-unit recordings and are summarized on the right side of Fig. 2. Inhibitory inputs seem to be mediated by GABA and excitatory ones via an endogenous glutamate receptor agonist. Probable but not clearly documented afferents to these cells also include inputs from the cerebellum (probably polysynaptic, McAllen, 1985), the parabrachial nuclei and the area surrounding the nucleus ambiguus at more caudal medullary levels (so-called "A_1" or "depressor" area, for refs. see Guyenet et al., 1987). These inputs are also represented in Fig. 2. The nature of these inputs indicates that RVLM reticulospinal sympathoexcitatory neurons, as a group, represent an essential hub for the integration of virtually all known sympathetic reflexes. This view is reinforced by the repeated observation that many sympathetic reflexes or responses evoked by CNS stimulation can be blocked by injections of selective antagonists of GABA- or glutamate-receptors restricted to the immediate vicinity of RVLM sympathoexcitatory neurons (e.g. Sun and Guyenet, 1987).

Heterogeneity of the reticulospinal sympathoexcitatory cells of the RVL: identification of putative adrenergic cells

As alluded to in the introduction, neuroanatomical data has amply demonstrated that RVLM reticulospinal neurons constitute a neurochemically heterogeneous group of cells since up to 50% of them display no immunoreactivity for catecholamine-synthesizing enzymes. Furthermore, the C_1 adrenergic cell group itself is neurochemically heterogeneous judging from the presence in some of these neurons of immunoreactive substance P (Loewy, 1987), neuropeptide Y (Everitt et al., 1984), perhaps also dynorphin (Menetrey and Basbaum, 1987). Electrophysiological evidence for heterogeneity within the reticulospinal barosen-

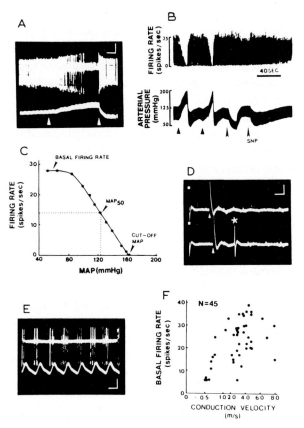

Fig. 3. Characteristics of reticulospinal barosensitive neurons of RVLM "in vivo" (A – C) Relationship between unit discharge and arterial pressure. (A) Oscilloscope record of spikes and carotid pressure; (B) relationship between discharge rate (integrated rate histogram) and AP; (C) plot of firing rate versus mean arterial pressure; (D) antidromic activation from spinal cord (collision test); (E) pulse-synchronous activity (carotid pressure shown as lower trace); (F) plot of basal discharge rate (baroreceptor unloaded) versus antidromic latency from spinal cord (one dot, one cell). (From Sun and Guyenet, 1985 with permission from the Am. J. Physiol.)

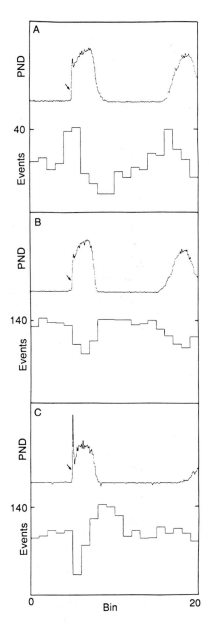

Fig. 4. Central respiratory generator-related modulation of the discharges of RVLM sympathoexcitatory neurons. Histograms representing the firing probability of RVLM reticulospinal barosensitive neurons (events) throughout the respiratory cycle in halothane-anesthetized, debuffered, vagotomized, paralyzed rats supplemented with CO_2 (endtidal CO_2 8 – 9%). PND: digitally averaged rectified phrenic nerve discharge recorded with bipolar electrodes and band pass of 100 – 3000 Hz. The computer was triggered on the rising phase of the PND (at arrows). Each histogram represents 50 sweeps; bin size is 100 msec. Three cells are shown which represent the three main patterns of respiratory modulation in rats (unpublished results of Haselton and Guyenet).

sitive neurons of RVLM is also gradually accumulating. The first evidence has been the bimodal distribution of the conduction velocity of their spinal axons (observed in rat and rabbit; peaks centered around 0.5 m/sec, and 3 m/sec, Brown and Guyenet, 1985; Terui et al., 1986) and the fact that every slow-conducting cell is inhibited by low hypotensive doses of clonidine (10 – 20 μg/kg i.v.) while only very few of the faster-conducting neurons are sensitive to this agent (Sun and Guyenet, 1985). The bimodal distribution of the axonal conduction velocity of RVLM barosensitive neurons is in perfect congruence with the observation that electrical stimulation of the RVLM produces two waves of sympathoexcitation in lumbar (Guyenet and Brown, 1986) and renal nerves (Morrison et al., 1988).

Since the turnover of brain epinephrine is greatly reduced by systemic administration of clonidine (Scatton and Bartholini, 1980), the hypothesis has been formulated that the slow-conducting RVLM barosensitive cells belong to the C_1 subgroup while the faster-conducting ones belong in majority to a non-catecholaminergic pathway (Sun and Guyenet, 1986). More recent experimentation indicates that a slow conduction velocity (0.3 – 0.8 m/sec) is actually not a diagnostic feature of all catecholaminergic RVLM barosensitive cells. Based on the result of a triple-labelling neuroanatomical study indicating that at least 88% of reticulospinal RVLM neurons with an ascending collateral in the pontine central tegmental tract are immunoreactive for PNMT and thus belong to the C_1 adrenergic cell cluster, we performed single-unit recordings on these neurons with pontine collaterals and compared their properties with those of RVLM barosensitive neurons with exclusive projections to the spinal cord (Haselton and Guyenet, in press). The spontaneously-active collateralized RVLM neurons were found to belong to the barosensitive cell population; they had a low rate of discharge (mean of 9 spikes/sec below baroreceptor threshold, silent cells not included) and were uniformly inhibited by i.v. clonidine (65% inhibition with 20 μg/kg). The conduction velocity of their spinal axonal process was bimodally distributed with 50% exhibiting a velocity below 1 m/sec and the rest a velocity between 1 and 4 m/sec. In contrast, RVLM barosensitive neurons with exclusive projection to the cord had much higher discharge rates (mean of 22 spikes/sec below baroreceptor threshold) and were uniformly insensitive to clonidine i.v. The conduction velocity of their spinal axon had a unimodal distribution and all belonged to the fast-conducting cell group (2 – 8 m/sec; mean 4 m/sec). This study (Haselton and Guyenet, in press) led us to conclude that (1) a very large majority of C_1 adrenergic cells project to both the lateral horn and one or more supramedullary structures; (2) these cells are specifically inhibited by clonidine; (3) their discharge rate is rather low and many are probably silent; and (4) axons of C_1 adrenergic neurons are either unmyelinated (conduction velocity 0.5 m/sec) or lightly myelinated (conduction velocity 1 – 4 m/sec). This last conclusion is congruent with the electron microscopic observation from the Cornell group which describes PNMT-immunoreactive axons of the lateral funiculus as either unmyelinated or lightly myelinated (Morrison et al., 1988).

The pacemaker neurons represent the subgroup of fast-conducting clonidine insensitive barosensitive neurons of RVLM

The evidence in support of this assertion relies in large part on the behavior of the highly active reticulospinal barosensitive RVLM neurons after intracisternal administration of the glutamate-receptor antagonist kynurenate. When administered i.c.v. to rats in such a way as to prevent diffusion of the blocker to the spinal subdural space, kynurenate blocked or largely attenuated a large variety of sympathetic reflexes while the resting sympathetic nerve discharge was maintained or slightly elevated (Sun and Guyenet, 1988a). The effectiveness of kynurenate is probably attributable to the fact that all supraspinal sympathetic reflexes are multisynaptic and include at least one synaptic relay which is critically dependent on the release of an endogenous glutamate-

receptor agonist. This is documented in the case of the baroreflex (Guyenet et al., 1987), vagosympathetic reflexes (Sun and Guyenet, 1987) and sympathoexcitatory effects triggered by posterior hypothalamic stimulation (Sun and Guyenet, 1986). Unit recording in the RVLM before and during kynurenate administration indicates that the drug slightly increases the discharge rate of RVLM barosensitive reticulospinal neurons and of course eliminates their barosensitivity. However, the most obvious effect of kynurenate is the transformation of the pattern of discharge of the fast-conducting highly active reticulospinal neurons. This pattern is changed from a rather irregular one into an extremely regular pacemaker-like discharge (Sun and Guyenet, 1988a). Resetting of this pacemaker-like discharge by antidromic activation from the spinal cord is always observed although cord stimulation delivered within the critical latency for collision produces no resetting whatsoever (Sun et al., 1988a). This evidence suggests that after kynurenic acid, the pacemaker discharges of these cells are due to intrinsic properties and moreover that collateral interactions between the cells are not observed in the presence of the glutamate antagonist.

Table I compares the properties of the non-catecholaminergic RVL pacemaker cells ''in vitro'' and that of the fast-conducting, highly active barosensitive reticulospinal neurons ''in vivo'' after kynurenate blockade. The remarkable congruence of the data argues strongly that the same cell population was recorded ''in vitro'' and ''in vivo''.

In the course of these experiments, a few slow-conducting barosensitive neurons were also recorded before and after kynurenate (putative adrenergic cells). Although these neurons were still active after kynurenate, their discharge pattern did not develop the striking regularity of their fast-conducting counterparts. Thus neither ''in vivo'' nor ''in vitro'' is there any clear indication that C_1 neurons might be endowed with intrinsic pacemaker properties but this possibility is by no means excluded yet, especially in view of the fact

TABLE I

Comparison between the properties of rat RVLM pacemaker "in vitro" and those of a subgroup of fast-conducting reticulospinal RVLM sympathoexcitatory (SE) neurons "in vivo"

	SE neurons "in vivo"	Pacemaker cells "in vitro"
Triphasic AP	+	+
Extracellular AP duration	1.5 – 2 msec	1.5 – 2 msec
Spinal axon	+	+
Firing rate at 37°C	22 spikes/sec	21 spikes/sec
Kynurenate-resistant pacemaker activity	+	+
Sensitivity to clonidine	–	–
Collateral interaction	None[a]	None[b]

[a] After i.c.v. kynurenate (Sun et al., 1988a).

[b] In the absence of kynurenate, intracellular depolarization produces no evidence of recurrent activity (Sun et al., 1988b). Furthermore, after intracellular labelling no axonal collateral in RVLM was ever observed (unpublished data of Sun and Guyenet).

that all other types of monoaminergic neurons in the CNS display pacemaker properties (dopaminergic, noradrenergic of locus coeruleus and serotonergic of raphe dorsalis). It is also possible that the discharges of these cells are largely if not exclusively synaptically driven under usual anesthetic conditions. A rigorous test of this hypothesis will be crucial to our understanding of the genesis of the vasomotor output.

Neurotransmitters released by RVLM sympathoexcitatory neurons in the intermediolateral cell column

This is a complex issue which has not received a definitive answer at this time. Neuroanatomical data indicate that C_1 neurons make monosynaptic contact with preganglionic neurons (Milner et al., 1988) but it is not known whether these postsynaptic targets have an exclusively vasoconstrictor or even vasomotor function. Since these cells synthesize noradrenaline and perhaps epinephrine plus various peptides (substance P, neuropeptide Y) which can all exert effects on some preganglionic neurons, each of the above substances may play some role in neurotransmission. Substance P may be particularly important since the sympathetic outflow is greatly reduced by the introduction of antagonists to this peptide in the spinal subarachnoid space (see review by Loewy, 1987). Another line of evidence supports the notion that an endogenous glutamate-receptor agonist could be a neurotransmitter of the RVLM-IML sympathoexcitatory pathway. This is based on several observations. First, intrathecal administration of the glutamate-receptor antagonist kynurenate eliminates the sympathetic outflow and the sympathoexcitation produced by RVLM stimulation (Guyenet et al., 1987). Second, iontophoretic application of the same substance decreases the spontaneous activity of individual preganglionic neurons and their driving from RVLM (Morrison and Reis, 1988). Finally, in coronal slices of the spinal cord, stimulation of the lateral funiculus produces EPSPs in preganglionic neurons which are blocked by kainate/quisqualate receptor antagonist (Nishi et al., 1987). None of the experiments mentioned in this section have produced mutually exclusive results and the participation of many different transmitters may be necessary to bring sympathetic preganglionic neurons beyond their firing threshold. The way in which the presence of a catecholamine can amplify the response to a standard intracellular depolarizing pulse (Fig. 5 insert) is a good illustration of the biasing influence that many neuromodulators could have on the effect produced by a more traditional ionophore-coupled transmitter such as glutamate. Taking this speculation one step further (Fig. 5) one can imagine that the effect of the pacemaker neurons on preganglionic neurons is to trigger, by way of glutamate release, a depolarizing membrane current of uniform amplitude in a wide number of vasomotor preganglionic neurons thereby producing the equivalent of the intracellular current pulse of Yoshimura et al. (1987; see insert Fig. 5). However, the frequency encoding of this

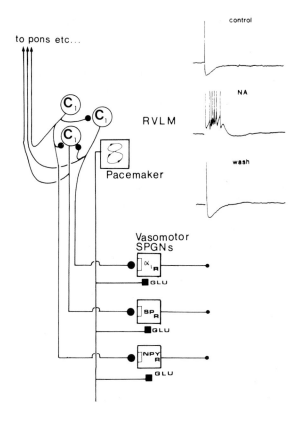

Fig. 5. Role of the RVLM in sympathetic vasomotor control: a hypothetical model. This theoretical construct incorporates the results of numerous lines of experimentation from several laboratories (summarized in the text). The pacemaker reticulospinal projection is viewed as a tone-generating perhaps glutamate-releasing pathway dedicated to contributing a background excitatory drive to numerous vasomotor efferent pathways. C_1 adrenergic neurons, perhaps numerically the majority, may have more topographically organized projections, and probably have local collaterals. These cells also project to a variety of rostral structures. It is hypothesized here that the various neurotransmitters which C_1 cells presumably release (catecholamines, substance P, NPY) may amplify or reduce the effect of the glutamate-induced depolarization of SPGNs thus producing differential control of the various vasomotor output channels. As an illustration of this type of control, the insert illustrates the effect of noradrenaline (perhaps through α_1-receptors) on the discharge of a cat sympathetic preganglionic neuron (SPGN, after Yoshimura et al., 1987; reproduced with permission of the J. Neurophysiol.). Norepinephrine, by altering the intrinsic membrane properties of the SPGN dramatically alters the frequency encoding of a standard intracellular depolarizing current which "in vivo" could be a glutamate receptor-dependent synaptic current. There is no evidence yet that C_1 cells have intrinsic pacemaker activity although this

depolarizing event (i.e. number of spikes triggered per EPSP) could be modulated to a great extent by catecholamines and peptide transmitters released by C_1 adrenergic neurons, raphe spinal neurons, etc. Such a framework could easily explain how both pacemaker and C_1 neurons (and maybe other cells such as the raphe spinal projection) could contribute significantly to the basal vasomotor tone. This theory could also explain that glutamate-receptor blockade in the cord antagonized both short- and long-latency excitation of preganglionic neurons when RVLM is stimulated (Morrison and Reis, 1987) and could account for the pronounced sympathoinhibitory effects of clonidine which occurs despite its selective action on C_1 neurons (Haselton and Guyenet, in press).

Summary and conclusions

In summary, a substantial portion of the excitatory drive to vasomotor sympathetic preganglionic neurons originates from reticulospinal tonically active cells located in the RVLM. This interpretation does not exclude the possible contribution of other tonically active bulbospinal or propriospinal inputs in generating the vasomotor outflow but under usual anesthetic conditions it seems that these alternative inputs are simply insufficient to bring the vasomotor preganglionic neurons to their firing threshold. Such may not be the case after plastic rearrangements consecutive to complete spinalization or chronic lesions of large portions of the RVLM have occurred (Cochrane and Nathan, 1987; for review see Schramm, 1986).

It is also clear at present that the RVLM is not merely a final common pathway consisting of premotoneurons passively driven by tonic synaptic in-

hypothesis is not excluded either. The source of their excitatory drive "in vivo" remains to be determined. Abbreviations: SPGN = sympathetic preganglionic neuron; $\alpha 1R$ = alpha-one adrenergic receptor, SPR = receptor to substance P; NPYR = receptor to neuropeptide Y; C_1 = adrenergic neurons of rostral ventrolateral medulla (RVLM).

puts originating elsewhere. Indeed the existence of a population of reticulospinal neurons with intrinsic pacemaker activity indicates that the RVLM contains at least one major intrinsic source of tonic activity. These neurons may release a glutamate-like substance and are not phenotypically adrenergic. They have no *documented* projections outside the cord and could subserve a tone-generating function specific to the sympathetic outflow, e.g. providing a background excitatory input to a large number of preganglionic neurons with vasoconstrictor of cardioaccelerator function. Strong anatomical evidence backed by weaker electrophysiological evidence also support the notion that C_1 adrenergic neurons may have a vasomotor role and contribute an excitatory drive to preganglionic neurons. This could be mediated via α_1-adrenergic receptors or by receptors to substance P or neuropeptide Y. There is no evidence yet that C_1 cells might have intrinsic pacemaker activity. The origin of the ongoing activity of many of these cells "in vivo" is therefore unclear and could depend on an excitatory drive from outside the RVLM. One might speculate that because these cells appear to have collateral interactions (PNMT-immunoreactive boutons synapse on C_1 cells, Milner et al., 1987), they could play a role in synchronizing the sympathetic vasomotor outflow (an unexplained phenomenon observable even in the absence of baroreceptor input). Because of the large variety of peptides which they contain, another speculative view could be that they make rather specific connections with subsets of preganglionic neurons and therefore might be responsible for the differential control of regional blood flows by the rostral medulla (Dampney and McAllen, 1988). C_1 cells are inhibited by low systemic doses of clonidine and therefore may be in part responsible for the hypotensive effect of this drug. The majority of C_1 cells also have rostral projections and thus convey cardiorespiratory information simultaneously to the cord and to many supramedullary structures which they innervate.

Collectively it is certain that both types of RVLM barosensitive reticulospinal neurons (non-aminergic pacemakers and C_1 cells) represent a hub for the integration of numerous vasomotor reflexes including baroreflexes, various viscero- and somatosympathetic reflexes. These cells also receive inputs from the hypothalamus, the central respiratory generator and indirectly from many other structures such as the central gray and cerebellum.

References

Andrezik, T.A., Chan-Palay, V. and Palay, S.L. (1981a) The nucleus paragigantocellularis lateralis in the rat: conformation and cytology. *Anat. Embryol.,* 161: 355–371.

Andrezik, J.A., Chan-Palay, V. and Palay, S.L. (1981b) The nucleus paragigantocellularis lateralis in the rat: demonstration of afferents by the retrograde transport of HRP. *Anat. Embryol.,* 161: 373–390.

Barman, S.M. and Gebber, G.L. (1985) Axonal projection patterns of ventrolateral medullospinal sympathoexcitatory neurons. *J. Neurophysiol.,* 53: 1567–1582.

Barman, S.M. and Gebber, G.L. (1987) Lateral tegmental field neurons of cat medulla: a source of basal activity of ventrolateral medullospinal sympathoexcitatory neurones. *J. Neurophysiol.,* 57: 1410–1425.

Bieger, D. and Hopkins, D.A. (1987) Viscerotopic representation of the alimentary tract in the medulla oblongata in the rat: the nucleus ambiguus. *J. Comp. Neurol.,* 262: 546–562.

Brown, D.L. and Guyenet, P.G. (1985) Electrophysiological study of cardiovascular neurons in the rostral ventrolateral medulla. *Circ. Res.,* 56: 359–369.

Cochrane, K.L. and Nathan, M.A. (1987) Normotension in conscious rats after lesion of rostral ventrolateral medulla (RVLM). *Soc. Neurosci. Abstr.,* 13: 276.

Dampney, R.A.L. and McAllen, R.M. (1988) Differential control of sympathetic fibers supplying kindlimb, skin, and muscle by subretrofacial neurones in the cat. *J. Physiol. (Lond.),* 395: 41–56.

Everitt, B.J., Hokfelt, T., Terenius, L., Takemoto, K., Mutt, V. and Goldstein, M. (1984) Differential coexistence of neuropeptide Y-(NPY)-like immunoreactivity with catecholamines in the central nervous system of the rat. *Neuroscience,* 11: 443–462.

Feldman, J.L. (1986) Neurophysiology of breathing in mammals. In F.E. Bloom (Ed.), *Handbook of Physiology: The Nervous System IV, Intrinsic Regulatory Systems of the Brain.* Am. Physiol. Soc. Bethesda, Md., pp. 463–524.

Guyenet, P.G. and Brown, D.L. (1986) Nucleus paragigantocellularis lateralis and lumbar sympathetic discharge in the rat. *Am. J. Physiol.*, 250: R1081 – R1094.

Guyenet, P.G., Sun, M.-K. and Brown, D.L. (1987) Role of GABA and excitatory aminoacids in medullary baroreflex pathways. In J. Ciriello, F.R. Calaresu, L.P. Renaud and C. Polosa (Eds.), *Organization of the Autonomic Nervous System: Central and Peripheral Mechanisms,* Alan R. Liss, Inc., New York, pp. 215 – 225.

Guyenet, P.G. and Young, B.S. (1987) Projections of nucleus paragigantocellularis lateralis to locus coeruleus and other structures in rat. *Brain Res.,* 406: 171 – 184.

Haselton, J.R. and Guyenet, P.G. (1989) Electrophysiological characterization of putative C_1 adrenergic neurons in the rat. *Neuroscience,* 30: 199 – 214.

Loewy, A.D. and McKellar, S. (1981) Serotonergic projections from the ventral medulla to the intermediolateral cell column in the rat. *Brain Res.,* 211: 146 – 152.

Loewy, A.D. (1987) Substance P neurons of the ventral medulla: their role in the control of vasomotor tone. In R. Hainsworth, R.J. Linden, P.N. McWilliam and D.A.S.G. Mary (Eds.), *Cardiogenic Reflexes,* Oxford University Press, London, pp. 269 – 284.

McAllen, R.M. (1985) Mediation of the fastigial pressor response and a somatosympathetic reflex by ventral medullary neurons in the cat. *J. Physiol. (Lond.),* 368: 423 – 434.

McCall, R.B. (1988) GABA-mediated inhibition of sympathoexcitatory neurons by midline medullary stimulation. *Am. J. Physiol.,* 255: R605 – R615.

Menetrey, D. and Basbaum, A.I. (1987) The distribution of substance P-, enkephalin-, and dynorphin-immunoreactive neurons in the medulla of the rat and their contribution to bulbospinal pathways. *Neuroscience,* 23: 173 – 187.

Milner, T.A., Pickel, V.M., Park, D.H. Joh, T.H. and Reis, D.J. (1987) Phenylethanolamine *N*-methyl transferase-containing neurons in the rostral ventrolateral medulla of the rat. I. Normal ultrastructure. *Brain Res.,* 411: 28 – 45.

Milner, T.A., Morrison, S.F., Abate, C. and Reis, D.J. (1988) Phenylethanolamine *N*-methyltransferase containing terminals synapse directly on sympathetic preganglionic neurons in the rat. *Brain Res.,* 448: 205 – 222.

Morrison, S.F., Milner, T., Pickel, V. and Reis, D.J. (1986) Reticulospinal sympathoexcitatory neurons in the C_1 region of the rostral ventrolateral medulla (RVL) may mediate the supraspinal component of the somatosympathetic reflex. *Soc. Neurosci. Abstr.,* 12: Part 12, 1157.

Morrison, S.F. and Reis, D.J. (1987) Glutamate receptor antagonist blocks the response of sympathetic preganglionic neurons (SPN) to stimulation of the C_1 area of the rostral ventrolateral medulla (RVL). *Soc. Neurosci. Abstr.,* 13: Part 2, 808.

Morrison, S.F., Milner, T.A., Pickel, B.M. and Reis, D.J. (1988) Reticulospinal vasomotor neurons of the rat rostral ventrolateral medulla (RVL): relationship to sympathetic nerve activity and the C_1 adrenergic cell group. *J. Neurosci.,* 8: 1286 – 1301.

Nishi, S., Yoshimura, M. and Polosa, C. (1987) Synaptic potentials and putative transmitter actions in sympathetic preganglionic neurons. In J. Ciriello, F.R. Calaresn, L.P. Renard and C. Polosna (Eds.), *Organization of the Autonomic Nervous System,* Alan R. Liss, Inc., New York, pp. 15 – 26.

Ross, C.A., Ruggiero, D.A., Joh. T.H., Park, D.H. and Reis, D.J. (1984a) Rostral ventrolateral medulla: selective projections to the thoracic autonomic cell column from the region containing C_1 adrenaline neurons. *J. Comp. Neurol.,* 228: 168 – 185.

Ross, C.A. Ruggiero, D.A., Park, D.H., Joh, T.H., Sved, A.F., Fernandez-Pardal, J., Saavedra, J.M. and Reis, D.J. (1984b) Tonic vasomotor control by the rostral ventrolateral medulla: effect of electrical or chemical stimulation of the area containing C_1 adrenaline neurons on arterial pressure, heart rate, and plasma catecholamines and vasopressin. *J. Neurosci.,* 4: 474 – 494.

Ross, C.A., Ruggiero, D.A. and Reis, D.J. (1985) Projections from the nucleus tractus solitarii to the rostral ventrolateral medulla. *J. Comp. Neurol.,* 242: 511 – 534.

Saeki, Y., Terui, N. and Kumada, M. (1988) Participation of ventrolateral medullary neurons in the renal-sympathetic reflex in rabbits. *Jpn. J. Physiol.,* 38: 267 – 281.

Scatton, B. and Bartholini, G. (1980) Effect of antihypertensives and other drugs on central adrenaline utilization. In K. Fuxe, M. Goldstein, B. Hökfelt, and T. Hökfelt (Eds.), *Central Adrenaline Neurons,* Pergamon Press, Oxford, pp. 183 – 197.

Schramm, L.P. (1986) Spinal factors in sympathetic regulation, In A. Magro, W. Osswald, D.S. Reis and P. Vanhoutte (Eds.), *Central and Peripheral Mechanisms of Cardiovascular Regulation,* Plenum Publ. Co., New York, pp. 303 – 352.

Sun, M.-K. and Guyenet, P.G. (1985) GABA-mediated baroreceptor inhibition of reticulospinal neurons. *Am. J. Physiol.,* 249: R672 – R680.

Sun, M.-K. and Guyenet, P.G. (1986) Effect of clonidine and GABA on the discharges of medullospinal sympathoexcitatory neurons in the rat. *Brain Res.,* 368: 1 – 17.

Sun, M.-K. and Guyenet, P.G. (1987) Arterial baroreceptor and vagal inputs to sympathoexcitatory neurons in rat medulla. *Am. J. Phsyiol.,* 252: R699 – R709.

Sun. M.-K., Hackett, J.T. and Guyenet, P.G. (1988a) Sympathoexcitatory neurons of rostral ventrolateral medulla exhibit pacemaker properties in presence of a glutamate-receptor antagonist. *Brain Res.,* 438: 23 – 40.

Sun, M.-K., Young, B.S., Hackett, J.T. and Guyenet, P.G. (1988b) Reticulospinal pacemaker neurons of the rat rostral ventrolateral medulla with putative sympathoexcitatory function: an intracellular study in vitro. *Brain Res.,* 442: 229 – 239.

Sun, M.-K., Young, B.S., Hackett, J.T. and Guyenet, P.G. (1988c) Rostral ventrolateral medullary neurons with intrinsic pacemaker properties are not catecholaminergic. *Brain Res.*, 451: 345–349.

Terui, N., Saeki, Y. and Kumada, M. (1986) Barosensory neurons in the ventrolateral medulla in rabbits and their responses to various afferent inputs from peripheral and central sources. *Jpn. J. Physiol.*, 36: 1148–1164.

Tucker, D.C., Saper, C.B., Ruggiero, D.A. and Reis, D.J. (1987) Organization of central adrenergic pathways. 1. Relationships of ventrolateral medullary projections to the hypothalamus and spinal cord. *J. Comp. Neurol.*, 259: 591–603.

Yoshimura, M., Polosa, C. and Nishi, S. (1987) Noradrenaline-induced afterdepolarization in cat sympathetic preganglionic neurons in vitro. *J. Neurophysiol.*, 57: 1314–1324.

Willette, R.N., Krieger, A.J., Barcas, P.P. and Sapru, H.N. (1983) Medullary-aminobutyric acid (GABA) receptors and the regulation of blood pressure in the rat. *J. Pharmacol. Exp. Therapeut.*, 226: 893–899.

Williams, J.T., North, R.A., Shefner, S.A., Nishi, S. and Egan, T.M. (1984) Membrane properties of rat locus coeruleus neurones. *Neuroscience*, 13: 136–156.

J. Ciriello, M.M. Caverson and C. Polosa (Eds.)
Progress in Brain Research, Vol. 81
© 1989 Elsevier Science Publishers B.V. (Biomedical Division)

CHAPTER 8

Basis for the naturally occurring activity of rostral ventrolateral medullary sympathoexcitatory neurons

Susan M. Barman[1] and Gerard L. Gebber[1,2]

Departments of [1]Pharmacology and Toxicology, and of [2]Physiology, Michigan State University, East Lansing, MI 48824, U.S.A.

Introduction

Sympathetic nerves that control the heart, vasculature and other visceral organs are tonically active under a variety of conditions in man and animals. Such activity is critical for the maintenance of blood pressure within normal limits. Although this was established over one hundred years ago (cf., Gebber, 1984) the central origin and mechanisms that account for the generation of background sympathetic nerve discharge (SND) remain controversial issues. The purpose of this chapter is to review recent research that has dealt with these fundamental issues. There is general agreement that neurons in the rostral ventrolateral medulla (RVLM) whose axons project to the thoraco-lumbar intermediolateral nucleus (IML) constitute the primary source of SND (cf. Ciriello et al., 1986; Millhorn and Eldridge, 1986; Calaresu and Yardley, 1988). The origin of the naturally occurring discharges of these neurons, however, is a hotly debated subject. One theory is that RVLM-spinal sympathoexcitatory (SE) neurons are driven by their antecedent inputs (Gebber and Barman, 1985). The neurons comprising these inputs are thought to form, either by themselves or in conjunction with RVLM-spinal SE neurons, a network oscillator capable of generating one of the major components of SND, the 2- to 6-Hz rhythm (see below). That is, it has been proposed that the 2- to 6-Hz component in SND arises from an ensemble of neurons of different types interconnected in such a way to generate rhythmic activity (Gebber and Barman, 1989). Such a circuit could be devoid of pacemaker neurons and still generate rhythmic activity (Selverston and Moulins, 1985).

The second theory on the origin of the naturally occurring discharges of RVLM-spinal SE neurons is that they possess pacemaker properties that account for most if not all of their activity (Sun et al., 1988a,b). The rhythmic activity (i.e. near constant interspike or interburst intervals) of a pacemaker neuron is attributed to the intrinsic properties (activation and/or inactivation of specific ionic currents) of its membrane rather than to periodic synaptic input (Connor, 1985).

Network oscillator theory

The network oscillator theory on the origin of SND is based on data from the cat. In this species, most (> 80%) of SND is in the form of a 2- to 6-Hz rhythm. This rhythm is cardiac-related before baroreceptor denervation and free-running after section of the carotid sinus, aortic depressor and vagus nerves (Barman and Gebber, 1980). The 2- to 6-Hz rhythm is ubiquitous to postganglionic sympathetic nerves with cardiovascular function (Gebber and Barman, 1980), and it persists in SND after midcollicular decerebration (Barman and Gebber, 1980). Importantly, the precipitous fall in blood pressure following transection of the cervical spinal cord is accompanied by loss of this sympathetic nerve rhythm (Ardell et al., 1982). Thus, the rhythm can be viewed as the signature of brain stem circuits responsible for a significant component of SND and, thereby, cardiovascular tone (Gebber, 1984).

In this section, we review those experiments performed in our laboratory that have led to the following proposals: (1) the 2- to 6-Hz rhythm in SND arises from a network oscillator rather than from a group of pacemaker neurons; (2) the 2- to 6-Hz rhythm is generated by neurons that are antecedent to RVLM-spinal SE neurons.

As a first step in understanding how the 2- to 6-Hz rhythm is generated, we used spike-triggered averaging to identify single brain stem neurons whose naturally occurring discharges are synchronized to this component in SND (Barman and Gebber, 1981, 1983; Morrison and Gebber, 1982). For this purpose, the extracellularly recorded action potentials (i.e. spikes) of the neuron (i.e. unit) serve as reference signals for computation of an average of accompanying changes in SND. Postganglionic SND is recorded with a wide preamplifier bandpass (1 – 1000 Hz) so that bursts of activity (i.e. envelopes of spikes) appear as slow waves (Gebber and Barman, 1985). SND occurring in a time window (e.g. ± 500 msec) surrounding each of the unit spikes is digitized and subsequently averaged by a computer. An example of the results obtained with this method is shown in Fig. 1D1. The spike-triggered average shows renal SND that preceded (left of zero lag) and followed (right of zero lag) the action potential of a neuron in the RVLM. The average of SND contains a rhythmic component whose period was 340 msec. Thus, the activity of this RVLM neuron was synchronized to a rhythm in renal SND in the 2- to 6-Hz range. A randomly generated series of pulses (same number and frequency as for the unit spike train) also is used to compute an average of SND. Such averages are termed "dummy" averages, and the one shown

in Fig. 1D2 was basically flat. Single neurons are considered to have sympathetic nerve-related activity when the amplitude of the first peak to the right of zero lag in the spike-triggered average exceeds that of the largest deflection in the "dummy" average by at least a factor of three.

Since the 2- to 6-Hz component in SND is synchronized to the cardiac cycle in baroreceptor-innervated cats (Barman and Gebber, 1980; Gebber, 1984), brain stem unit activity correlated to

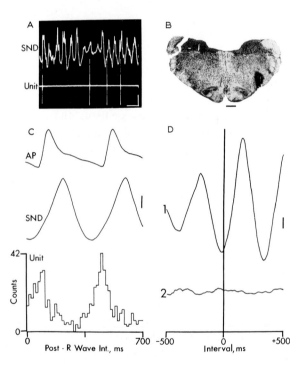

Fig. 1. Cat ventrolateral medullary neuron with cardiac- and sympathetic nerve-related discharges. (A) Oscilloscopic records of renal sympathetic nerve discharge (SND) (top) and medullary unit spikes (bottom). Vertical calibration is 50 μV for SND and 200 μV for unit spikes; horizontal calibration is 500 msec. (B) Frontal section through medulla approximately 2 mm posterior to caudal border of trapezoid body. Arrow marks site of unit recording. Calibration is 1 mm. (C) Post-R wave averages of arterial pulse (AP) wave (top) and SND (middle), and histogram of unit spikes (bottom). Number of trials was 1500. Mean blood pressure was 140 mmHg. Bin width for averages was 1.4 msec and for unit histogram was 14 msec. Vertical calibration for SND is 20 μV. (D) Spike-triggered average of SND (trace 1) and "dummy" pulse-triggered average of SND (trace 2). Unit spikes and "dummy" pulses are at zero lag. Number of trials is 700. Bin width was 1 msec. Vertical calibration is 5 μV. (Reprinted from Barman and Gebber, 1983.)

this rhythm should also be cardiac-related. That such is the case was demonstrated with post-R wave (ECG) analysis. Averages of the arterial pulse wave and SND, and a histogram of the occurrences of brain stem unit spikes are constructed by using the R wave as the reference signal. The cardiac-related discharge pattern of an RVLM neuron with sympathetic nerve-related activity is shown in Fig. 1C.

Brain stem neurons with cardiac-related activity might be contained in circuits directly involved in generating SND. Alternatively, they might be interneurons in the afferent limb of the baroreceptor reflex arc. One can distinguish between these two neuronal types by comparing the relationship between unit activity and SND at control blood pressure with that after blood pressure is lowered to a level at which synchronization of the 2- to 6-Hz sympathetic nerve rhythm to the cardiac cycle is disrupted due to reduced baroreceptor nerve activity (Gebber and Barman, 1985). The discharges of neurons directly responsible for SND should remain correlated to the 2- to 6-Hz rhythm when blood pressure is lowered while those of baroreceptor interneurons should not. In the case shown in Fig. 2, the activity of a single neuron located in the lateral tegmental field (LTF) of the cat medulla was recorded. The spike-triggered average in panel IA1 shows that unit activity was correlated to a 2- to 6-Hz rhythm in inferior cardiac SND. As demonstrated with post-R wave analysis, this rhythm had the period of the cardiac cycle when mean blood pressure was 135 mmHg (IB). Blood pressure was then lowered to disrupt the synchronization of SND and unit activity to the cardiac cycle. This is indicated by the flat post-R wave average of SND and histogram of unit spike occurrences shown in panel IIB. As demonstrated with spike-triggered averaging (IIA1), LTF unit activity remained correlated to SND at this time. Thus, the discharges of this LTF neuron were more closely associated with SND than with baroreceptor afferent nerve activity. It should also be noted that the interval (132 msec) between unit spike occurrence and the peak of the next sympathetic nerve

slow wave was unchanged when blood pressure was lowered from 135 to 90 mmHg (see spike-triggered averages in IA1, IIA1). This observation supports the view that unit activity was correlated to the same component in SND at the two levels of blood pressure.

Neurons with the properties illustrated in Fig. 2 are presumed to comprise central circuits responsible for the 2- to 6-Hz rhythm in SND. The distribution of such neurons in the cat medulla is shown in Fig. 3. They were located in three regions − the LTF, RVLM and raphe nuclei. LTF neurons with

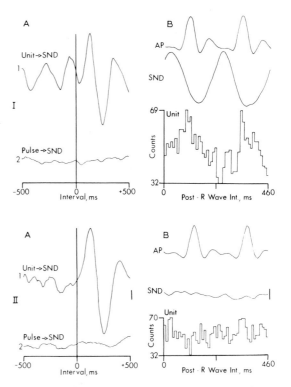

Fig. 2. Sympathetic nerve-related activity of a neuron in lateral tegmental field of cat medulla at two levels of mean blood pressure. Mean blood pressure was 135 mmHg in I and 90 mmHg in II. IA, IIA: spike-triggered (trace 1) and "dummy" pulse-triggered (trace 2) averages of inferior cardiac sympathetic nerve discharge (SND). Unit spikes and "dummy" pulses are at zero lag. Number of trials was 340 (IA) and 363 (IIA). Bin width was 1 msec. Vertical calibration is 10 μV. IB, IIB: post-R wave averages of arterial pulse (AP, top) and SND (middle), and histogram of unit spikes. Number of trials was 653 (IB) and 725 (IIB). Bin width was 920 μsec for averages and 9.2 msec for histogram. Vertical calibration for SND is 20 μV. (Reprinted from Gebber and Barman, 1985.)

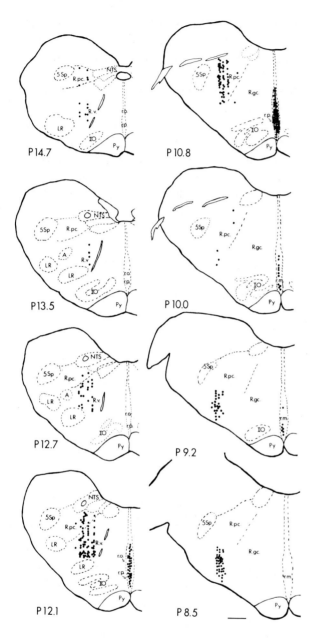

Fig. 3. Anatomical distribution of cat medullary neurons with sympathetic nerve-related activity. Frontal sections 8.5 – 14.7 mm posterior to the interaural line are shown. A = nucleus ambiguus; IO = inferior olive; LR = lateral reticular nucleus; NTS = nucleus of tractus solitarius; Py = pyramid; R.gc. = nucleus reticularis gigantocellularis; R.pc. = nucleus reticularis parvocellularis; R.v. = nucleus reticularis ventralis; r.m. = nucleus raphe magnus; r.o. = nucleus raphe obscurus; r.p. = nucleus raphe pallidus; 5Sp = spinal nucleus of trigeminal nerve. Calibration is 1 mm. (Reprinted from Gebber and Barman, 1985.)

sympathetic nerve-related activity were found in nucleus reticularis parvocellularis and nucleus reticularis ventralis 10.0 – 14.7 mm posterior to the interaural line (stereotaxic planes P10 – P14.7). RVLM neurons were located caudal to the facial nucleus (stereotaxic planes P8.5 – P10) in a region ventral to nucleus reticularis parvocellularis and ventrolateral to nucleus reticularis gigantocellularis. Medullary neurons with sympathetic nerve-related activity located on or near the midline (stereotaxic planes P9.2 – P12.1) were located in nuclei raphe magnus, pallidus and obscurus.

Forty-five percent of the neurons sampled in the cat RVLM had activity correlated to the 2- to 6-Hz rhythm in SND (Barman and Gebber, 1983). The corresponding values for LTF (Barman and Gebber, 1981) and raphe (Morrison and Gebber, 1982) neurons were 28% and 24%, respectively. Neurons with and those without sympathetic nerve-related activity were intermingled throughout the RVLM, LTF and raphe nuclei. The discharges of both types of neurons often appeared in the recording field of the same microelectrode (Gebber et al., 1987). Thus, the brain stem regions containing neurons with sympathetic nerve-related activity are functionally heterogeneous. The importance of correlational techniques (e.g. spike-triggered averaging) used to characterize the relationships between the activity of single brain stem neurons and sympathetic nerves becomes clearer in this light.

Baroreceptor reflex activation was used to determine which brain stem neurons with sympathetic nerve-related activity subserve excitatory function and which subserve inhibitory function. For this purpose, changes in the firing rate of the brain stem neuron are monitored when baroreceptor afferent nerve traffic is increased. Neurons mediating SE effects should be inhibited by baroreceptor reflex activation. Neurons exerting sympathoinhibitory (SI) actions should be excited by baroreceptor reflex activation. In the case shown in Fig. 4C, baroreceptor reflex activation was accomplished by raising pressure in a carotid sinus that had been reversibly isolated from the systemic circulation. SND and RVLM neuronal activity were inhibited in parallel during the rise in carotid sinus pressure. Thus, this RVLM-spinal

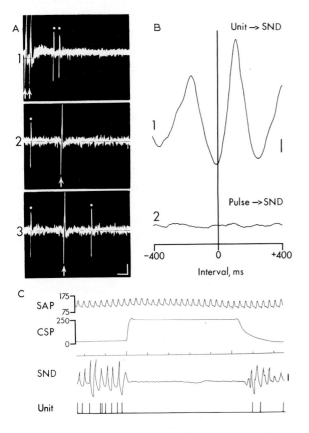

Fig. 4. Discharge characteristics of a cat ventrolateral medullospinal sympathoexcitatory neuron. (A) Antidromic responses initiated by stimulation in gray matter of second thoracic spinal segment. Four superimposed traces appear in each panel. Dots mark spontaneous and stimulus-induced action potentials; arrows mark spinal stimuli. Panel 1: estimation of axonal refractory period with paired stimuli. Panels 2 and 3: time-controlled collision test for antidromic activation (see text for details). Stimulus current was 1.5 × threshold. Horizontal calibration is 10 msec; vertical calibration is 50 μV. (B) Spike-triggered (trace 1) and "dummy" pulse-triggered (trace 2) averages of inferior cardiac sympathetic nerve discharge (SND) each based on 700 trials. Unit spikes and "dummy" pulses are at zero lag. Bin width is 0.8 msec and vertical calibration is 30 μV. (C) Baroreceptor reflex response. Traces show (top to bottom): systemic arterial pressure (SAP; mmHg), carotid sinus pressure (CSP; mmHg), time base (1 sec/division), SND, and standardized pulses derived from action potentials of the neuron. Vertical calibration is 100 μV. (Reprinted from Barman and Gebber, 1985.)

neuron likely subserved a SE function. Using this test, we found that the RVLM and raphe contain primarily SE and SI neurons, respectively, whereas the LTF contains a more equal mixture of both neuronal types (Morrison and Gebber, 1984, 1985; Barman and Gebber, 1985, 1987; Gebber and Barman, 1985, 1988).

The second step towards understanding how the 2- to 6-Hz rhythm is generated is to define the connections of those brain stem neurons whose naturally occurring discharges are synchronized to this component of SND. One of the techniques that we have used for this purpose is antidromic mapping. One applies an electrical stimulus through a microelectrode placed in a region suspected to contain the axon or terminal field of the neuron. When the electrical stimulus excites the axon or a terminal, the action potential travels antidromically to the cell body (i.e., the neuron is backfired). Such responses are proven to be antidromic in nature by colliding them with spontaneously occurring action potentials of the same cell travelling in the orthodromic direction (Lipski, 1981). When the electrical stimulus is applied too soon after the occurrence of a spontaneous spike, the antidromic and orthodromic spikes collide somewhere along the axon. As a consequence, the antidromic response fails to reach the cell body. The antidromic spike can again be recorded at the cell body when the interval between the spontaneous spike and the electrical stimulus is lengthened to a value equal to the sum of the latency of the antidromic spike (L) and the refractory period of the axon (R). This is the critical delay (CD) for antidromic activation: CD = L + R. R (period of reduced excitability following an action potential) is estimated by determining the minimum interval between paired electrical stimuli producing two action potentials.

The collision test for antidromic activation of an RVLM-SE neuron by microstimulation in the second thoracic spinal segment (T2) is shown in Fig. 4A. This neuron was activated with a constant onset latency (26 msec) and faithfully followed paired T2 stimuli separated by 3.8 msec (A1). The response to electrical stimulation failed to occur (A2) when the interval (28 msec) between a spontaneous spike and the spinal stimulus was less than the critical delay for antidromic activation (29.8 msec), but a response was recorded when the interval was 30 msec (A3). Thus, the response elicited by spinal stimulation was antidromic in nature. It follows that the axon of this RVLM-SE neuron projected to T2.

The use of the antidromic mapping technique to locate the terminal field of an RVLM-spinal SE neuron is illustrated in Fig. 5. In this case, the neuron was antidromically activated by microstimulation in T2. The stimulating microelectrode was moved vertically in 200-μm steps through a series of tracks separated by 500 – 1000 μm in the mediolateral and rostrocaudal directions. Twelve tracks (four in each of three rostrocaudal planes) were made in this experiment. One of these planes is shown on the left side of Fig. 5. Threshold current for antidromic activation of the RVLM neuron, response onset latency and the depth of the electrode tip below the dorsal surface of T2

were recorded at each site of stimulation. Depth-threshold curves were constructed from these data. The main axon of the RVLM neuron was assumed to be near the site in the white matter (track A) from which the shortest latency (15 msec) antidromic response was initiated with the lowest threshold current (28 μA). The site (track C) from which the longest latency (19 msec) antidromic response was elicited with the lowest stimulus current (10 μA) was in the IML. This site presumably was near the terminal field of either the main axon or one of its branches. Antidromic mapping was continued until it was demonstrated that this point was surrounded by sites requiring the application of higher current to elicit an antidromic response with the same latency. The antidromic response of intermediate onset latency (18 msec) likely monitored activation of the main axon or one of its branches en route to the IML. It can be noted that the stimulus current needed to antidromically activate the neuron from sites in track D was higher than those needed in track C. This indicates that the axon did not cross the midline at this level.

Currently available information (Barman and Gebber, 1985, 1987, 1988; Morrison and Gebber, 1985) on the connections made by medullary neurons with activity synchronized to the 2- to 6-Hz rhythm in SND is summarized in Fig. 6A. RVLM-SE and raphe-SI neurons send their axons to innervate the IML of the thoracic spinal cord. In contrast, the axons of LTF-SE and LTF-SI neurons do not project to the spinal cord. Rather, LTF-SE neurons project to the region of the RVLM containing SE neurons with spinal axons whereas LTF-SI neurons project to the region of the raphe containing SI neurons with spinal axons. Finally, the axons of RVLM-spinal SE and raphe spinal-SI neurons branch in the medulla. The branches of RVLM-spinal SE neurons course to the region of the LTF whereas those of raphe spinal-SI neurons ascend to the region of the RVLM.

Our experiments on cats have not revealed signs of pacemaker activity for LTF, RVLM or raphe neurons whose discharges are synchronized to the 2- to 6-Hz rhythm in SND. The firing rates of these

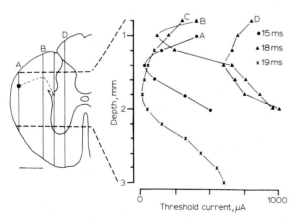

Fig. 5. Dorsolateral funicular axon (filled circle) of a cat ventrolateral medullospinal sympathoexcitatory neuron projecting to the ipsilateral intermediolateral nucleus (IML) of the second thoracic spinal segment (T2). The presumed path of a branch from the main axon to the IML is shown as a broken line. T2 cross-section with electrode tracks (A – D) is on the left. Calibration is 1 mm. Corresponding depth-threshold curves for antidromic activation of the neuron are on the right. Dashed lines show extent of ordinate relative to the cross-section. Depth below dorsal surface on the ordinate relates to track C. (Reprinted from Barman and Gebber, 1985.)

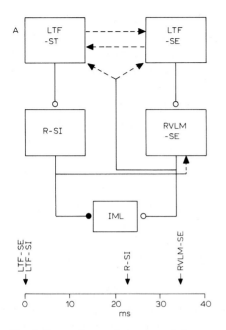

Fig. 6. Connections made by cat medullary neurons with activity correlated to 2- to 6-Hz sympathetic nerve discharge. (A) Circuit diagram: LTF-SE is sympathoexcitatory neuron in lateral tegmental field. LTF-SI is sympathoinhibitory neuron in lateral tegmental field. RVLM-SE is sympathoexcitatory neuron in rostral ventrolateral medulla. R-SI is sympathoinhibitory neuron in medullary raphe. IML is intermediolateral spinal sympathetic nucleus. Solid lines are established pathways. Dotted lines are hypothetical pathways. Open circle is excitatory connection. Closed circle is inhibitory connection. Arrow head is connection of unknown sign (see text for details). (B) Time line depicting sequence of firing of medullary neurons relative to peak of next inferior cardiac sympathetic nerve slow wave.

responsible for the 2- to 6-Hz rhythm in SND of the cat. Furthermore, only a small and continuously changing segment of the population of neurons comprising the network oscillator accounts for each 2- to 6-Hz sympathetic nerve slow wave. This is evident since the individual brain stem neuron does not participate in every cycle of SND. Thus, we refer to the generator of 2- to 6-Hz SND as a probabilistic oscillator. A detailed physiologically based model of the probabilistic oscillator is presented in another paper in this volume (Gebber and Barman, 1989).

A corollary to our network oscillator hypothesis is that the 2- to 6-Hz rhythm is generated by neurons that are antecendent to RVLM-spinal SE neurons. One approach to the problem of identifying the region of origin of the 2- to 6-Hz rhythm in SND is to compare the firing times of different groups of brain stem neurons with this activity pattern (Gebber and Barman, 1985). Those neurons which fire earliest during the 2- to 6-Hz cycle of SND should be the source of such activity. The reference point used to compare the firing times of LTF, RVLM and raphe neurons was the lag between unit spike occurrence and the peak of the next 2- to 6-Hz slow wave recorded from the postganglionic inferior cardiac sympathetic nerve. This interval, measured from spike-triggered averages, is unchanged when synchronization of the 2- to 6-Hz sympathetic nerve slow wave to the cardiac cycle is disrupted by lowering blood pressure (see Fig. 2) or when the period of the cardiac cycle and, thus, the slow wave in SND is changed by pacing the heart (Morrison and Gebber, 1982; Barman and Gebber, 1983).

The time line in Fig. 6B shows the sequence of firing of the four groups of medullary neurons. LTF neurons fired earliest during the sympathetic nerve slow wave. On the average, LTF-SE and LTF-SI neurons fired 116 ± 6 msec and 116 ± 7 msec, respectively, before the peak of the accompanying slow wave in the inferior cardiac nerve. RVLM-spinal SE and raphe spinal-SI neurons fired significantly later than LTF neurons (Gebber and Barman, 1985; Barman and Gebber, 1987).

neurons generally are lower than the frequency of occurrence of 2- to 6- Hz slow waves in SND. It is because of the low firing rates of these cells that averaging techniques must be used to demonstrate their sympathetic nerve-related activity. A representative example of the discharge pattern of a cat brain stem neuron with sympathetic nerve-related activity is shown in Fig. 1A. This RVLM-spinal SE neuron failed to fire during the majority of 2- to 6-Hz sympathetic nerve slow waves and the number of cycles missed varied. Thus, the interspike intervals of the neuron were variable. These are not the properties of intrinsic pacemaker neurons. Thus, the currently available information favors the hypothesis that a network oscillator is

These data support the view that the 2- to 6-Hz rhythm in SND is generated not by bulbospinal neurons, but rather by their antecedent inputs. Regarding this proposal, Barman and Gebber (1987) found that the difference in the firing times of LTF-SE and RVLM-spinal SE neurons relative to the peak of the 2- to 6-Hz sympathetic nerve slow wave was close to the modal onset latency of synaptic activation of the latter neurons by microstimulation in the LTF. This observation is consistent with the view that LTF-SE neurons are an important source of the driving input to RVLM-SE neurons innervating the IML. The same types of comparisons have also led us to propose that LTF-SI neurons are an important source of the background discharges of raphe spinal-SI neurons (Barman and Gebber, 1988). Whether local circuits of LTF neurons comprise the generator of 2- to 6-Hz SND remains to be tested. It is also possible that LTF neurons are driven by inputs from a 2- to 6-Hz rhythm generator located elsewhere or that LTF neurons are part of a network oscillator that is anatomically distributed. Regarding the lattermost possibility, it is worth reiterating that the axons of some RVLM-spinal SE and raphe spinal-SI neurons emit branches in the medulla (Fig. 6A). Although we have not yet determined the sites of termination of the medullary branches of these neurons, those emitted by RVLM-SE neurons appear to feedback to the LTF. This is consistent with the possibility that the 2- to 6-Hz rhythm is an emergent property of an antomically distributed system of reciprocally connected neurons.

Pacemaker theory

The pacemaker theory on the origin of SND is based on data from the rat. Sun et al. (1988a) recorded from RVLM-spinal neurons with cardiac-related activity that were inhibited during baroreceptor reflex activation. Following the intracisternal (i.c.) administration of the glutamate-receptor antagonist, kynurenate (KYN), these neurons develop pacemaker-like activity (i.e. nearly constant interspike intervals) with a beating frequency near 20 Hz. At this time, a variety of excitatory and inhibitory synaptic responses of these neurons are eliminated or markedly attenuated. In a subsequent study, Sun et al. (1988b) found that the regular discharge pattern of rat RVLM neurons in slice arises from typical pacemaker potentials. Intracellular injection of hyperpolarizing current silenced these neurons without unmasking excitatory or inhibitory postsynaptic potentials. While the evidence for the existence of pacemaker neurons in the rat RVLM is convincing, it has not yet been established whether these neurons are involved in the control of SND. First, Sun et al. did not determine whether the axons of RVLM pacemaker neurons terminate in the IML or other spinal sympathetic regions. Moreover, whether RVLM pacemaker neurons have activity related to SND after baroreceptor denervation (in the absence of KYN) was not tested by Sun et al. This is an important point since the cardiac-related activity of these neurons before i.c. KYN does not necessarily prove that they were contained in pathways controlling SND. Their cardiac-related activity may simply reflect the sharing of pulse synchronous baroreceptor nerve input with the sympathetic system. It is well known that baroreceptor reflex influences are distributed to non-autonomic as well as autonomic networks (cf. Gebber, 1980).

Sun et al. (1988a) reported that in the presence of KYN, the rhythmic activity of RVLM pacemaker neurons is reset by spinal stimulation only when an antidromic spike is elicited. This observation led Sun et al. to propose that these neurons are subject neither to feedback inhibition nor excitation from their neighbors, at least after glutamate-receptor blockade with KYN. On this basis, we reasoned that i.c. KYN should desynchronize SND (i.e. eliminate its rhythmic components) if, as Sun et al. (1988b) state, "vasoconstrictor and cardioaccelerator sympathetic tone is due in large part to the intrinsic pacemaker activity of a small group of reticulospinal excitatory neurons located at the extreme anterior tip of the ventrolateral medulla".

Desynchronization would be expected since RVLM pacemaker neurons discharging independently of each other would provide a limited-band (> 20 Hz) white noise input to spinal preganglionic sympathetic neurons. The results of our experiments on rats are not consistent with the pacemaker hypothesis on the generation of SND.

The i.c. dose of KYN used by Sun et al. (1988a) to uncover pacemaker activity in the rat RVLM was 5 μmol. Five times this amount (delivered in divided doses) failed to desynchronize rat splanchnic SND in our experiments. In agreement with

Sun et al. (1988a), i.c. KYN (5 μmol in 20 μl of phosphate buffer; pH 7.4) blocked the baroreceptor reflexes. This was manifested in two ways. First, i.c. KYN prevented the reflex inhibition of SND accompanying the rise in blood pressure produced by i.v. injection of norepinephrine (Fig. 7). Note that this occurred without a marked change in the resting levels of SND and blood pressure. Second, i.c. KYN eliminated the cardiac-related rhythm in SND. As demonstrated with post-R wave averaging, splanchnic nerve slow waves were related 1:1 to the arterial pulse before i.c. KYN (Fig. 8C). This relationship disappeared following i.c. KYN as indicated by the flat average of SND (Fig. 8D). It is important to note that although no longer cardiac-related, sympathetic nerve slow waves persisted following i.c. KYN. This is shown in the oscilloscopic traces of SND in Fig. 8B. The failure of KYN to desynchronize SND was formally demonstrated with power density spectral analysis.

Power density spectral analysis performed by fast Fourier transform converts a time series of SND into a plot of power (voltage^2) of the signal

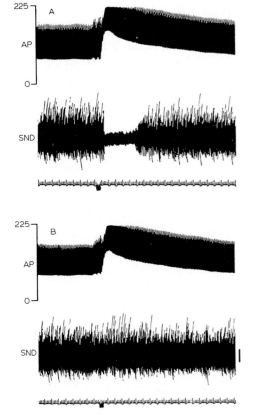

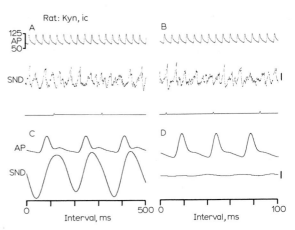

Fig. 7. Blockade of baroreceptor reflex-induced inhibition of rat splanchnic sympathetic nerve discharge (SND) by intracisternal (i.c.) kynurenate (KYN). Traces in each panel are arterial blood pressure (AP in mmHg; top) and SND (bottom). (A) Reflex inhibition of SND during pressor response elicited by i.v. norepinephrine (1 μg/kg). Norepinephrine was injected at downward deflection of time base. (B) Blockade of this response by i.c. KYN (5 μmol). Vertical calibration is 100 μV for SND. Time base is 1 sec/division.

Fig. 8. Loss of cardiac-related component in rat splanchnic sympathetic nerve discharge (SND) following intracisternal (i.c.) administration of kynurenate (KYN). Traces in each panel are arterial blood pressure (AP in mmHg; top) and SND (bottom). (A,B) Oscillographic records before and after i.c. KYN (5 μmol). (C,D) Post-R wave averages (100 sweeps) before and after i.c. KYN. Bin width is 1 msec. Vertical calibration is 100 μV for SND in (A,B) and 20 μV in (C,D). Time base is 1 sec/division in (A,B).

126

against its frequency components (Bendat and Piersol, 1971). As shown in Fig. 9, most of the power in rat splanchnic SND before KYN administration was contained between 2 and 10 Hz. The largest peak in the power density spectra (PDS) of SND from baroreceptor-innervated rats corresponded to the cardiac-related rhythm (Fig. 9IA). As expected, doses of KYN (5 μmol) that blocked the baroreceptor reflexes eliminated or markedly attenuated this peak (Fig. 9IB). Nonetheless, SND was not desynchronized as evidenced by the fact that most of the power in the PDS remained in the 2- to 10-Hz band. Desynchronization would have been manifested by a uniform distribution of power in the PDS. Additional i.c. doses of KYN (10 μmol in Fig. 9IC and in Fig. 9ID) also failed to desynchronize SND. In

the example shown, the total power in SND was increased following the second i.c. injection of KYN.

As was the case in baroreceptor-innervated preparations, KYN did not desynchronize SND in baroreceptor-denervated rats. In the case shown, the PDS of splanchnic SND before KYN injection contained two sharp peaks at 1 and 2 Hz (Fig. 9IIA). These peaks corresponded to the rate of artificial ventilation and its first harmonic. Note that the respiratory-related component in SND was eliminated following the first dose (5 μmol) of i.c. KYN (Fig. 9IIB). As a consequence, the PDS of SND was sharper following i.c. KYN. Additional doses of i.c. KYN produced no further change in the shape of the PDS of SND.

There are at least four ways to explain why KYN failed to desynchronize SND. The first and most

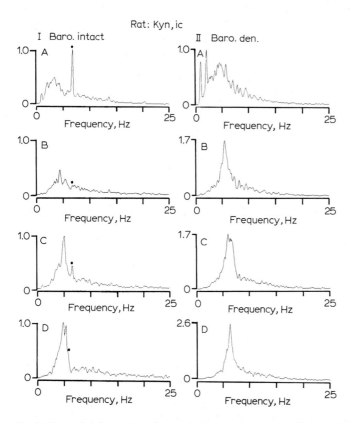

Fig. 9. Power density spectra of splanchnic sympathetic nerve discharge in baroreceptor-innervated (I) and -denervated (II) rat (A) before, and 10 min after intracisternal (i.c.) injection of each of three doses (5 μmol for B; 10 μmol for C; 10 μmol for D) of kynurenate. Power (relative to a value of one for largest peak in control spectrum) is plotted against frequency. Each spectrum is average of 24 10-sec data blocks. Frequency resolution is 0.1 Hz. Dots in I placed at frequency corresponding to heart rate.

obvious explanation is that RVLM pacemaker neurons do not have a role in generating the major component of SND in the rat, i.e. the 2- to 10-Hz rhythm. The second potential explanation is that the white noise output of independently acting RVLM pacemaker neurons is transformed at a spinal level to a 2- to 10-Hz activity pattern. That is, white noise might engage a 2- to 10-Hz spinal sympathetic generator. Currently, there is no evidence available pointing to the existence of such a spinal generator in the rat. Moreover, Morrison et al. (1988) have identified rat RVLM-spinal neurons whose naturally occurring activity precedes and is locked to the 2- to 10-Hz rhythm in SND. Thus, we view the second potential explanation for the failure of KYN to desynchronize SND as unlikely.

A third potential explanation for the failure of KYN to desynchronize SND is that the discharges of the population of RVLM pacemaker neurons are synchronized by a KYN-insensitive feedforward synaptic mechanism. If so, spinal sympathetic neurons would have to act as frequency dividers to account for the predominance of the 2- to 10-Hz component in rat SND. This is because the beating frequency of rat RVLM pacemaker neurons is near 20 Hz (Sun et al., 1988a). While attractive, this explanation does not fit the results obtained with electrical stimulation. We recorded the rat splanchnic nerve responses produced by electrical stimulation of the second cervical spinal segment (C2). Following spinal transection at C1, square wave pulses (0.5 msec duration, 100–200 μA) were applied to sites in C2 from which increases in SND could be elicited. The results from one experiment are illustrated in Fig. 10. Panel A shows the increase in rat splanchnic SND (averaged response) elicited by single shocks applied once every second to C2. Both a small early (onset latency, 40 msec) and a larger late (onset latency, 100 msec) increase in SND were observed. The PDS of SND during higher frequency stimulation (10 Hz in Fig. 10B and 21 Hz in Fig. 10C) are also shown. These spectra contain sharp peaks corresponding to the frequency of stimulation and in panel B, its

first harmonic. The PDS of SND was flat below 10 Hz. This reflects elimination of the 2- to 10-Hz rhythm by spinal transection and the inability of spinal sympathetic circuits to act as frequency dividers of input volleys provided by spinal stimulation. Such volleys in descending spinal pathways would simulate the synchronized discharge of a population of pacemaker neurons beating at 20 Hz.

The fourth potential explanation for the failure of KYN to desynchronize SND is that whereas rat RVLM pacemaker neurons are involved in sym-

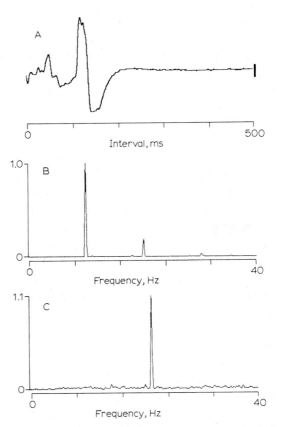

Fig. 10. Splanchnic sympathetic nerve responses of spinal rat [transection of first cervical segment (C1)] to electrical stimulation (100 μA) in second cervical spinal segment (C2). (A) Averaged splanchnic nerve response (40 trials) produced by single shocks applied once every second in C2. Vertical calibration is 100 μV. (B) Power density spectrum of sympathetic nerve discharge during 10 Hz stimulation in C2. (C) Same, but during 21 Hz stimulation. Each spectrum is average of 6 10-sec data blocks. Frequency resolution is 0.1 Hz.

pathetic nerve control, their function is not directly related to generation of the 2- to 10-Hz activity pattern. Rather, the white noise emanating from a population of independently acting pacemaker neurons might help to set the gain of the responses of preganglionic sympathetic neurons to 2- to 10-Hz rhythmic input supplied by a second system of brain stem neurons. Providing that the rhythm generator does not contain a KYN-sensitive process, desynchronization of SND would not be expected. As already discussed, evidence is available that the 2- to 6-Hz rhythm in cat SND is generated at a site antecedent to the RVLM. Whether this holds for the 2- to 10-Hz activity pattern in rats remains to be determined. If so, a group of non-pacemaker RVLM neurons might relay the 2- to 10-Hz activity pattern from the generator to spinal sympathetic networks. Regarding this possibility, Sun et al. (1988a) have identified a second group of rat RVLM-spinal neurons whose discharges are less regularly spaced after i.c. KYN than those of neighboring pacemaker cells. These neurons have slower axonal conduction velocities and lower discharge rates than the pacemaker cells. As is the case for pacemakers before i.c. KYN administration, the second group of RVLM-spinal neurons have cardiac-related activity and are inhibited by baroreceptor reflex activation (Guyenet and Brown, 1986; Morrison et al., 1988). Unlike the pacemaker neurons, it appears that the non-pacemaker neurons are not tonically active in slice preparations (Sun et al., 1988b).

Summary

This chapter entertains two theories (network oscillator vs. intrinsic pacemaker) on the generation of the major component of SND — the 2- to 6-Hz rhythm in the cat and the 2- to 10-Hz rhythm in the rat. Evidence from experiments on cats strongly supports the hypothesis that the 2- to 6-Hz rhythm is an emergent property of a network oscillator located in the brain stem. Specifically, we propose that the 2- to 6-Hz component in SND arises from an ensemble of neurons of different types interconnected in such a way to generate the rhythm. There is no evidence for the existence of intrinsic pacemaker neurons in this network. Our experiments on cats also indicate that the rhythm is generated by neurons in the brain stem that are antecedent to RVLM-spinal SE and raphespinal-SI neurons.

Our experiments on rats are not consistent with the hypothesis of Sun et al. (1988b) that "vasoconstrictor and cardioaccelerator sympathetic tone is due in large part to the intrinsic pacemaker activity of a small group of reticulospinal excitatory neurons located at the extreme anterior tip of the ventrolateral medulla". Rat RVLM pacemaker neurons act independently of each other following i.c. injection of the glutamate-receptor antagonist, KYN (Sun et al., 1988a). Thus, they would as a group provide white noise input to spinal neurons. It follows that i.c. KYN should have desynchronized SND if, as proposed by Sun et al., RVLM pacemakers are primarily responsible for SND in the rat. This was found not to be the case. The most likely explanation is that the 2- to 10-Hz rhythm in rat SND is not generated by intrinsic pacemaker neurons in the RVLM.

Acknowledgements

The authors are grateful to Ms. Diane Hummel for typing the manuscript. This study was supported by National Institutes of Health grants HL13187 and HL33266.

References

Ardell, J.L., Barman, S.M. and Gebber, G.L. (1982) Sympathetic nerve discharge in chronic spinal cat. *Am. J. Physiol.*, 243: H463 – H470.

Barman, S.M. and Gebber, G.L. (1980) Sympathetic nerve rhythm of brain stem origin. *Am. J. Physiol.*, 239: R42 – R47.

Barman, S.M. and Gebber, G.L. (1981) Brain stem neuronal types with activity patterns related to sympathetic nerve discharge. *Am. J. Physiol.*, 40: R335 – R347.

Barman, S.M. and Gebber, G.L. (1983) Sequence of activation of ventrolateral and dorsal medullary sympathetic neurons. *Am. J. Physiol.*, 245: R438 – R447.

Barman, S.M. and Gebber, G.L. (1985) Axonal projection patterns of ventrolateral medullospinal sympathoexcitatory neurons. *J. Neurophysiol.,* 53: 1551–1566.

Barman, S.M. and Gebber, G.L. (1987) Lateral tegmental field neurons of cat medulla: a source of basal activity of ventrolateral medullospinal sympathoexcitatory neurons. *J. Neurophysiol.,* 57: 1410–1424.

Barman, S.M. and Gebber, G.L. (1988) Lateral tegmental field sympathoinhibitory (LTF-SI) neurons project to medullary raphe nuclei. *Soc. Neurosci. Abstr.,* 14: 327.

Bendat, J.S. and Piersol, A.G. (1971) *Random Data: Analysis and Measurement Procedures,* Wiley, New York, 407 pp.

Calaresu, F.R. and Yardley, C.P. (1988) Medullary basal sympathetic tone. *Ann. Rev. Physiol.,* 50: 511–524.

Ciriello, J., Caverson, M.M. and Polosa, C. (1986) Function of the ventrolateral medulla in the control of the circulation. *Brain Res. Rev.,* 11: 359–391.

Connor, J.A. (1985) Neural pacemakers and rhythmicity. *Ann. Rev. Physiol.,* 47: 17–28.

Gebber, G.L. (1980) Central oscillators responsible for sympathetic nerve discharge. *Am. J. Physiol.,* 239: H143–H155.

Gebber, G.L. (1984) Brainstem systems involved in cardiovascular regulation. In W.C. Randall (Ed.), *Nervous Control of Cardiovascular Function,* Oxford, New York, pp. 346–368.

Gebber, G.L. and Barman, S.M. (1980) Basis for 2-6 cycle/s rhythm in sympathetic nerve discharge. *Am. J. Physiol.,* 239: R48–R56.

Gebber, G.L. and Barman, S.M. (1985) Lateral tegmental field neurons of cat medulla: a potential source of basal sympathetic nerve discharge. *J. Neurophysiol.,* 54: 1498–1512.

Gebber, G.L. and Barman, S.M. (1988) Studies on the origin and generation of sympathetic nerve activity. *Clin. Exp. Hypertension,* A10 (Suppl. 1): 33–44.

Gebber, G.L. and Barman, S.M. (1989) A physiologically-based model of the brain stem generator of sympathetic nerve discharge. In J. Ciriello, C. Polosa and M.M. Caverson (Eds.), *Function of the Ventrolateral Medulla in the Control of the Circulation, Progress in Brain Research, Vol.*

81, Elsevier, Amsterdam, pp. 131–139.

Gebber, G.L., Barman, S.M. and Morrison, S.F. (1987) Electrophysiological evidence for the modular organization of the reticular formation: sympathetic controlling circuits. *Brain Res.,* 410: 106–110.

Guyenet, P.G. and Brown, D.L. (1986) Nucleus paragigantocellularis lateralis and lumbar sympathetic discharge in the rat. *Am. J. Physiol.,* 250: R1081–R1094.

Lipski, J. (1981) Antidromic activation of neurones as an analytic tool in the study of the central nervous system. *J. Neurosci. Methods,* 4: 1–32.

Millhorn, D.E. and Eldrigde, F.L. (1986) Role of ventrolateral medulla in regulation of respiratory and cardiovascular systems. *J. Appl. Physiol.,* 61: 1249–1263.

Morrison, S.F. and Gebber, G.L. (1982) Classification of raphe neurons with cardiac-related activity. *Am. J. Physiol.,* 243: R49–R59.

Morrison, S.F. and Gebber, G.L. (1984) Raphe neurons with sympathetic-related activity: baroreceptor responses and spinal connections. *Am. J. Physiol.,* 246: R338–R348.

Morrison, S.F. and Gebber, G.L. (1985) Axonal branching patterns and funicular trajectories of raphespinal sympathetic neurons. *J. Neurophysiol.,* 53: 759–772.

Morrison, S.F., Milner, T.A. and Reis, D.J. (1988) Reticulospinal vasomotor neurons of the rat rostral ventrolateral medulla: relationship to sympathetic nerve activity and the C1 adrenergic cell group. *J. Neurosci.,* 8: 1286–1301.

Selverston, A.I. and Moulins, M. (1985) Oscillatory neural networks. *Ann. Rev. Physiol.,* 47: 29–48.

Sun, M.-K., Hackett, J.T. and Guyenet, P.G. (1988a) Sympathoexcitatory neurons of rostral ventrolateral medulla exibit pacemaker properties in the presence of a glutamate-receptor antagonist. *Brain Res.,* 438: 23–40.

Sun, M.-K., Young, B.S., Hackett, J.T. and Guyenet, P.G. (1988b) Reticulospinal pacemaker neurons of the rat rostral ventrolateral medulla with putative sympathoexcitatory function: an intracellular study in vitro. *Brain Res.,* 442: 229–239.

J. Ciriello, M.M. Caverson and C. Polosa (Eds.)
Progress in Brain Research, Vol. 81
© 1989 Elsevier Science Publishers B.V. (Biomedical Division)

CHAPTER 9

A physiologically-based model of the brain stem generator of sympathetic nerve discharge

Gerard L. Gebber[1,2] and Susan M. Barman[1]

Departments of [1]Pharmacology and Toxicology, and of [2]Physiology, Michigan State University, East Lansing, MI 48824, U.S.A.

Introduction

As demonstrated with power density spectral analysis (Barman and Gebber, 1980; Gebber and Barman, 1980), sympathetic nerve discharge (SND) in anesthetized cats contains a prominent 2- to 6-Hz rhythm. This rhythm is cardiac-related before baroreceptor denervation and free-running after baroreceptor denervation (Barman and Gebber, 1980; Gebber and Barman, 1980). The 2- to 6-Hz rhythm is ubiquitous to postganglionic sympathetic nerves from which we have recorded (e.g. inferior cardiac, renal). The rhythm persists after midcollicular decerebration in baroreceptor-denervated cats but is eliminated acutely by cervical spinal cord transection (Barman and Gebber, 1980; Ardell et al., 1982). On this basis, we view the 2- to 6-Hz rhythm as the signature of a brain stem generator that is responsible for a significant component of the background discharges of sympathetic nerves and, thus, cardiovascular tone. The purpose of this chapter is to present a model of the generator of 2- to 6-Hz SND based on physiological data.

Studies on invertebrates have provided much of what we know about the generation of neural rhythms (Kristan, 1980; Selverston and Moulins, 1985). Neuronal oscillators in invertebrates often are comprised of a few cells. As a consequence, it is relatively easy to identify the neuronal types and synaptic connections that are responsible for rhythmogenesis. Moreover, the small number of neurons in invertebrate oscillators dictates that each cell must act in a highly reliable manner. Thus, it is not surprising that the discharge pattern of individual invertebrate neurons provides explicit information on the phase and period of the rhythm as might be monitored from a motor nerve or muscle. Vertebrate neural oscillators contain many cells. In some cases, their individual components also are highly reliable. For example, individual inspiratory neurons of the mammalian respiratory oscillator begin and end their firing at nearly the same points in successive respiratory cycles (Cohen, 1979; Richter, 1982; Feldman, 1986). Thus, the phase and period of the respiratory rhythm are represented at the level of the single brain stem neuron. As we shall see, such is not the case for brain stem neurons that comprise the network responsible for the 2- to 6-Hz rhythm in SND. Rather, the 2- to 6-Hz rhythm is an emergent property of the brain stem sympathetic generator as a whole. We hypothesize that the 2- to 6-Hz rhythm in SND reflects the near coincident firing of a small and continuously changing segment of the total population of neurons comprising the brain stem oscillator. We refer to the generator of 2- to 6-Hz SND as a probabilistic oscillator.

Experimental data

Our model of a probabilistic oscillator is based on an analysis of the discharge patterns of three groups of neurons whose naturally occurring activity is synchronized to the 2- to 6-Hz rhythm in postganglionic inferior cardiac or renal SND of the cat (as demonstrated with spike-triggered averaging). These are brain stem neurons located in the medullary lateral tegmental field (LTF) and the rostral ventrolateral medulla (RVLM), and preganglionic sympathetic neurons of the thoracic spinal intermediolateral nucleus (IML). The discharges of the medullary neurons are inhibited during baroreceptor reflex activation (Barman and Gebber, 1985, 1987; Gebber and Barman, 1985). Thus, we refer to them as sympathoexcitatory (SE) neurons. The three groups of neurons are serially connected (Fig. 1). As demonstrated with antidromic mapping, the spinal axons of RVLM-SE neurons innervate the thoracic IML (Barman and Gebber, 1985) while the axons of LTF-SE neurons project to the region of the RVLM containing SE neurons with spinal axons (Barman and Gebber, 1987). On the average, LTF-SE neurons fire 31 msec earlier during the 2- to 6-Hz burst of inferior cardiac SND than their counterparts in the RVLM (Barman and Gebber, 1987). This difference coincides closely with conduction time in the pathway from the LTF to the RVLM. Regarding this point, the modal onset latency of synaptic activation of RVLM-spinal SE neurons produced by LTF microstimulation is 26 ± 3 msec (Barman and Gebber, 1987). The axons of some RVLM-spinal SE neurons emit branches in the vinicity of the LTF (Barman and Gebber, 1987). This raises the possibility that RVLM-spinal SE neurons provide feedback to their antecedent inputs (i.e. LTF-SE neurons; see Fig. 1). Although the LTF also contains sympathoinhibitory neurons, we describe the discharge patterns of only SE neurons in this chapter.

Discharge properties of brain stem neurons. The discharge patterns of LTF-SE and RVLM-SE neurons in baroreceptor-innervated cats are similar in two respects. First, these neurons do not fire during each 2- to 6-Hz burst of SND. Second, the number of cycles of SND missed varies. Thus, these neurons have inconstant interspike intervals. Typical examples are shown in Figs. 2A and 3A. Bursts of SND in these figures appear as slow waves after preamplification with the bandpass set at 1 – 1000 Hz. The experiments were performed on Dial-urethane anesthetized cats.

We used power density spectral analysis to examine more closely the irregular discharge patterns of LTF-SE and RVLM-SE neurons. Power density

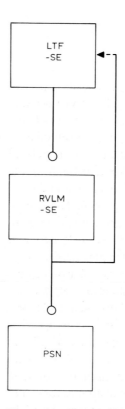

Fig. 1. Sympathoexcitatory neurons and their connections. LTF-SE is a sympathoexcitatory neuron in the lateral tegmental field of the medullary reticular formation. RVLM-SE is a sympathoexcitatory neuron in the rostral ventrolateral medulla. PSN is a preganglionic sympathetic neuron. Solid lines are established pathways. Dotted line from axonal branch of RVLM-SE neuron is presumed to terminate on LTF-SE neuron in this scheme. Open circles are excitatory connections. Arrow head is connection of unknown sign.

spectral analysis performed by fast Fourier transform separates the frequency components in a signal and quantifies the proportion of total activity contained within designated frequency bands (Bendat and Piersol, 1971). Standardized pulses (2 msec in duration) derived from the action potentials of individual brain stem neurons were filtered (0 – 100 Hz) and then subjected to fast Fourier transform. Under the conditions of our analysis, the region of the power density spectra (PDS) of

unit activity below 100 Hz is dominated by interspike interval statistics rather than by the shape of the pulse derived from the neuronal action potential (Richardson and Mitchell, 1982). PDS of sympathetic nerve activity were also constructed in these experiments. We found that while the PDS of inferior cardiac or renal SND contained a sharp peak corresponding to the frequency of the cardiac-related rhythm (Figs. 2D and 3D), those of LTF-SE (Fig. 2E) and RVLM-SE (Fig. 3E)

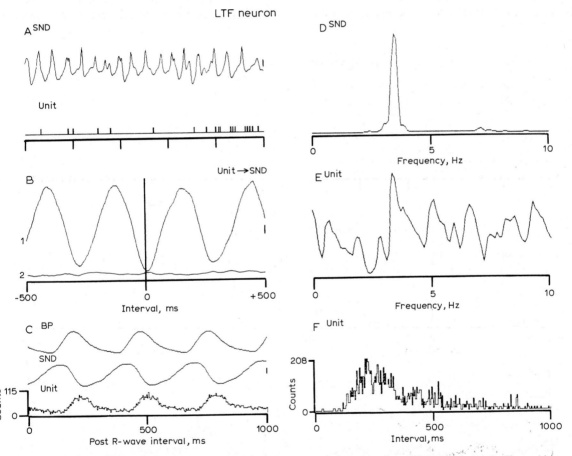

Fig. 2. Discharge characteristics of sympathoexcitatory neuron in medullary lateral tegmental field (LTF). (A) Oscillographic traces of inferior cardiac sympathetic nerve discharge (SND; top) and standardized pulses derived from unit spikes (bottom). Vertical calibration is 100 μV for SND. Time base is one sec/division. (B) LTF unit spike-triggered average (633 sweeps) of SND is shown in trace 1; trace 2 shows "dummy" average of SND. Bin width is 4 msec. Vertical calibration is 5 μV. (C) Post-R wave-triggered averages (2442 sweeps) of blood pressure wave (BP; top), SND (middle) and histogram of LTF unit spike occurrences (bottom). Bin width is 4 msec. Vertical calibration is 100 μV for SND. (D) Power density spectrum of SND. (E) Power density spectrum of LTF unit discharges. Each spectrum is average of 35 10-sec data blocks. Frequency resolution is 0.1 Hz. (F) Interspike interval histogram for LTF unit. Bin width is 4 msec; 875 intervals are plotted.

134

neuronal activity did not have or showed only a hint of such a peak. That is, the PDS of unit activity were basically flat. Such PDS are indicative of irregularly spaced action potentials.

The irregular firing pattern of LTF-SE and RVLM-SE neurons was also formally demonstrated by using interspike interval analysis. The interspike interval histograms (ISIH) for these neurons contained one broad peak. Typical examples are shown in Figs. 2F and 3F. Note that the interspike intervals comprising the peaks in these histograms were spread over a period of more than 500 msec. Such ISIH are to be expected for ir-

regularly firing neurons (Stein, 1980).

Due to their irregular firing patterns, averaging techniques must be used to demonstrate the sympathetic nerve-related activity of LTF-SE and RVLM-SE neurons. One of these techniques is spike-triggered averaging. The extracellularly recorded action potentials of the neuron serve as reference signals for computation of an average of accompanying changes in postganglionic SND. SND occurring in the window (e.g. ± 500 msec) surrounding each of the unit spikes is digitized and several hundred sweeps are averaged. Examples of the results obtained with this method are shown in

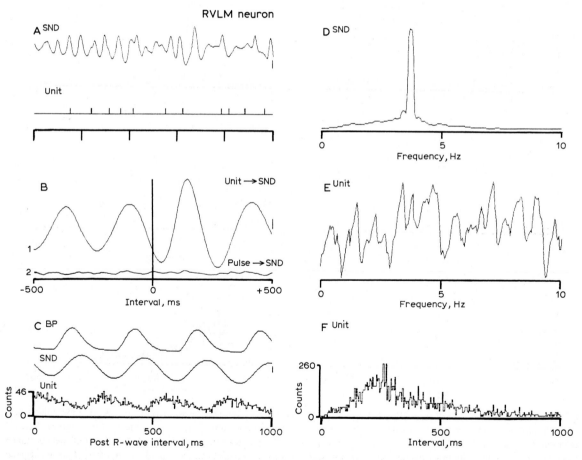

Fig. 3. Discharge characteristics of sympathoexcitatory neuron in rostral ventrolateral medulla (RVLM neuron). Recordings of renal sympathetic nerve discharge were made in this experiment. (A – F) Same sequence, bin widths and calibrations as in Fig. 2. Number of sweeps averaged was 1542 in (B) and 2257 in (C). Data blocks and frequency resolution in (D) and (E) same as in Fig. 2. Interspike interval histogram in (F) contains 1477 intervals.

Figs. 2B1 and 3B1. The spike-triggered averages show inferior cardiac or renal SND that preceded (left of zero lag) and followed (right of zero lag) the action potential of the brain stem neuron. The averages of SND contain a rhythmic component in the 2- to 6-Hz range. A randomly generated series of pulses (same number and frequency as for unit spike train) also is used to compute an average of SND (Figs. 2B2 and 3B2). Such averages are termed "dummy" averages. Single neurons are considered to have sympathetic nerve-related activity when the amplitude of first peak to the right of zero lag in the spike-triggered average exceeds that of the largest deflection in the "dummy" average by at least a factor of three.

Although the PDS of LTF-SE and RVLM-SE unit discharges did not contain a sharp peak corresponding to the heart rate, post-R wave analysis revealed that these neurons had cardiac-related activity. Averages of the arterial pulse wave and SND, and a histogram of the occurrence of LTF-SE or RVLM-SE unit spikes are constructed using the R wave of the electrocardiogram as the reference signal. Typical examples of the results obtained using post-R wave analysis are shown in Figs. 2C and 3C. Note that both brain stem unit activity and SND contained a prominent cardiac-related rhythm. The period of the cardiac-related rhythm was the same as that in the corresponding spike-triggered average of SND (Figs. 2B and 3B).

The irregular discharge pattern of LTF-SE and RVLM-SE neurons is only partly related to the fact that these cells miss firing in some cardiac cycles. A second factor involves the position during the 2- to 6-Hz sympathetic nerve slow wave at which these neurons fire. The position shifts from cycle to cycle. This was formally demonstrated by constructing a histogram of the intervals between the spikes of individual brain stem units and the peaks of surrounding 2- to 6-Hz sympathetic nerve slow waves. SND was passed through an analog differentiator. The peak of each sympathetic nerve slow wave was marked by a pulse at $dv/dt = 0$. Representative histograms for a LTF-SE and a RVLM-SE neuron are shown in Figs. 4A and 4B,

respectively. Note the absence of zero counts in the histograms. Particular attention should also be paid to the broadness of the first peak to the right of zero lag in each histogram. The counts comprising this peak represent lags between unit spike occurrence and the point of maximal activity in the next cycle of SND. These characteristics of the histograms indicate that LTF-SE and RVLM-SE neurons can fire at any point during the 2- to 6-Hz

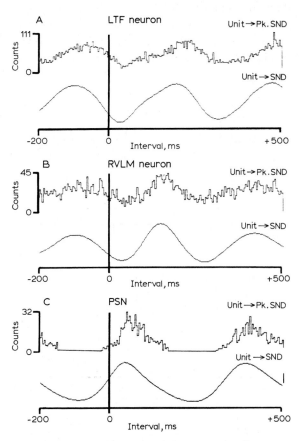

Fig. 4. Histograms of the intervals between unit spike occurrence (at zero lag) and peaks of surrounding 2- to 6-Hz sympathetic nerve slow waves. Corresponding spike-triggered averages of sympathetic nerve discharge (SND) are shown below each histogram. Bin width for histograms and averages is 4 msec. (A) Lateral tegmental field sympathoexcitatory (LTF) neuron. (B) Rostral ventrolateral medullary sympathoexcitatory (RVLM) neuron. (C) Preganglionic sympathetic neuron (PSN). Histograms and averages based on 3548 unit spikes in (A), 1544 spikes in (B) and 631 spikes in (C). Inferior cardiac SND was recorded in (A), renal SND in (B) and external carotid SND in (C). Vertical calibration is 5 μV for SND.

136

sympathetic nerve slow wave. Corresponding spike-triggered averages of SND are shown below each histogram.

Discharge properties of preganglionic sympathetic neurons (PSNs). The discharge patterns of PSNs are similar to those of LTF-SE and RVLM-SE neurons in some respects but are quite different in others. As was the case for brain stem neurons, PSNs did not fire during every 2- to 6-Hz sympathetic nerve slow wave and the number of cycles missed varied. A representative experiment is shown in Fig. 5A. The recordings were made from the

postganglionic external carotid nerve (top) and the axon of a single PSN teased from the contralateral cervical sympathetic nerve (bottom). The latter nerve provides the preganglionic input to ganglion cells whose axons form the external carotid nerve. As might be expected, spike-triggered averaging revealed that the discharges of the PSN were probabilistically related to SND (Fig. 5B). Also, post-R wave analysis showed that the PSN had cardiac-related activity (Fig. 5C). However, unlike the PDS of the discharges of LTF-SE and RVLM-SE neurons, those for PSNs (Fig. 5E) contained a sharp peak corresponding to the frequency of the

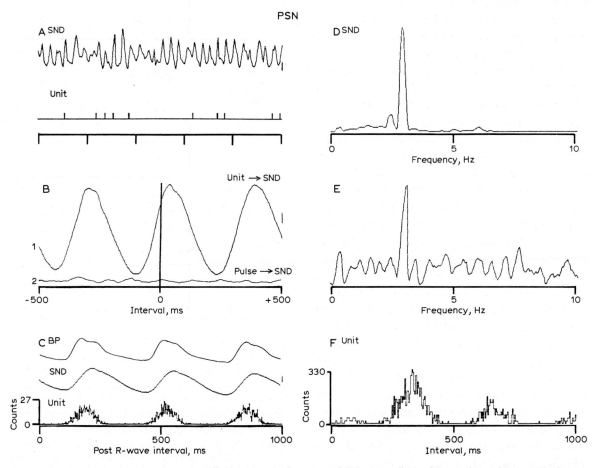

Fig. 5. Discharge characteristics of a preganglionic sympathetic neuron (PSN). Recordings of external carotid sympathetic nerve discharge were made in this experiment. (A – F) Same sequence, bin widths and calibrations as in Fig. 2. Number of sweeps averaged was 500 in (B) and 1609 in (C). Data blocks and frequency resolution in (D) and (E) same as in Fig. 2. Interspike interval histogram in (F) contains 578 intervals.

cardiac-related rhythm in SND (Fig. 5D). Moreover, while the ISIH of LTF-SE and RVLM-SE neurons were unimodal and dispersed, those of PSNs contained at least two sharp peaks that were separated by the period of the cardiac cycle. In the example shown in Fig. 5F, the first modal interval denotes instances when the PSN fired in successive cardiac cycles. The second and third modal intervals signify instances when the PSN fired in every other or every third cardiac cycle. The sharpness of these peaks suggests that, in contrast to LTF-SE and RVLM-SE neurons, PSNs fire at about the same time in those cycles of SND in which they are active. This was demonstrated by constructing histograms of the intervals between the spikes of individual PSNs and the peaks of surrounding 2- to 6-Hz sympathetic nerve slow waves (Fig. 4C). These histograms contained zero counts during a significant proportion of the cardiac-related cycle of SND. Thus, the firing times of PSNs during the sympathetic nerve slow wave are restricted to a relatively narrow window.

Model of the probabilistic oscillator

The discharge patterns of LTF-SE and RVLM-SE neurons lead us to model the brain stem circuits responsible for the 2- to 6-Hz rhythm in SND as a probabilistic network oscillator. These neurons exhibit irregular discharge patterns (i.e. inconstant interspike intervals). This suggests that neuronal interactions rather than endogenous pacemaker neurons are responsible for the 2- to 6-Hz rhythm. That is, we propose that the 2- to 6-Hz sympathetic nerve rhythm is an emergent property of a network oscillator, i.e. an ensemble of neurons interconnected in such a way so as to generate periodic activity.

We use the term probabilistic network oscillator since only a small and continuously changing segment of the population of neurons comprising the generator accounts for each 2- to 6-Hz sympathetic nerve slow wave. This is evident since individual brain stem neurons with activity probabilistically related to the 2- to 6-Hz rhythm in SND (as demonstrated with spike-triggered averaging and post-R wave analysis) do not fire in every cycle. Thus, the processes involved in generating individual 2- to 6-Hz sympathetic nerve slow waves include the dynamic and instantaneous formation and dissolution of subsets of active brain stem neurons.

We also propose that a single brain stem neuron can be part of n subsets. This is suggested by the variability of the lag between the spikes of LTF-SE or RVLM-SE neurons and the peak of the next 2- to 6-Hz sympathetic nerve slow wave. We hypothesize that each interval (or more likely a set of intervals) denotes the temporal position of the neuron in a different subset of the network. The shifting in time of unit firing relative to peak SND plus the fact that the neuron is not part of every subset (it does not fire in every cycle of SND) explains why the 2- to 6-Hz sympathetic nerve rhythm is not reflected in the PDS or ISIH of unit activity. Thus, individual LTF-SE or RVLM-SE neurons do not reliably reflect the behavior of the network oscillator as a whole. Rather, the highly rhythmic pattern of SND apparently is obtained by using a network composed of many more individual components than are necessary to produce each cycle of activity. We suggest that the reliability of the system is derived from the redundancy of its unreliable elements.

PSNs discharge at about the same time during those cycles of SND in which they are active. Thus, PSNs more reliably reflect the behavior of the network oscillator than do its individual components in the brain stem. We propose that this property of PSNs reflects the convergence onto them of the outputs of a large number of brain stem neurons. That is, it is hypothesized that individual PSNs receive cardiac-related excitatory input at about the same time in each cycle of SND independent of the subset of active brain stem neurons involved. Pulse synchronous baroreceptor nerve activity in this system would act as a timing signal to entrain the discharges of the ever changing subset of active brain stem neurons to the cardiac cycle.

The manner in which the probabilistic network

138

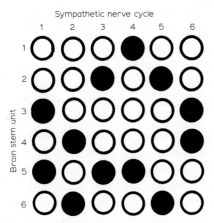

Sympathetic nerve cycle

Fig. 6. Schematic depiction of operation of the probabilistic network oscillator responsible for 2- to 6-Hz rhythm in sympathetic nerve discharge. Closed circles depict active state of individual brain stem neurons (1–6) in six sympathetic nerve cycles. Open circles depict inactive state of individual neurons (see text for details).

oscillator is hypothesized to generate the 2- to 6-Hz rhythm in SND is schematically depicted in Fig. 6. The active (closed circles) and inactive (open circles) states of six brain stem neurons are shown during six cardiac-related cycles of SND. In this model, the coincident firing of two neurons is required to generate a sympathetic nerve slow wave. For example, cycle 1 arises from the coincident firing of units 3 and 5 whereas cycle 2 arises from the simultaneous discharges of units 4 and 6. Thus, cycles 1 and 2 arise from entirely different subsets of brain stem neurons. The subsets responsible for cycles 3 and 4 are also different, but they share a common element (i.e. unit 5). Although the discharges of each of the six neurons are probabilistically related to SND, the sympathetic nerve rhythm is not directly reflected in their irregular discharge patterns. Thus, the 2- to 6-Hz rhythm in SND is an emergent property of the network as a whole. The network functions as a probabilistic oscillator since the subset of active brain stem neurons changes from cycle to cycle. Why the network functions in this way remains obscure. One possibility is that the ability of the network to engage different active subsets of neurons at dif-

ferent times represents a mechanism by which the brain stem reticular formation selects between patterns of spinal sympathetic outflow, each best suited to a particular behavioral state. For example, the cardiovascular component of the defence reaction involves a complex and highly differentiated pattern of spinal sympathetic outflow that is quite different from that accompanying the state of desynchronized sleep (Hilton, 1982; Gebber, 1989). Perhaps the switching from one active subset of brain stem neurons to another in the anesthetized cat reflects the scanning by the reticular formation of all possible programs of spinal sympathetic outflow available to it. On the other hand, such switching might more simply reflect the continual search for responsive members of the network that maintains basal sympathetic nerve activity.

Acknowledgements

The authors are grateful to Ms. Diane Hummel for typing the manuscript. This study was supported by National Institutes of Health grants HL13187 and HL33266.

References

Ardell, J.L., Barman, S.M. and Gebber, G.L. (1982) Sympathetic nerve discharge in chronic spinal cat. Am. J. Physiol., 243: H463 – H470.

Barman, S.M. and Gebber, G.L. (1980) Sympathetic nerve rhythm of brain stem origin. Am. J. Physiol., 239: R42 – R47.

Barman, S.M. and Gebber, G.L. (1985) Axonal projection patterns of ventrolateral medullospinal sympathoexcitatory neurons. J. Neurophysiol., 53: 1551 – 1566.

Barman, S.M. and Gebber, G.L. (1987) Lateral tegmental field neurons of cat medulla: a source of basal activity of ventrolateral medullospinal sympathoexcitatory neurons. J. Neurophysiol., 57: 1410 – 1424.

Bendat, J.S. and Piersol, A.G. (1971) Random Data: Analysis and Measurement Procedures, Wiley, New York, 407 pp.

Cohen, M.I. (1979) Neurogenesis of respiratory rhythm in the mammal. Physiol. Rev., 59: 1105 – 1173.

Feldman, J.L. (1986) Neurophysiology of breathing in mammals. In F.E. Bloom (Ed.), Handbook of Physiology, Section 1: The Nervous System, Vol. IV, Intrinsic Regulatory

Systems of the Brain, Am. Physiol. Soc., Bethesda, pp. 463 – 524.

Gebber, G.L. (1989) Central determinants of sympathetic nerve discharge. In A.D. Loewy and K.M. Spyer (Eds.), *Central Regulation of Autonomic Functions,* Oxford University New York (in press).

Gebber, G.L and Barman, S.M. (1980) Basis for 2-6 cycle/s rhythm in sympathetic nerve discharge. *Am. J. Physiol.,* 239: R48 – R56.

Gebber, G.L. and Barman, S.M. (1985) Lateral tegmental field neurons of cat medulla: a potential source of basal sympathetic nerve discharge. *J. Neurophysiol.,* 54: 1498 – 1512.

Hilton, S.M. (1982) The defence-arousal system and its relevance for circulatory and respiratory control. *J. Exp. Biol.,* 100: 159 – 174.

Kristan, W.B. (1980) Generation of rhythmic motor patterns. In H.M. Pinsker and W.D. Willis (Eds.), *Information Processing in the Nervous System,* Raven Press, New York, pp. 241 – 261.

Richardson, C.A. and Mitchell, R.A. (1982) Power spectral analysis of inspiratory nerve activity in the decerebrate cat. *Brain Res.,* 233: 317 – 336.

Richter, D.W. (1982) Generation and maintenance of the respiratory rhythm. *J. Exp. Biol.,* 100: 93 – 107.

Selverston, A.I. and Moulins, M. (1985) Oscillatory neural networks. *Ann. Rev. Physiol.,* 47: 29 – 48.

Stein, R.B. (1980) *Nerve and Muscle: Membranes, Cells, and Systems.* Plenum Press, New York, 265 pp.

SECTION III

Effect of Ventrolateral Medullary Inputs on Sympathetic Preganglionic Neuron Activity

J. Ciriello, M.M. Caverson and C. Polosa (Eds.)
Progress in Brain Research, Vol. 81
© 1989 Elsevier Science Publishers B.V. (Biomedical Division)

CHAPTER 10

Some properties of the sympathoinhibition from the caudal ventrolateral medulla oblongata in the cat

K. Dembowsky, J. Czachurski and H. Seller

I. Physiologisches Institut, Universität Heidelberg, Im Neuenheimer Feld 326, 6900 Heidelberg, F.R.G.

Introduction

Neurones in the caudal ventrolateral medulla oblongata (CVLM) play an important role in the control of sympathetic activity. Excitation of these neurones by small injections of excitatory amino acids causes an inhibition of sympathetic activity and a fall in arterial blood pressure (Blessing and Reis, 1982; Willette et al., 1983; McAllen, 1986a). Since inhibition of these neurones by injections of inhibitory amino acids or lesions of this area produce an increase in blood pressure which is partly due to an augmented sympathetic activity, these sympathoinhibitory neurones in the CVLM are probably tonically active (Blessing et al., 1981b; Blessing and Reis, 1982; Willette et al., 1983; Pilowsky et al., 1985; Blessing and Willoughby, 1987). This sympathoinhibitory area in the CVLM partly overlaps with the noradrenergic A1 cell group in the lower brainstem and the lateral reticular nucleus (Blessing and Reis, 1982).

The pathway of this sympathoinhibition from the CVLM to sympathetic preganglionic neurones (SPNs) in the spinal cord is not fully understood. There may be a descending inhibitory pathway to SPNs originating in the CVLM, although this pathway does not arise from neurones of the A1 cell group (Blessing et al., 1981a; Loewy and Neil, 1981; McKellar and Loewy, 1982). The inhibitory response from the CVLM would then be due to post-synaptic inhibition of SPNs. Alternately,

there is evidence suggesting that this sympathoinhibition is relayed to SPNs through the rostral ventrolateral medulla oblongata (RVLM) (Willette et al., 1984; Granata et al., 1985, 1986; Blessing, 1988). Here bulbospinal, sympathoexcitatory neurones have been localized which provide a tonic excitatory input to SPNs (Amendt et al., 1979; Dembowsky et al., 1981; Dampney et al., 1982; Barman and Gebber, 1985; Brown and Guyenet, 1985; McAllen, 1986b). In this latter case, the sympathoinhibition from CVLM would be caused via a short inhibitory projection from CVLM to these sympathoexcitatory neurones in RVLM and thus be due to a removal of a tonic excitatory input to SPNs, e.g. to a disfacilitation of SPNs. It has been suggested that this projection from the CVLM to the RVLM arises from the noradrenergic A1 neurones (Granata et al., 1985, 1986), although this could not be confirmed by anatomical techniques (Sun and Guyenet, 1986; Blessing et al., 1987a) and in a study using microstimulation in CVLM (Day et al., 1983).

The present study was designed to clarify the question whether the sympathoinhibition from CVLM is due to post-synaptic inhibition or disfacilitation of SPNs by first studying the spinal pathway of this inhibitory response. If its pathway in the spinal cord could be dissociated from the descending pathway of the sympathoexcitatory neurones in RVLM which runs in the dorso- and ventrolateral funiculus of the spinal cord (Barman and Gebber, 1985; Dampney et al., 1987) this would be strong evidence against disfacilitation of SPNs. Since more direct evidence for either disfacilitation or post-synaptic inhibition should be provided by intracellular recordings of SPNs, this question was also addressed by recording SPNs intracellularly and studying the effects of glutamate injections into CVLM on their membrane potential. It was also studied if noradrenaline acting on α_2-adrenergic receptors is involved as transmitter in this inhibition and if this sympathoinhibition involves an afferent projection from the CVLM to the hypothalamus (McKellar and Loewy, 1982) or cerebellum (Batton et al., 1977).

Methods

All experiments were performed on cats anaesthetized with α-chloralose (70 mg/kg i.v.) after induction with ether. A tracheotomy was performed and a femoral artery and vein were catheterized. The animals were vagotomized, paralyzed with pancuronium bromide and artificially ventilated. Ventilation was adjusted to an end-tidal CO_2 of 3.8 – 4.5%. Respiratory movements of the spinal cord were prevented by a bilateral pneumothorax. Body temperature was maintained at 38.5 $\pm$ 0.2°C by an infrared lamp.

The following nerves were exposed for recording or stimulation on the left side: white rami of the second to fourth thoracic segment (WR-T2 to WR-T4), the inferior cardiac nerve (CN), the renal nerve (RN) and the fifth cervical rootlet of the phrenic nerve (PN). Except for WR which were left in continuity with the sympathetic chain, the nerves were cut peripherally and activity was recorded from the central end by using bipolar platinum electrodes. Preganglionic sympathetic activity in WR was passed through a window discriminator and the normalized impulses were counted in intervals of 1 – 3 sec. Phrenic nerve activity was integrated with a time constant of 100 msec. Postganglionic sympathetic activity in CN and RN was monitored as the raw signal.

After a laminectomy from C8-T6 and fixation of the spinal cord by clamps on spinous processes above and below the laminectomy, intracellular recordings from SPNs of the third thoracic segment were obtained by using glass microelectrodes filled with a 3 M KCl solution and conventional electrophysiological techniques; DC-resistance of these electrodes ranged from 20 to 70 MΩ. Neurones were identified by recording the antidromic action potential in response to stimulation of WR-T3 (for further details see Dembowsky et al., 1985).

In some experiments an additional laminectomy was performed at C3/C4 for subsequent lesions of the spinal cord with small knife cuts. The extent of the lesions was assessed histologically. Anaemic decerebration was performed in one experiment by occluding both common carotid arteries and the basilar artery.

The ventral or dorsal surface of the brainstem was exposed in different experiments for pressure microinjections of L-glutamate (0.2 M, pH 7.4, 30 – 60 nl) into the left ventrolateral medulla oblongata. Injections were made from either the ventral or dorsal surface with glass microelectrodes having a tip diameter of 10 – 20 μm. Using the ventral approach, the most cranial rootlet of the hypoglossal nerve was used as a landmark to localize the inhibitory area in the CVLM: it was located 0.5 – 1 mm lateral and 0.8 – 1.5 mm caudal to this rootlet and at a depth of 1 mm from the ventral surface. Using the dorsal approach, the dorsal surface was aligned horizontally and the obex was used as the reference point: the inhibitory area was located 4 – 5 mm lateral and 1.5 – 2.5 mm cranial to the obex and 5 – 5.5 mm below the dorsal surface. For injections at these coordinates the cerebellum was either removed by suction or gently pushed cranially. Between successive glutamate injections an interval of at least 15 min was allowed for recovery. In the majority of the experiments the inhibitory area was readily located according to these stereotactic coordinates. In some animals, however, no inhibitory response was evoked from these sites in the CVLM; in these experiments a much larger area of the ventrolateral medulla (both in the mediolateral and the craniocaudal direction) was mapped with repeated glutamate injections in an attempt to localize this area. In some experiments the inhibitory area in the CVLM was also stimulated electrically with a bipolar concentric stainless steel microelectrode (diameter 250 μm).

The activity in different nerves, the membrane potential of SPNs and arterial blood pressure were monitored on a Brush pen recorder and were also stored on magnetic tape for further analysis.

Results

In two thirds of the experiments a sympathoinhibitory response was readily evoked by unilateral injections of 30–60 nl glutamate (total dose 15–30 nM) into the left CVLM. The response was characterized by a complete suppression of the background activity in sympathetic pre- and post-ganglionic nerves which was followed within a few seconds by a profound fall in blood pressure to 40–60 mmHg (Figs. 1A and 5A). In some experiments this fall in blood pressure was accompanied by a bradycardia (Figs. 7 and 8A). The duration of this complete suppression of sympathetic activity ranged in different experiments from 5 to 30 sec; in some experiments it was considerably longer in the RN than CN (Fig. 5A). Recovery of sympathetic activity was mostly complete within 1–2 min after injection. In some cats the accompanying fall in blood pressure outlasted the inhibition of sympathetic activity for several minutes and even persisted, although sympathetic activity had almost returned to control levels (Fig. 1A); in this animal blood pressure was only restored to control levels after an i.v. injection of noradrenaline (3 μg/kg). Glutamate injections at sites from where this sympathoinhibitory and depressor response was evoked also had very characteristic and reproducible effects on PN activity: the sympathoinhibitory response was mostly associated with a strong, tonic excitation of PN activity (Figs. 1, 5, 7 and 8). In some cats, this tonic

excitation was followed by a complete inhibition of phrenic activity before control rhythmic activity was restored. This phrenic response was highly specific for the inhibitory area in CVLM; it was only occasionally observed when glutamate was injected into adjacent sites in the CVLM from which no sympathoinhibitory and depressor response could be evoked. Glutamate injections outside of

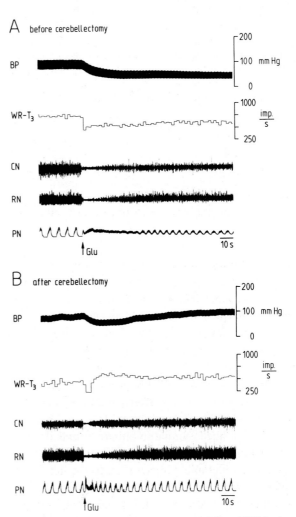

Fig. 1. Effects of a glutamate injection (60 nl) into CVLM using the dorsal approach before (A) and after removing the cerebellum by suction (B). Traces are from top to bottom: arterial blood pressure (BP), activity in white ramus T3 (WR-T3), inferior cardiac nerve (CN), renal nerve (RN) and phrenic nerve (PN). Note the long-lasting fall in blood pressure although sympathetic activity in WR-T3, CN and RN had returned almost to control levels.

146

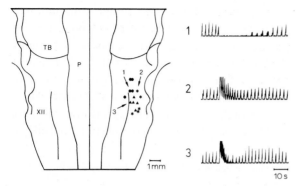

Fig. 2. Glutamate injections into the ventrolateral medulla oblongata at different sites have distinct effects on phrenic nerve activity. The injection sites are shown on a schematic drawing of the ventral surface of the brainstem. Abbreviations: TB = trapezoid body; P = pyramids; XII = exit of the hypoglossal rootlets; the small dot in the midline indicates the level of the obex. Arrows 1 – 3 indicate the sites from which the responses shown on the right side were evoked. From all sites marked with the same symbol qualitatively similar responses were evoked. In other experiments it could be shown that the small medial strip from which an inhibition of phrenic activity was evoked extended more caudally than shown in this figure.

the inhibitory area evoked completely different phrenic responses. Injections of glutamate into CVLM at more medial sites resulted in an inhibition of PN activity (Fig. 2-1), whereas injections into more lateral sites evoked a tachypnoeic response associated with an increase of each phrenic burst (Fig. 2-2). The inhibition of phrenic activity evoked from CVLM at more medial sites was similar to that seen after glutamate injections into RVLM (Fig. 2-1; see also McAllen, 1986a).

The described sympathoinhibitory and depressor response was only evoked in two thirds of the animals by glutamate injections into the inhibitory area in CVLM. In the remainder of the experiments in addition to the usual effects on PN activity (e.g. tonic excitation), a sympathoexcitatory rather than an inhibitory response was evoked by injections of glutamate into corresponding sites in CVLM (Figs. 3 and 4A). The sympathoexcitatory response from CVLM was often associated with an increase in blood pressure and closely resembled the excitatory response that is

usually evoked from RVLM (Fig. 3). Despite an extensive mapping of the ventrolateral medulla no sympathoinhibitory response could be evoked from any point in the ventrolateral medulla in these experiments. The only difference that could be detected so far between these two groups of animals was related to the degree of respiratory

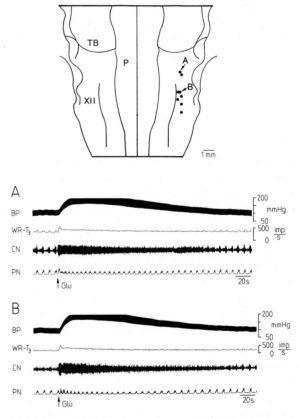

Fig. 3. Glutamate injections into CVLM evoked a sympathoexcitatory rather than an inhibitory response in this experiment (B). This response was very similar to the excitatory response evoked from RVLM (A). Traces are from top to bottom: blood pressure (BP), activity in white ramus (WR-T3), inferior cardiac nerve (CN) and phrenic nerve (PN). All injection sites from which similar sympathoexcitatory responses were elicited are shown in a schematic drawing of the ventral surface of the brainstem (abbreviations as in Fig. 2). Arrows indicate the sites from which the responses in (A) and (B) were evoked. In this animal no sympathoinhibitory response was evoked from any of the injections into CVLM. Note the respiratory modulation of sympathetic background activity in this animal. The tonic excitation of PN was not as pronounced as in other experiments (see Fig. 10A).

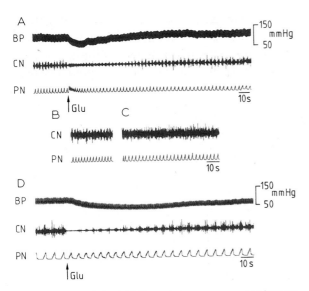

Fig. 4. Change of the initially excitatory response (A) into an inhibitory response (D) after sympathetic background activity has changed from an inspiratory-related to a more irregular discharge pattern during the course of the experiment. Two intervening states of sympathetic activity are shown in (B) and (C). Glutamate was injected in (A) and (D) at exactly the same site in CVLM. The fall in blood pressure in (A) might be caused by a net decrease of sympathetic activity despite the excitation in response to the glutamate injection. The initially very prominent respiratory modulation of sympathetic activity was not completely lost during this experiment. It was still evident during the recovery of sympathetic activity after the glutamate injection in (D). The respiratory modulation of sympathetic activity in (D) prior to the glutamate injection was due to an incomplete recovery after a previous glutamate injection. Note that the glutamate injection in (A) also evoked a tonic excitation of phrenic nerve activity.

modulation of sympathetic background activity. In animals in which sympathetic background activity in WR, CN and RN showed a pronounced, inspiratory-related discharge pattern a sympathoexcitatory response was evoked from CVLM (Fig. 3). In contrast, in experiments in which a sympathoinhibitory response was readily evoked from CVLM, sympathetic background activity was not or only a little modulated by the central respiratory drive and showed an irregular discharge pattern (Figs. 1 and 5). In two experiments sympathetic background activity initially showed an inspiratory-related discharge pattern

and a sympathoexcitatory response was evoked by glutamate injections into CVLM (Fig. 4A). In these two animals, sympathetic background activity changed slowly over hours during the course of the experiment to an irregular pattern (Fig. 4B,C); when the glutamate injections were then repeated at identical sites in CVLM a sympathoinhibitory response was evoked (Fig. 4D). Neither the initial respiratory modulation of sympathetic background activity nor the excitatory response from CVLM could be restored in these two animals by an additional injection of chloralose (20 mg/kg i.v.).

In animals in which the sympathoinhibitory response was evoked from CVLM some of its properties were studied. Both the sympathoinhibitory and depressor response and the tonic excitation of PN activity persisted after removal of the cerebellum (Fig. 1) and in one cat after anaemic decerebration.

The involvement of catecholamines acting on α_2-adrenergic receptors in this inhibitory response was tested by evoking the response before and after an i.v. injection of the selective α_2-adrenergic antagonist rauwolscine (50–100 μg/kg) (Fig. 5). At this low dose, rauwolscine had only small or no effects on sympathetic background activity (Fig. 5C). The sympathoinhibitory response from CVLM, however, was not affected at all (Fig. 5). Rauwolscine also had no effect on the tonic excitation of PN activity in response to glutamate injections into the inhibitory area in CVLM (Fig. 5).

The spinal pathway of this sympathoinhibitory response was studied by evoking the response before and after various lesions in the cervical spinal cord (Fig. 6). The response persisted after right (contralateral to the side of recording) hemisections (Fig. 6D), after lesions of the left ventral quadrant (Fig. 6B) and small lesions in the left dorsal root entry zone (Fig. 6E). These lesions which only left intact the left dorsolateral funiculus also did not substantially affect sympathetic background activity (Fig. 6). The inhibitory response could only be abolished when the lesions included the left (ipsilateral) dorsolateral

148

funiculus of the spinal cord. These lesions, however, also disrupted all major descending excitatory pathways to SPNs of the left side and thus, also abolished sympathetic background activity. However, as long as sympathetic background activity was not completely abolished, for example after partial lesions of the dorsolateral funiculus as in Fig. 6F, an inhibitory response

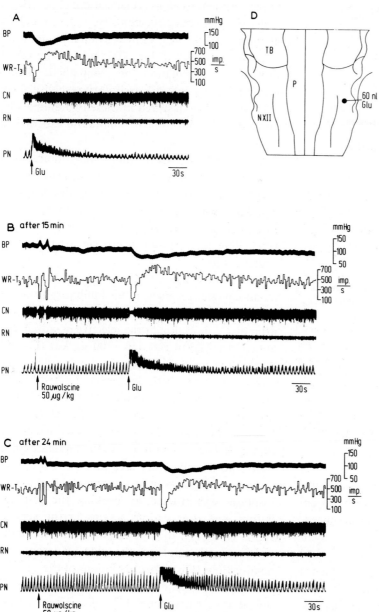

Fig. 5. Rauwolscine has no effect on the sympathoinhibitory and depressor response from the CVLM (A – C). (A) Control injection; (B) glutamate injection after i.v. injection of rauwolscine (15 min after A); (C) glutamate injection after a second i.v. injection of rauwolscine (24 min after B). Traces are from top to bottom: blood pressure (BP), activity in white ramus T3 (WR-T3), inferior cardiac nerve (CN), renal nerve (RN) and phrenic nerve (PN). The injection site is shown in (D). Note the slight increase in sympathetic activity after rauwolscine (C) and that the tonic excitation of phrenic activity was also not affected by rauwolscine.

could still be evoked. With this method it was not possible to abolish selectively only the inhibitory response from CVLM leaving descending excitatory pathways intact.

Due to difficulties in obtaining stable intracellular recordings of SPNs during the depressor response from CVLM the effects of

glutamate injections on the membrane potential of SPNs could only be analyzed in a small number of neurones. For this reason the synaptic input from CVLM to SPNs was also studied in some experiments by electrical stimulation of this area.

In four SPNs, a glutamate injection into CVLM had no effect on the membrane potential or synap-

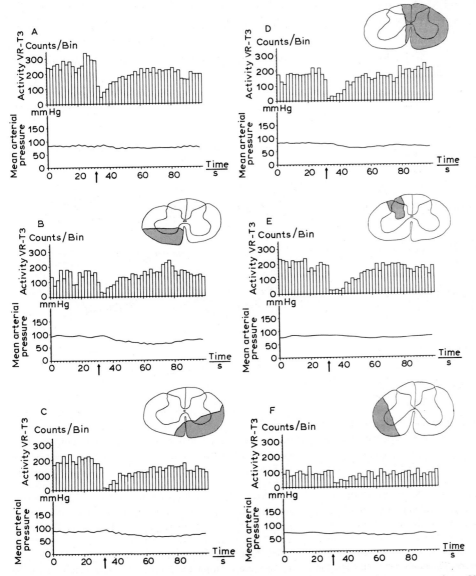

Fig. 6. Effects of lesions in the cervical spinal cord at C3/C4 (B – F) on the inhibitory response from CVLM. (A) Control response. In this experiment only white ramus T3 (WR-T3) and mean arterial blood pressure were recorded. The extent of the lesions was assessed from histological sections. The pathway of the inhibitory response could not be separated from the major descending excitatory pathways running in the dorsolateral funiculus.

150

tic activity, although a fall in blood pressure and a tonic excitation of PN activity was evoked by these injections. In the remainder of the neurones in which this stimulation could be tested a reversible reduction or abolition of excitatory postsynaptic potentials (EPSPs) of the ongoing synaptic activity was observed (Figs. 7B and 8). In some neurones this was associated with a membrane hyperpolarization (Figs. 7A and 8). A common feature of both responses (reduction of EPSPs and hyper-

polarization) was the rather short duration (1 – 5 sec) if compared to the duration of the effects on the activity in pre- and postganglionic nerves and PN and on blood pressure. Similar results were obtained with electrical rather than chemical stimulation of this area in CVLM (Fig. 9), although in this case the evoked hyperpolarization was invariably contaminated by some EPSPs (Figs. 9 and 10).

Since a membrane hyperpolarization in combination with a reduction of the ongoing synaptic activity can result from either disfacilitation or post-synaptic inhibition it was necessary to deter-

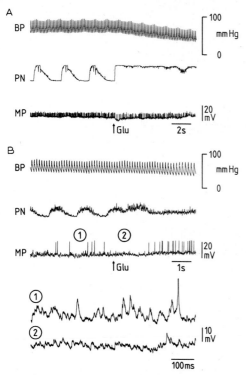

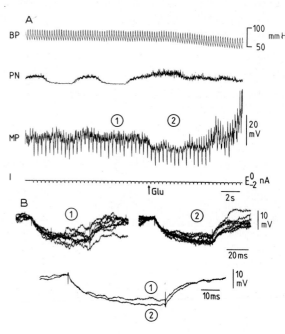

Fig. 7. Effects of glutamate injections into CVLM on the membrane potential of two different SPNs (A,B) recorded in two different cats. Traces show from top to bottom: blood pressure (BP), phrenic nerve activity (PN, saturating in A) and membrane potential (MP). (A) Although this SPN was seriously damaged by the impaling microelectrode and displayed a high frequency injury discharge, a glutamate injection into CVLM evoked a hyperpolarization and inhibition of this injury discharge. (B) In this neurone, the glutamate injection caused a reduction of the ongoing synaptic activity. From some EPSPs of this ongoing activity, action potentials were initiated, the amplitude of which was not faithfully reproduced by the pen recorder. The ongoing synaptic activity before (1) and after the glutamate injection (2) is also shown at a faster time scale and higher gain.

Fig. 8. An injection of glutamate into CVLM evoked a hyperpolarization in this SPN which was associated with an increase in input resistance. (A) Traces are from top to bottom: blood pressure (BP), phrenic nerve activity (PN), membrane potential (MP) and the current (I) injected into the neurone through the recording microelectrode. This neurone was lost shortly after the injection of glutamate probably due to the evoked fall in blood pressure. The discharge of action potentials from the ongoing synaptic activity was prevented by the injection of a DC-current of − 1.5 nA. Input resistance was measured with short (50 msec) hyperpolarizing current pulses (−0.5 nA). (B) The voltage drop during these hyperpolarizing current pulses is shown as superimposed sweeps (top) and after averaging 10 consecutive sweeps (bottom); 1: before, 2: after the glutamate injection. The input resistance was 26 MΩ before and 31 MΩ after the glutamate injection.

mine both the neuronal input resistance and the reversal potential of the evoked hyperpolarization in order to differentiate between these two mechanisms. In four SPNs, the input resistance could be measured with short hyperpolarizing current pulses before and after a glutamate injection into CVLM: In two neurones, the input resistance was reversibly decreased after an injection of glutamate (by 17 and 18%); in both neurones, however, this response was not associated with any change in membrane potential. The decrease in input resistance indicates that this response might be due to post-synaptic inhibition of these SPNs. Since in both neurones an additional negative DC-current was injected to prevent the discharge of action potentials, the observation that no hyperpolarization was evoked by these inhibitory post-synaptic potentials (IPSPs) might be the result of the current-induced hyperpolarizing shift of membrane potential to a level close to the reversal

potential of these IPSPs; since the electromotive force for these IPSPs would then be abolished or at least greatly reduced, these IPSPs should not cause any change in membrane potential. In another two SPNs, a membrane hyperpolarization was evoked in response to a glutamate injection into CVLM which in these neurones was associated with an increase of the input resistance by 17 and 19% (Fig. 8).

The reversal potential of the evoked hyperpolarization could not be determined with glutamate injections since this requires repeated injections at different levels of the membrane potential; many SPNs, however, were lost after the first

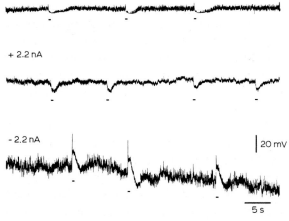

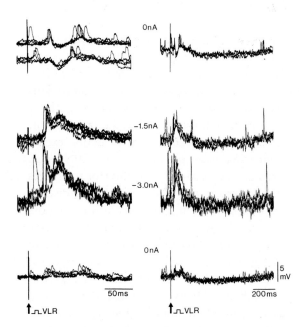

Fig. 9. Demonstration of IPSPs in a SPN by electrical stimulation in CVLM with a short train of impulses (100 Hz, 50 impulses, 3 V, 0.5 msec; period of stimulation is marked by bar). This SPN was seriously damaged by the impaling microelectrode and displayed a high frequency injury discharge. CVLM stimulation evoked a hyperpolarization (top trace) which was enhanced by the injection of a depolarizing DC-current of +2.2 nA (middle trace) and nullified by the injection of a hyperpolarizing DC-current of −2.2 nA (lower trace). The depolarizing potentials that were recorded during the injection of negative current most probably represent EPSPs and action potentials which were also evoked by this stimulation and were enhanced by this membrane hyperpolarization.

Fig. 10. Single shock stimulation in CVLM (VLR) evokes an IPSP and additional EPSPs in this SPN. Superimposed sweeps are shown at two different time scales (left and right hand side) (top traces). The IPSP was reversed into a depolarizing potential by the injection of negative DC-current (−1.5 and −3.0 nA) (middle traces). Since SPNs were recorded with microelectrodes filled with a 3 M KCl solution, the injection of negative current resulted in an increase of the intracellular chloride concentration and thus, a small depolarizing IPSP at the end of the current injection (lower trace). Note that the IPSP and EPSPs evoked by this stimulation are followed by a small, long-lasting hyperpolarization which was only decreased, but not reversed by the injection of negative current (right side); this late, long-lasting hyperpolarization was not studied in detail.

glutamate injection due to the accompanying fall in blood pressure (Fig. 8). However, using electrical stimulation in CVLM a nullification or even reversal of the initially hyperpolarizing response into a depolarizing potential was accomplished in a few neurones by the injection of hyperpolarizing DC-current (Figs. 9 and 10), indicating that this response is evoked by IPSPs. In one of these SPNs the latency of the IPSP was measured with single shock stimulation in CVLM: it ranged from 42 to 47 msec. The conduction velocity of this descending inhibitory pathway to SPNs was calculated to range from 2.1 to 2.4 m/sec.

Discussion

The results of this study demonstrate that the sympathoinhibition from CVLM is due to both disfacilitation and post-synaptic inhibition of SPNs. The evidence for disfacilitation of SPNs is twofold. First, the spinal pathway of the sympathoinhibition is confined to the same area in the spinal cord through which all major excitatory bulbospinal pathways project onto SPNs, e.g. the ipsilateral dorsolateral funiculus (for references see Dembowsky et al., 1985). By placing discrete lesions in the cervical spinal cord it was not possible to abolish selectively the inhibitory response without simultaneously affecting sympathetic background activity; the inhibitory response was only abolished by lesions which also abolished sympathetic activity. Although this finding indicates that the inhibition of sympathetic activity from CVLM takes place in the brainstem and acts by reducing a tonic excitatory input to SPNs, it does not exclude a descending inhibitory pathway running in the same area in the spinal cord intermingled with descending excitatory pathways. Second, more direct evidence for disfacilitation, however, was provided by intracellular recordings of SPNs. Glutamate injections into CVLM produced a reversible abolition of EPSPs of the ongoing synaptic activity which in some SPNs was associated with a hyperpolarization of the membrane potential and an increase of the input resistance. This increased input resistance during the hyperpolarizing response is inconsistent with a post-synaptic inhibition of SPNs in which case the response would have been associated with a decreased input resistance due to the opening of receptor-gated chloride or potassium channels. It is possible that this disfacilitation of SPNs results from an inhibition of sympathoexcitatory neurones in RVLM which provide a tonic excitatory input to SPNs (Dembowsky et al., 1981). Blessing (1988) has shown that the sympathoinhibitory response from CVLM is completely abolished after blockade of GABA-receptors in RVLM. A direct projection from CVLM to RVLM, however, could not be demonstrated in a recent anatomical study from our laboratory (Dampney et al., 1987) in which the afferent projections to RVLM have been studied by the retrograde transport of horseradish peroxidase (HRP). After HRP injections into RVLM retrogradely labelled neurones were only very rarely found in CVLM in this study (Dampney et al., 1987). To account for these conflicting results it is suggested that the projection from CVLM to RVLM is made up of a chain of neurones rather than a single neurone or that this projection is comprised of only a very small number of neurones.

Disfacilitation, however, is not the only mechanism by which sympathetic activity may be inhibited by CVLM. Certainly, in some SPNs inhibition is achieved by post-synaptic inhibition readily identified by standard criteria. First, a decrease in input resistance and second, a nullification or conversion of the hyperpolarizing response into a depolarizing potential by negative current injection. Although post-synaptic inhibition was more readily evoked by electrical than by chemical stimulation and might be due to stimulation of axons passing through this area, it could also be demonstrated by glutamate injections into CVLM. In addition, it would be very difficult to explain the hyperpolarization and inhibition of abortive spikes in seriously damaged neurones in response to a glutamate injection into CVLM as in

Fig. 7A solely on the basis of disfacilitation. Thus, it is concluded that at least in some SPNs the sympathoinhibition from CVLM is also accomplished by post-synaptic inhibition. This post-synaptic inhibition might arise from bulbospinal, non-noradrenergic neurones in CVLM (McKellar and Loewy, 1982). Recently, bulbospinal GABAergic and thus inhibitory neurones have been demonstrated in the ventrolateral medulla (Millhorn et al., 1987) and in vestibular nuclei (Blessing et al., 1987b). Since bulbospinal neurones of CVLM, however, do not project directly to the intermediolateral cell column (Amendt et al., 1979), the possibility must also be considered that the post-synaptic inhibition from CVLM is mediated by inhibitory spinal interneurones located outside of the intermediolateral cell column. Regardless of the anatomical organization of this inhibitory pathway, its conduction velocity is slow and ranges from 2 to 3 m/sec. A descending inhibitory pathway with a similar conduction velocity has been localized in dorsal parts of the dorsolateral funiculus and the dorsal root entry zone (Coote and MacLeod, 1975; Dembowsky et al., 1985). Since lesions of this area, however, did not abolish the suppression of extracellularly recorded sympathetic activity evoked from CVLM (Fig. 6E), it seems possible that the post-synaptic inhibition from CVLM only acts on silent SPNs. As discussed previously (Dembowsky et al., 1985), it is very difficult to ascertain, on the basis of intracellular recordings, whether the SPN under study is spontaneously active or silent. The suggestion that post-synaptic inhibition from CVLM might preferentially act on silent SPNs is in agreement with the conclusion derived from extracellular recordings of the activity of spontaneously active sympathetic postganglionic fibres in the renal nerve that the inhibition of this activity by glutamate injections into CVLM is exclusively due to disfacilitation (Blessing, 1988).

At present, the functional significance of this post-synaptic inhibition of SPNs remains unclear. A similar dual control of SPNs by disfacilitation and post-synaptic inhibition, however, has also been shown for the inhibition of sympathetic activity by baroreceptor afferents (Dembowsky et al., 1986). With respect to this finding it would be interesting to know whether the inhibition of sympathetic activity by neurones in CVLM and by baroreceptor afferents is caused in the same SPNs by the same mechanism.

The finding of the present study that the sympathoinhibitory response from CVLM is not abolished by the selective α_2-adrenergic antagonist rauwolscine provides another piece of evidence that noradrenergic neurones of the A1 area are not involved in this sympathoinhibition (see also Day et al., 1983; Sun and Guyenet, 1986; Blessing et al., 1987a; Blessing, 1988). The sympathoexcitatory action of α_2-adrenergic antagonists (McCall et al., 1983) must therefore be due to blockade of the effects of some other catecholaminergic cell groups in the brainstem.

Recently, it has been shown that microinjections of excitatory amino acids into the cerebellar fastigial nucleus evoke a depressor rather than a pressor response which is only seen with electrical stimulation (Chida et al., 1986). Since the fastigial nucleus receives an afferent projection from the lateral reticular nucleus which partly overlaps with the inhibitory area in CVLM (Blessing and Reis, 1982) and also projects back to this brainstem nucleus (Batton et al., 1977), it might be possible that the inhibitory response from CVLM is relayed through the fastigial nucleus. The present study has shown that this possibility can be ruled out since the response persisted after removal of the cerebellum. The question whether the CVLM is an integral part of the efferent pathway of the fastigial depressor response, however, was not addressed.

The sympathoinhibitory response was mostly accompanied by a tonic excitation of PN activity. This phrenic response was very specific for the inhibitory area in CVLM and was only rarely evoked at sites from which no sympathoinhibitory response was elicited. Although the location of the injection sites was not assessed histologically in the present study, the effects on PN activity are most likely attributed to excitation of neurones located dorsally to the injection site in the para-ambigualis region, the intermediate portion of the ventral respiratory group (VRG) between the obex and the retrofacial nucleus (Kalia, 1981). In this part of the VRG bulbospinal and brainstem intrinsic neurones discharging synchronously with PN activity are concentrated (Kalia, 1981). Fairly large glutamate injections into CVLM at depths of 1 mm below the ventral surface might well affect the activity of these more dorsally located neurones in VRG by diffusion. Day et al. (1983) have shown that the inhibitory response from CVLM is evoked from an area immediately dorsal to the A1 region. Using very small glutamate injections in the picomolar range, McCrimmon et al. (1986) were able to evoke distinct responses of PN activity from VRG. Similar to the findings of the present study they found that glutamate injections into medial aspects of VRG caused an inhibition of PN activity, whereas more lateral injections caused an excitation (McCrimmon et al., 1986a). Although they have used much smaller injection volumes than we did, they have also described that at some injection sites the effect on PN activity was associated with a marked depressor response. Interestingly, the largest depressor responses were evoked at sites from which PN activity was excited (McCrimmon et al., 1986b). The nature of this close association of an excitatory response of PN discharge and an inhibitory response of sympathetic activity is unknown. A possible link between the two responses might be provided by the post-inspiratory neurones of the respiratory network in the brainstem. The post-inspiratory phase (or stage I expiration) of the respiratory cycle which is defined as the phase of declining phrenic activity before the beginning of the expiration (Richter, 1982) is associated with a short inhibition of sympathetic background activity (Bainton et al., 1985); the mechanism of this post-inspiratory inhibition of sympathetic activity, however, is unknown. If the tonic excitation of PN activity after injections of picomoles of glutamate into VRG (McCrimmon et al., 1986a,b) or as in the present study after injections of nanomoles of glutamate into CVLM represents post-inspiratory activity, an inhibition of sympathetic activity might be expected. Intracellular recordings of neurones in this part of the VRG have revealed the existence of post-inspiratory neurones (Remmers et al., 1986). It should be possible to test this assumption by studying the effects of glutamate injections into CVLM on the membrane potential of expiratory bulbospinal neurones in the caudal VRG. Some of these neurones receive post-inspiratory IPSPs during the early part of the expiratory depolarization which are affected by a variety of stimuli known to influence post-inspiratory activity (Ballantyne and Richter, 1986; Ballantyne et al., 1988). With respect to this hypothesis, it would be of great interest to know the mechanism of the post-inspiratory inhibition of sympathetic activity (Bainton et al., 1985) and whether it is also relayed through sympathoexcitatory neurones in RVLM.

A puzzling observation in the present study was the finding that in some animals no sympathoinhibitory response could be evoked from any site in CVLM. On the contrary, in these animals a sympathoexcitatory response was evoked by glutamate injections into CVLM. This observation raises some questions. Prior to any discussion about the functional implications of this result it must be ascertained that the excitatory response indeed results from excitation of the same set of neurones in CVLM which in other animals causes an inhibitory response. Since the injection sites were not localized in histological sections of the brainstem it cannot be excluded definitely that different pools of neurones are involved in these two responses. For several reasons, however, this seems unlikely. First, although in experiments in which an excitatory response was evoked from CVLM a large area of the ventrolateral medulla was explored with repeated glutamate injections, an inhibitory response was never observed. Second, large injection volumes of 30 – 60 nl were used which should affect the activity of neurones in a large area. Using 50 nl injections of a dye, it has been shown that the injected dye spread over an area of 0.5 – 0.7 mm in diameter (Gordon and McCann, 1988). Third, the tonic excitation of PN activity which was very specific for the inhibitory area in CVLM was readily evoked in animals in which an excitatory response was elicited from CVLM; this indicates that the microinjections were placed in both groups of animals at very similar sites. Fourth, in two animals the nature of the response evoked by glutamate injections into the same site in CVLM changed during the course of the experiment from an initial excitation to an inhibition. It is most unlikely that the excitatory and pressor response results from injections into the caudal pressor area which has been recently identified caudal to the inhibitory area in CVLM (Gordon and McCann, 1988). This caudal pressor area is localized 1 – 1.5 mm caudal to the obex, in the present study, however, all glutamate injections were placed cranial to the obex. Likewise, an activation of neurones in RVLM by diffusion of the glutamate injected into CVLM seems unlikely because of the large distance involved (more than 2 mm) and the opposite nature of the phrenic response evoked from both areas.

The occurrence of a sympathoexcitatory response from CVLM was correlated with a prominent inspiratory-related discharge pattern of sympathetic background activity. Furthermore, when this activity pattern of sympathetic activity was changed to a more irregular and tonic type of pattern during the course of an experiment this was associated with a conversion of the CVLM response from excitation to inhibition. So far, no reasonable explanation can be given for this correlation between the nature of the response and the degree of respiratory modulation of sympathetic background activity and also for the large variability in the respiratory modulation of sympathetic background activity among different animals. One parameter that may influence both this interrelationship and the respiratory modulation of sympathetic activity certainly is the depth of anaesthesia. Anaesthesia-dependent effects on blood pressure by the topical application of leptazol to an area of the ventral surface of the brainstem which is caudal to, but greatly overlaps the inhibitory area in CVLM have recently been reported by Feldberg and Guertzenstein (1986). While during light anaesthesia a depressor response was evoked, this response was changed to a pressor reaction when anaesthesia was deepened (Feldberg and Guertzenstein, 1986). With respect to the present study, the reverse argument may apply. It may be possible that the change from an inspiratory-related discharge pattern of sympathetic background activity to a more irregular, tonic activity pattern and thus the change of the CVLM response from an excitation to inhibition results from the decreasing effects of the anaesthetic during the course of these long experiments. This, however, is unlikely since this change could not be reversed by injecting additional amounts of chloralose. It is more likely that other factors which also strongly affect the state of the animal and consequently sympathetic activity and its discharge pattern are involved, for example blood loss during the preparation, substitution of fluid, and acid-base status. Nonetheless, these findings indicate that neurones in CVLM and in the adjacent VRG may be crucial for the central coupling of sympathetic and respiratory activity. The result of the present experiments that the degree of respiratory modulation of sympathetic background activity, for whatsoever reason, determines the nature of the response from CVLM might be tested in future experiments by studying this response during normo- and hypercapnia; recent experiments in our laboratory have shown that an irregular discharge pattern of sympathetic background activity can readily be converted to an inspiratory-related discharge pattern during hypercapnia (Katona et al., 1989).

Acknowledgements

This work was supported by the Deutsche Forschungsgemeinschaft (De 364/1-2 and SFB 320). The technical assistance of Miss Andrea Zobel and Miss Bärbel Phillipin is gratefully acknowledged. Thanks are also due to Dr. D. Ballantyne for

156

discussions about the organization of the respiratory network in the brainstem.

References

Amendt, K., Czachurski, J., Dembowsky, K. and Seller, H. (1979) Bulbospinal projections to the intermediolateral cell column; a neuroanatomical study. *J. Auton. Nerv. Syst.,* 1: 103 – 117.

Bainton, C.R., Richter, D.W., Seller, H., Ballantyne, D. and Klein, J.P. (1985) Respiratory modulation of sympathetic activity. *J. Auton. Nerv. Syst.,* 12: 77 – 90.

Ballantyne, D. and Richter, D.W. (1986) The non-uniform character of expiratory synaptic activity in expiratory bulbospinal neurones of the cat. *J. Physiol. (Lond.),* 370: 433 – 456.

Ballantyne, D., Jordan, D., Spyer, K.M. and Wood, L.M. (1988) Synaptic rhythm of caudal medullary expiratory neurones during stimulation of the hypothalamic defence area of the cat. *J. Physiol. (Lond.),* 405: 527 – 546.

Barman, S.M. and Gebber, G.L. (1985) Axonal projection patterns of ventrolateral medullospinal sympathoexcitatory neurons. *J. Neurophysiol.,* 53: 1551 – 1566.

Batton, R.R., Jayaraman, A., Ruggiero, D. and Carpenter, M.B. (1977) Fastigial efferent projections in the monkey: an autoradiographic study. *J. Comp. Neurol.,* 174: 281 – 306.

Blessing, W.W. (1988) Depressor neurons in rabbit caudal medulla act via GABA receptors in rostral medulla. *Am. J. Physiol.,* 254: H686 – H692.

Blessing, W.W. and Reis, D.J. (1982) Inhibitory cardiovascular function of neurons in the caudal ventrolateral medulla of the rabbit: relationship to the area containing A1 noradrenergic cells. *Brain Res.,* 253: 161 – 171.

Blessing, W.W. and Willoughby, J.O. (1987) Depressor neurons in rabbit caudal medulla do not transmit the baroreceptor-vasomotor reflex. *Am. J. Physiol.,* 253: H777 – H786.

Blessing, W.W., Goodchild, A.K., Dampney, R.A.L. and Chalmers, J.P. (1981a) Cell groups in the lower brain stem of the rabbit projecting to the spinal cord, with special reference to catecholamine-containing neurons. *Brain Res.,* 221: 35 – 55.

Blessing, W.W., West, M.J. and Chalmers, J.P. (1981b) Hypertension, bradycardia and pulmonary edema in the conscious rabbit after brainstem lesions coinciding with the A1 group of catecholamine neurons. *Circ. Res.,* 49: 949 – 958.

Blessing, W.W., Hedger, S.C., Joh, T.H. and Willoughby, J.O. (1987a) Neurons in the area postrema are the only catecholamine-synthesizing cells in the medulla or pons with projections to the rostral ventrolateral medulla (C_1-area) in the rabbit. *Brain Res.,* 419: 336 – 340.

Blessing, W.W., Hedger, S.C. and Oertel, W.H. (1987b) Vestibulospinal pathway in rabbit includes GABA-synthesizing neurons. *Neurosci. Lett.,* 80: 158 – 162.

Brown, D.L. and Guyenet, P.G. (1985) Electrophysiological study of cardiovascular neurons in the rostral ventrolateral medulla in rats. *Circ. Res.,* 56: 359 – 369.

Chida, K., Iadecola, C., Underwood, M.D. and Reis, D.J. (1986) A novel vasodepressor response elicited from the rat cerebellar fastigial nucleus: the fastigial depressor response. *Brain Res.,* 370: 378 – 383.

Coote, J.H. and MacLeod, V.H. (1975) The spinal route of sympatho-inhibitory pathways descending from the medulla oblongata. *Pflügers Arch.,* 359: 335 – 347.

Dampney, R.A.L., Goodchild, A.K., Robertson, L.G. and Montgomery, W. (1982) Role of ventrolateral medulla in vasomotor regulation: a correlative anatomical and physiological study. *Brain Res.,* 249: 223 – 235.

Dampney, R.A.L., Czachurski, J., Dembowsky, K., Goodchild, A.K. and Seller, H. (1987) Afferent connections and spinal projections of the pressor region in the rostral ventrolateral medulla of the cat. *J. Auton. Nerv. Syst.,* 20: 73 – 86.

Day, T.A., Ro, A. and Renaud, L.P. (1983) Depressor area within caudal ventrolateral medulla of the rat does not correspond to the A1 catecholamine cell group. *Brain Res.,* 279: 299 – 302.

Dembowsky, K., Lackner, K., Czachurski, J. and Seller, H. (1981) Tonic catecholaminergic inhibition of the spinal somato-sympathetic reflexes originating in the ventrolateral medulla oblongata. *J. Auton. Nerv. Syst.,* 3: 277 – 290.

Dembowsky, K., Czachurski, J. and Seller, H. (1985) An intracellular study of the synaptic input to sympathetic preganglionic neurones of the third thoracic segment of the cat. *J. Auton. Nerv. Syst.* 13: 201 – 244.

Dembowsky, K., Czachurski, J. and Seller, H. (1986) Baroreceptor induced disfacilitation and postsynaptic inhibition in sympathetic preganglionic neurones of the cat. *Pflügers Arch.,* 406: R24.

Feldberg, W. and Guertzenstein, P.G. (1986) Blood pressure effects of leptazol applied to the ventral surface of the brain stem of cats. *J. Physiol. (Lond.),* 372: 445 – 456.

Gordon, F.J. and McCann, L.A. (1988) Pressor responses evoked by microinjections of L-glutamate into the caudal ventrolateral medulla of the rat. *Brain Res.,* 457: 251 – 258.

Granata, A.R., Kumada, M. and Reis, D.J. (1985) Sympathoinhibition by A1-noradrenergic neurons is mediated by neurons in the C1 area of the rostral medulla. *J. Auton. Nerv. Syst.,* 14: 387 – 395.

Granata, A.R., Numao, Y., Kumada, M. and Reis, D.J. (1986) A1 noradrenergic neurons tonically inhibit sympathoexcitatory neurons of C1 area in rat brainstem. *Brain Res.,* 377: 127 – 146.

Kalia, M.P. (1981) Anatomical organization of central respiratory neurons. *Ann. Rev. Physiol.,* 43: 105 – 120.

Katona, P.G., Dembowsky, K., Czachurski, J. and Seller, H. (1989) Chemoreceptor stimulation on sympathetic activity:

dependence on respiratory phase. *Am. J. Physiol.* (in press).

Loewy, A.D. and Neil, J.J. (1981) The role of descending monoaminergic systems in the central control of blood pressure. *Fed. Proc.,* 40: 2778 – 2785.

McAllen, R.M. (1986a) Location of neurones with cardiovascular and respiratory function, at the ventral surface of the cat's medulla. *Neuroscience,* 18: 43 – 49.

McAllen, R.M. (1986b) Identification and properties of sub-retrofacial bulbospinal neurones: a descending cardiovascular pathway in the cat. *J. Auton. Nerv. Syst.,* 17: 151 – 164.

McCall, R.B., Schuette, M.R., Humphrey, S.J., Lahti, R.A. and Barsuhn, C. (1983) Evidence for a central sympathoexcitatory action of alpha-2 adrenergic antagonists. *J. Pharmacol. Exp. Ther.,* 224: 501 – 507.

McCrimmon, D.R., Feldman, J.L. and Speck, D.F. (1986a) Respiratory motoneuronal activity is altered by injections of picomoles of glutamate into cat brain stem. *J. Neurosci.,* 6: 2384 – 2392.

McCrimmon, D.R., Feldman, J.L., Speck, D.F., Ellenberger, H.H. and Smith, J.C. (1986b) Functional heterogeneity of dorsal, ventral, and pontine respiratory groups revealed by micropharmacological techniques. In C. von Euler and H. Lagercrantz (Eds.), *Neurobiology of the Control of Breathing,* Raven Press, New York, pp. 201 – 208.

McKellar, S. and Loewy, A.D. (1982) Efferent projections of the A1 catecholamine cell group in the rat: an autoradiographic study. *Brain Res.,* 241: 11 – 29.

Millhorn, D.E., Hökfelt, T., Seroogy, K., Oertel, W., Verhofstad, A.A.J. and Wu, J.-Y. (1987) Immunohistochemical evidence for colocalization of γ-aminobutyric acid and serotonin in neurons of the ventral medulla oblongata projecting to the spinal cord. *Brain Res.,* 410: 179 – 185.

Pilowsky, P., West, M. and Chalmers, J. (1985) Renal sympathetic nerve response to stimulation, inhibition and destruction of the ventrolateral medulla in the rabbit. *Neurosci. Lett.,* 60: 51 – 55.

Remmers, J.E., Richter, D.W., Ballantyne, D., Bainton, C.R. and Klein, J.P. (1986) Reflex prolongation of stage I expiration. *Pflügers Arch.,* 407: 190 – 198.

Richter, D.W. (1982) Generation and maintenance of the respiratory rhythm. *J. Exp. Biol.,* 100: 93 – 107.

Sun, M.-K. and Guyenet, P.G. (1986) Effect of clonidine and γ-aminobutyric acid on the discharges of medullo-spinal sympathoexcitatory neurons in the rat. *Brain Res.,* 368: 1 – 17.

Willette, R.N., Barcas, P.P., Krieger, A.J. and Sapru, H.N. (1983) Vasopressor and depressor areas in the rat medulla. Identification by microinjection of L-glutamate. *Neuropharmacology,* 22: 1071 – 1079.

Willette, R.N., Punnen, S., Krieger, A.J. and Sapru, H.N. (1984) Interdependence of rostral and caudal ventrolateral medullary areas in the control of blood pressure. *Brain Res.,* 321: 169 – 174.

J. Ciriello, M.M. Caverson and C. Polosa (Eds.)
Progress in Brain Research, Vol. 81
© 1989 Elsevier Science Publishers B.V. (Biomedical Division)

CHAPTER 11

A glutamate mechanism in the intermediolateral nucleus mediates sympathoexcitatory responses to stimulation of the rostral ventrolateral medulla

Shaun F. Morrison, Paul Ernsberger, Teresa A. Milner, Janie Callaway, Anson Gong and Donald J. Reis

Division of Neurobiology, Department of Neurology and Neuroscience, Cornell University Medical College, 411 E. 69th Street, New York, NY 10021, U.S.A.

Introduction

The rostral ventrolateral medulla (RVL) contains a population of reticulospinal, sympathoexcitatory neurons (Brown and Guyenet, 1984; Barman and Gebber, 1985; Morrison et al., 1988). Regulation of the discharge of RVL-spinal vasomotor neurons by afferent pathways to the RVL underlies many of the reflex adjustments of the circulation in response to peripheral and central stimuli (Granata et al., 1985; Sun and Guyenet, 1986; Morrison and Reis, 1988). While vasomotor neurons of the RVL are presumed to exert their sympathoexcitatory effects over pathways terminating in the intermediolateral nucleus (IML) of the thoracolumbar spinal cord, little is known of the role played by specific spinal transmitter systems in mediating the increases in sympathetic nerve activity evoked by RVL neuronal discharge.

In the present studies, we combined electrophysiological, immunocytochemical and receptor autoradiographic techniques to test the hypothesis that an excitatory amino acid is the "fast" transmitter implicated in RVL-evoked excitation of sympathetic preganglionic neurons (SPNs). Our results suggest that RVL stimulation causes the release of glutamate from nerve terminals in the IML which interacts with glutamate receptors of

the kainate subtype to excite SPNs, thereby producing an increase in sympathetic nerve activity and arterial pressure.

Glutamate receptor antagonist blocks the SPN response to RVL stimulation

The ubiquity of excitatory amino acid neurotransmission in the central nervous system has only recently been recognized with the development of specific antagonists for glutamate-activated receptors. Glutamate receptors can be divided into the NMDA, the quisqualate, the kainate, and the calcium/chloride-dependent receptor (Foster and Fagg, 1984). In general, glutamate-induced depolarization of neurons exhibits a rapid onset and time course and is accompanied by a decrease in neuronal input resistance due to the opening of cation channels (Mayer and Westbrook, 1987).

A number of highly selective antagonists have been developed for the NMDA receptor, but not for the other glutamate receptor subtypes. Therefore, to determine if the RVL-evoked excitation of SPNs is mediated through activation of a specific class of glutamate receptors, we compared the amplitude of these responses during application of the broad spectrum glutamate receptor antagonist, kynurenic acid, with those elicited during applica-

160

tion of the selective NMDA receptor blockers, D-2,5-phosphonovaleric acid (APV) and ketamine.

The RVL-evoked responses of SPNs, the axons of which project to the splanchnic nerve, were studied in Sprague-Dawley rats anesthetized with an intraperitoneal injection of urethane (800 mg/kg) followed by i.v. administration of chloralose (70 mg/kg). The details of the surgical and recording procedures have been described (Morrison et al., 1988). Animals were placed in a stereotaxic apparatus and spinal investigation unit (David Kopf Instruments) with the bite bar 11 mm below the intraural line and the spinal clamp on the T8 and T9 vertebral processes. An occipital craniotomy and T5–T7 laminectomy were performed. Animals were paralyzed, artificially respirated and pneumothoracotomized.

The action potentials of SPNs were recorded extracellularly with the center barrel (2 M NaCl, 2–6 MΩ at 1000 Hz) of multibarrel glass micropipettes. The SPNs contributing to the splanchnic nerve were antidromically identified with stimuli (500 μA, 1 msec, 0.5 Hz) applied to the central end of the cut splanchnic nerve. In some experiments, the activity of splanchnic nerve bundles was recorded with bipolar platinum hook electrodes.

Bipolar concentric electrodes were used to deliver single or twin stimuli (50–400 μA, 1 msec) to the RVL. The stimulating electrode was positioned 300 μm caudal to the caudal pole of the facial nucleus, the region corresponding to the rostral pole of the C1 adrenergic cell group which contains a concentration of vasomotor neurons that project to the spinal cord (Brown and Guyenet, 1984; Morrison et al., 1988). With respect to the calamus scriptorius, the stimulation site was approximately 2.6 mm rostral, 2.0 mm lateral, and 2.4 mm ventral.

Kynurenic acid (Sigma, 200 mM, pH 8) and APV (Cambridge Research Biochemicals, 50 mM, pH 8) were iontophoretically applied to individual SPNs from the side barrels of multi-barrel micropipettes. Retaining currents of 5–10 nA were applied between ejection periods. One side barrel contained 2 M NaCl for current balancing.

Ketamine (Parke-Davis, 2 mg/kg) was administered intravenously.

Post-stimulus time averages and histograms of the RVL-evoked discharge of the splanchnic nerve and of SPNs, respectively, were computed using a Dell 286 computer with a Tecmar A/D board and ASYST software. Response histograms were analyzed to determine the response ratio (spikes/stimulus) of the SPNs. The significance of changes in the response ratio during drug administration was determined with the paired Student's t-test.

The response of the splanchnic nerve to single stimuli applied to the RVL consisted of an early and a late excitation (Fig. 1). The mean (± S.E.M.) onset latency of the early excitation was 33 ± 3 msec (n = 6). The peak increase in splanchnic nerve activity occurred 64 ± 2 msec and 160 ± 4 msec following RVL stimulation. These latencies correspond closely to the estimated spinal conduction times (plus peripheral conduction time) of the two populations of spinally-projecting, vasomotor neurons in the RVL (Brown

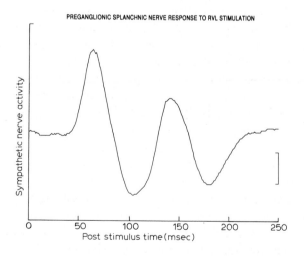

Fig. 1. Average response recorded from a splanchnic nerve bundle following 20 stimuli (100 μA, 1 msec, 0.5 Hz) applied to the region of the RVL containing reticulospinal, vasomotor neurons. Note the biphasic excitation. Bin width is 1 msec, calibration is 15 μV.

and Guyenet, 1984; Morrison et al., 1988). This finding suggests that the early and late peaks in the splanchnic nerve response to RVL stimulation arise from the activation of the rapidly and slowly conducting groups of RVL-spinal neurons, respectively.

To examine the RVL-evoked responses of individual SPNs, the IML of the seventh and eighth thoracic segments was explored for neurons that responded antidromically to stimuli applied to the splanchnic nerve. Figure 2A shows the antidromic response of an IML neuron to splanchnic nerve stimulation. Figure 2B illustrates the collision test. The antidromic onset latencies of 38 SPNs ranged from 8 to 46 msec and corresponded to a mean conduction velocity of 1 m/sec.

Spontaneously active SPNs (approximately 40%) had mean firing rates that rarely exceeded 5 Hz and responded to single RVL stimuli with single action potentials. Response ratios (evoked action potentials per stimulus) were approximately 1.0. Nearly half of the responsive neurons were excited with a short latency (mean: 25 msec) following RVL stimulation (Fig. 3A). One quarter of the responsive neurons exhibited a long latency (mean: 110 msec) response (Fig. 3B), while the remaining 25% were excited with both short and long latencies corresponding to those of the SPNs with unimodal response latencies.

The iontophoretic application of kynurenate (15 – 100 nA) blocked both the short (Fig. 4) and long latency (not shown) excitation following RVL stimulation. Prior to kynurenate iontophoresis, every RVL stimulus evoked at least one action potential from this SPN (Fig. 4A), yielding a response ratio of 1.08. Within 30 sec of applying kynurenate (60 nA), the same RVL stimuli only occasionally produced a response in the SPN (Fig. 4B), reducing the response ratio to 0.12. Similar results were obtained during iontophoresis of kynurenate onto SPNs which responded to RVL stimulation either at the long latency only, or at both the short and long latencies. These data suggest that the RVL-evoked excitation of SPNs is mediated by an excitatory amino acid transmitter

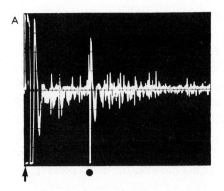

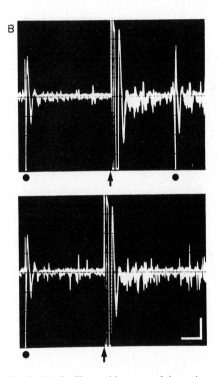

Fig. 2. (A) Oscillographic traces of the action potential evoked in a neuron in the intermediolateral nucleus of the seventh thoracic segment by stimuli (200 μA, 1 msec duration) applied to the splanchnic nerve. Note that the responses occurred at a constant onset latency (36 msec). (B) Collision test demonstrating antidromic activation. Neuron responds (upper panel) to splanchnic nerve stimuli when they are presented at least 43 msec (critical delay) after spontaneous spikes, but fails (lower panel) when the interval is less than 43 msec. Thus, the critical delay is approximately equal to the onset latency plus the axonal refractory period (6 msec), satisfying the collision test criteria. Arrows indicate splanchnic nerve stimuli, dots indicate extracellular action potentials. Vertical calibration is 200 μV, horizontal calibration is 10 msec.

162

activating a glutamate receptor in the SPN membrane.

To characterize the glutamate receptor subtype involved in the SPN response to RVL stimulation, we tested the effects of selective NMDA receptor antagonists on the RVL-evoked excitation of SPNs. Neither iontophoretic application of APV (20–100 nA), nor i.v. administration of ketamine (Fig. 5) was effective in blocking the excitation of SPNs. Ketamine did not alter the mean onset laten-

cy of the response (19 msec; Fig. 5A,B), nor was the response ratio significantly different before (0.95, Fig. 5A) and after (1.05, Fig. 5B) ketamine. On the basis of these results, it is unlikely that blockade of glutamate receptors of the NMDA subtype underlies the kynurenate antagonism of the RVL-evoked activation of SPNs. Rather, these data are consistent with an SPN excitation mediated by either a kainate or quisqualate receptor mechanism.

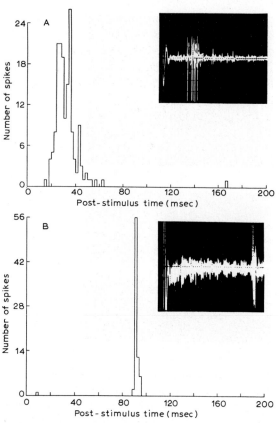

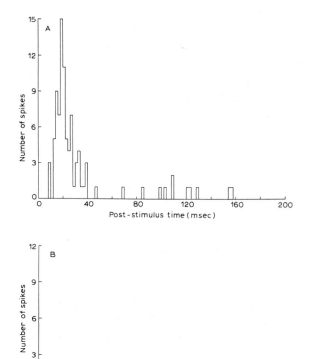

Fig. 3. Responses of two splanchnic preganglionic neurons (SPN) to single RVL stimuli. (A) Five superimposed oscillographic traces (inset) of the RVL-evoked action potentials of an SPN with a short response latency. Post-stimulus time histogram of the SPN response to 200 RVL stimuli (200 μA, 1 msec duration, 0.5 Hz), response ratio is 0.82. Mean latency is 30 msec, bin width is 2 msec. (B) Similar to (A) for a splanchnic SPN with a long response latency. Histogram constructed from 80 RVL stimuli (350 μA, 1 msec, 0.5 msec), response ratio is 0.96. Mean latency is 90 msec, bin width is 2 msec.

Fig. 4. Effect of iontophoretically applied kynurenate on the RVL-evoked response of a splanchnic SPN with a short response latency. (A) Post-stimulus time histogram of the SPN responses to 60 RVL stimuli (150 μA, 1 msec, 0.5 Hz) under control conditions. Mean latency is 29 msec, response ratio is 1.08, bin width is 2 ms. (B) Similar to (A) during kynurenate (200 mM) iontophoresis (60 nA), 60 RVL stimuli, response ratio is reduced to 0.12.

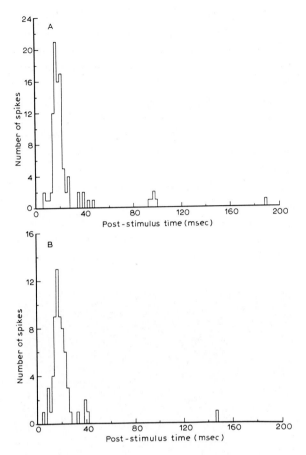

Fig. 5. Effect of intravenously administered ketamine on the RVL-evoked response of a splanchnic SPN with a short response latency. (A) Post-stimulus time histogram of the SPN responses to 100 RVL stimuli (300 μA, 1 msec. 0.5 Hz) under control conditions. Mean latency is 19 msec, response ratio is 0.95, bin width is 2 msec. (B) Similar to (A) following i.v. ketamine (2 mg/kg), 60 RVL stimuli, response ratio is 1.05.

The close correspondence between the orthodromic latencies of the SPN responses and the antidromic conduction velocities of reticulospinal, sympathoexcitatory neurons in the C1 region of the RVL (Brown and Guyenet, 1984; Morrison et al., 1988) suggests that the SPN excitation arose from stimulation of the RVL-spinal neurons whose descending excitatory input to the IML is known to play a critical role in the maintenance of basal sympathetic tone and arterial pressure (Ross et al., 1984).

Our findings are in agreement with results of Nishi et al. (1987) who demonstrated that both the fast excitatory post-synaptic potential (EPSP) evoked in SPNs by focal stimulation in cat spinal cord slices in vitro and the depolarization produced by glutamate superfusion were not affected by the application of APV which eliminated NMDA-induced depolarizations. In contrast, Mo and Dun (1987) suggest that the dorsal root stimulus-evoked responses of SPNs in neonatal rat spinal cord slices are mediated by NMDA-receptor activation. The present study also supports the observation of Guyenet et al. (1987) that intrathecal kynurenic acid application reduces the activation of lumbar sympathetic nerve following RVL stimulation. Our results suggest that this effect was produced by an action of kynurenic acid directly on SPNs, and that it involved blockade of either kainate or quisqualate receptor subtypes.

Localization of glutamate immunoreactivity in the IML

Recently developed antisera against glutamate have been used for the immunocytochemical localization of this excitatory amino acid in the central nervous system and in sensory ganglia (Ottersen and Storm-Mathisen, 1983; Hepler et al., 1988). In addition to its role as a putative neurotransmitter, however, glutamate is also used by cells within the brain for many metabolic functions. This fact precludes the identification of glutamatergic neurons solely on the basis of their staining for glutamate. In contrast, localization of glutamate immunoreactivity in axon terminals is indicative of the transmitter pool of glutamate, and suggests that glutamate may be released at synapses in which the presynaptic element is labelled. Thus, to identify the anatomical substrate underlying the kynurenic acid blockade of the RVL-evoked excitation of SPNs, we sought to determine if glutamate could be immunocytochemically localized in axon terminals within the IML.

Following anesthesia with pentobarbital (50 mg/kg, i.p.), male Sprague-Dawley rats were perfused with 4% paraformaldehyde in 0.1 M phosphate buffer (pH 7.4), the upper thoracic spinal cord was removed and postfixed for 8 – 12 h. Frozen (light microscopy) or vibratome (electron microscopy) sections were immunocytochemically labelled with a polyclonal antiserum to hemocyanin-conjugated glutamate (Hepler et al., 1988) using the method of Sternberger (1979), as modified by Pickel (1981).

For electron microscopy, glutamate immunocytochemistry was followed by further fixation of the sections in glutaraldehyde (1% in 0.1 M phosphate buffer, 20 min). The sections were then prepared for electron microscopy according to the procedure of Pickel (1981). The final preparations were examined with a Philips 201 electron microscope.

Tissue from the four animals with the best immunocytochemical labelling and preservation of ultrastructural morphology were used in the quantitative analysis. From each animal, at least 12 grids containing 3 – 6 thin (50 nm) sections were collected from the surface of three or more plastic-embedded vibratome sections. All labelled profiles within one section from each grid were photographed for analysis.

Low levels of glutamate-like immunoreactivity (GLU-LI) were found in cells throughout the grey matter of the thoracic spinal cord (Fig. 6). In contrast, GLU-LI was concentrated in neuronal processes in the superficial layers of the dorsal horn and in the IML, where it almost completely envelopes the SPN perikarya and their processes extending into the lateral funiculus. GLU-LI in sections of thoracic spinal cord was eliminated by preincubation of the antibody with low concentrations (130 μg/ml) of glutamate, but not aspartate. In addition, GLU-LI in the IML, but not in the dorsal horn could be greatly reduced by chronic transection of the spinal cord at a rostral segment. These results suggest that the antibody is specifically recognizing glutamate in the IML and that GLU-LI in the IML is dependent on descending inputs.

Ultrastructural examination of the IML revealed that under the fixation conditions used in these experiments, GLU-LI was localized primarily in lightly myelinated axons and in axon terminals. Terminals containing GLU-LI formed synaptic associations with dendritic processes (Fig. 7). The majority (59% of 105) of the synaptic contacts were asymmetric. Moreover, most (71% of 105) contacts occurred on the shafts of small (0.5 – 1.5 μm) dendrites. However, terminals with GLU-LI also formed symmetric contacts on the perikarya and processes of IML neurons. Asymmetric (Gray type I) synapses are thought to mediate excitation, based largely on the detection of enriched populations of thickened post-synaptic densities in re-

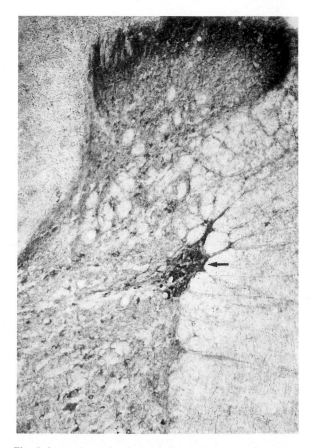

Fig. 6. Immunocytochemical labelling of a coronal section through the third thoracic spinal segment with an antibody to hemocyanin-conjugated glutamate. Glutamate-like immunoreactivity is concentrated in the superficial layers of the dorsal horn and in the sympathetic intermediolateral nucleus (arrow).

gions of the brain containing higher proportions of excitatory synapses. Similarly, symmetric (Gray type II) contacts are considered indicative of inhibitory synapses (Uchizono, 1965; Cohen et al., 1982).

The localization of GLU-LI in synaptic vesicles within axon terminals making asymmetric contacts with the dendrites of IML neurons suggests that glutamate could be released at excitatory synapses within the IML. This finding is consistent with the electrophysiological evidence described above indicating that the sympathoexcitation of RVL origin is mediated by release of an excitatory amino acid onto SPNs. Whether axon terminals containing GLU-LI also contain PNMT, and whether they synapse directly on SPNs remain to be determined.

The finding that some terminals containing GLU-LI made symmetric (inhibitory) synapses with dendrites of IML neurons is paradoxical. These instances may, however, have been dependent on the plane of ultrathin sectioning. In this regard, if a section were taken near the edge of an asymmetric synapse, the axodendritic contact might appear to be symmetric due to poorly developed post-synaptic density. This possibility will be investigated further by following such synaptic contacts in serial sections.

Autoradiographic visualization of glutamate receptors of the kainate subtype in the IML

The question arises as to which of the glutamate receptor subtypes mediates the excitation of SPNs.

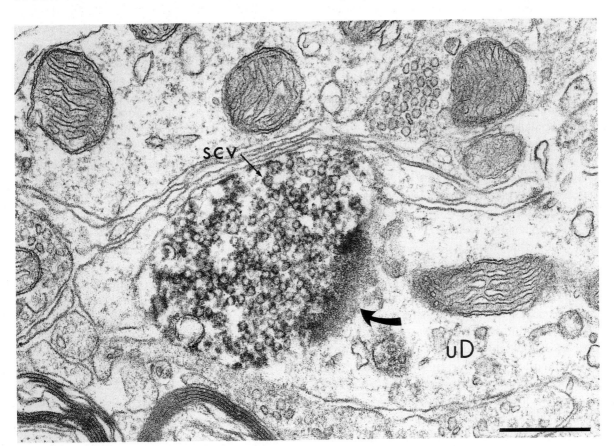

Fig. 7. Axon terminal containing glutamate-like immunoreactivity surrounding small clear vesicles (scv) forms an asymmetric (excitatory) synapse (arrow) on a distal dendrite (uD) of a neuron in the intermediolateral nucleus of the third thoracic spinal segment.

The in vivo electrophysiological data described earlier (p. 159) appear to rule out NMDA receptors, since the excitatory response of SPNs was not blocked by the potent and selective NMDA antagonists APV and ketamine. Furthermore, receptor autoradiographic studies have demonstrated that NMDA receptors in the spinal cord are almost entirely confined to superficial layers of the dorsal horn (Monaghan and Cotman, 1985). These findings suggest that the glutamatergic excitation of SPNs is mediated by a non-NMDA receptor.

RVL-evoked excitation of SPNs was completely and potently antagonized by kynurenic acid, which blocks kainate receptors with the greatest potency but also affects the quisqualate and NMDA subtypes at higher doses. Furthermore, the presence of kainate receptors on SPNs in the IML is suggested by the finding that one to two orders of magnitude lower doses of kainate than of glutamate were required to excite SPNs iontophoretically (data not shown). Therefore, we sought to determine whether kainate receptors in the IML can be visualized and characterized using receptor autoradiography.

Male Sprague-Dawley rats 10 – 12 weeks of age were anesthetized with pentobarbital (35 mg/kg) and perfused intracardially with 50 ml oxygenated Krebs' buffer at 20°C followed by 100 ml ice-cold sucrose (265 mM) buffered with 50 mM Hepes (pH 7.0). The thoracic spinal cord was rapidly removed, frozen in boiling Freon ($-25°C$), and stored at $-70°C$. Lengths of spinal cord were mounted on microtome chucks with mounting medium (Lipshaw M-1) and sectioned at 12 μm on a cryostat (Hacker). Sections were thaw-mounted onto glass slides precoated with 1% gelatin, dried in a vacuum desiccator for 1 h, and stored at $-20°C$ for 2 – 5 days to allow adhesion to the slide before being stored at $-70°C$ for up to 3 weeks.

[^{3}H]Kainate autoradiography was performed by an extensive modification of the methods of Unnerstall and Wamsley (1983) using techniques previously established in our laboratory (Ernsberger et al., 1988a,b,c). Slide-mounted sections of rat thoracic spinal cord were warmed to room temperature in a vacuum desiccator to prevent condensation, and preincubated for 15 min in Coplin jars containing 265 mM sucrose buffered with 50 mM Tris-acetate (pH 7.1) to which 0.5 mM EDTA had been added to remove endogenous glutamate and divalent cations, which inhibit [^{3}H]kainate binding (Braitman and Coyle, 1987). The sections were further preincubated in sucrose/Tris-acetate without EDTA for 15 min on ice, then incubated with 5 nM [^{3}H]kainate for 2 h on ice. Nonspecific binding was determined in adjacent sections incubated in parallel with 1 mM L-glutamate.

To remove unbound radioligand while minimizing dissociation of receptor-bound label, sections were washed in buffer for 2 min, dipped in distilled water to remove buffer salts, and briefly dipped in 2.5% glutaraldehyde in acetone. This latter step has been shown to speed the drying of sections, thus minimizing the diffusion of radioligand away from the receptor site, without altering binding characteristics (Greenamyre et al., 1984). In preliminary experiments, the glutaraldehyde/acetone rinse reduced nonspecific binding by 3-fold (59 ± 8 dpm/section versus 190 ± 60 dpm/section, $n = 2$). In initial experiments to characterize rat spinal cord [^{3}H]kainate binding, sections were wiped from the slide with a glass fiber filter (Whatman GF/B) following the glutaraldehyde/acetone rinse, placed in a scintillation vial, covered with cocktail (Beckman Ready-Solv) and counted at 50% efficiency.

Specific [^{3}H]kainate binding to slide-mounted spinal cord sections increased rapidly with increasing time of incubation ($t_{1/2}$ of approximately 40 min). The equilibrium binding kinetics of [^{3}H]kainate were determined by progressively increasing apparent radioligand concentration from 0.6 to 100 nM by isotopic dilution. Computerized nonlinear curve-fitting analysis (Munson and Rodbard, 1980) using six ligand concentrations revealed that kainate bound to a high density of specific saturable sites (B_{max} = 4.6 ± 0.8 fmol/section) in thoracic spinal cord sections with a high affinity (K_d = 12 ± 4 nM). L-Glutamate potently and completely inhibited specific [³H]kainate binding (IC$_{50}$ = 2.2 μM, n = 2).

For autoradiography, the sections were further dried after the glutaraldehyde/acetone rinse under a stream of cold air dehumidified by a gas-drying apparatus (Driaire Corp.) and then stored in a vacuum desiccator at 4°C for 48 h. Dried sections were arranged in an X-ray film cassette and apposed to tritium-sensitive film (Amersham Hyperfilm). After an exposure of 8 – 10 weeks at 4°C under low humidity, the film was developed for 4 min (Kodak D-19), fixed for 5 min, and rinsed in running water of 30 min. Prints were prepared directly from the autoradiogram, using it as a negative.

Autoradiograms of sections labelled with [³H]kainate showed a discrete distribution of autoradiographic grains, as shown in Fig. 8. Very high grain densities are localized over the laminae I and II of the dorsal horn, while the more ventral laminae III and IV are more sparsely labelled. A small compact cluster of grains is typically associated with the IML, indicating that the IML contains a higher density of kainate receptors than the surrounding spinal laminae or the ventral horn. A secondary accumulation of grains is also found over the intermediomedial column surrounding the

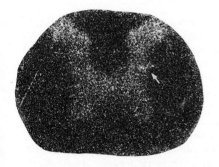

Fig. 8. Autoradiogram of [³H]kainate binding to glutamate receptors of the kainate subtype in the thoracic spinal cord of the rat. The section was incubated with 5 nM [³H]kainate for 2 h, rinsed, dried, and exposed to tritium-sensitive film for 10 weeks. The densest accumulation of grains overlies the superficial layers of the dorsal horn, while the white matter is indistinguishable from background. Note the discrete aggregation of grains over the IML, particularly on the right side (arrow).

central canal, which has also been implicated in the control of SPN discharge.

The present study is the first to map the distribution of glutamate receptors of the kainate subtype within the thoracic spinal cord. The two previous autoradiographic studies of [³H]kainate binding sites have either examined the cervical cord alone (Monaghan and Cotman, 1982) or excluded the spinal cord altogether (Unnerstall and Wamsley, 1983). Greenamyre and colleagues (1984) described [³H]glutamate binding sites in the thoracic cord, but they did not distinguish between glutamate receptor subtypes nor did they identify the IML or the intermediomedial column.

The K_d for [³H]kainate binding to slide-mounted sections of thoracic spinal cord in the present study agrees with the high-affinity component of [³H]kainate binding to striatal sections reported by Unnerstall and Wamsley (1983) (12 nM in both cases), but the K_d reported by Monaghan and Cotman (1982) was more than 5-fold higher. The IC$_{50}$ for L-glutamate reported here (2 μM) agrees reasonably well with that reported by Unnerstall and Wamsley (1983) (0.8 μM). These findings indicate that [³H]kainate binding sites in the thoracic spinal cord closely resemble those in the forebrain. Furthermore, under the present experimental conditions, high-affinity [³H]kainate sites were labelled, but not the low-affinity sites described in other studies (Monaghan and Cotman, 1982; Unnerstall and Wamsley, 1983; Foster and Fagg, 1984). This presumably reflects the relatively low radioligand concentration (5 nM) and the removal with EDTA of endogenous divalent cations, which selectively inhibit high-affinity binding (Braitman and Coyle, 1987).

The pattern of glutamatergic innervation, as revealed by GLU-LI, closely corresponded to the distribution of kainate receptors. Both GLU-LI and [³H]kainate binding were concentrated in the superficial laminae of the dorsal horn and in the IML. This extensive co-localization of GLU-LI and [³H]kainate binding sites is consistent with the proposal that kainate receptors are specific to glutamatergic synapses (Foster et al., 1981; Foster and Fagg, 1984). Subcellular fractionation studies show that [³H]kainate binding sites are enriched 20-fold in synaptic junctions containing post-synaptic densities (Foster et al., 1981). In the present study, asymmetric synapses with post-synaptic densities were associated with axon terminals containing GLU-LI. Thus, the distributions of GLU-LI and kainate receptors also appear to correspond at the subcellular level as well as at the level of regional organization. This correspondence is consistent with the finding that glutamate is the sole endogenous ligand for [³H]kainate receptors (Riveros and Orrego, 1982).

Although a strong relationship between transmitter and receptor distributions would appear to be an expected outcome, Herkenham (1987) has contended that "close transmitter/receptor matches are the exception rather than the rule for most well-characterized neurochemical systems". This conclusion was largely based on comparison of immunohistochemical and receptor autoradiographic studies reported by different authors. In our laboratory, we have recently shown strong correlations (r values ranging from 0.7 to 0.9) between the distribution of choline acetyltransferase, the synthetic enzyme for acetylcholine, and muscarinic acetylcholine receptor density (Ernsberger et al., 1988b). The present study now demonstrates a close correspondence between the distribution of glutamate and its receptors in the spinal cord. It is possible that major discrepancies between the localization of transmitters and their receptors may be widespread in other systems, while "fast" neurotransmitters such as acetylcholine and glutamate are closely colocalized with their receptors.

Kainate receptors may contribute significantly to the regulation of the neuronal activity of SPNs in the IML. The small number of cells contained within the IML, the relatively high density of [³H]kainate binding therein, and the strength of kainate receptor-mediated excitatory responses serve to amplify the importance of this small glutamatergic receptive field. Thus, although the total absolute amount of [³H]kainate binding

localized to the IML is relatively small, it nonetheless may be of considerable physiological importance.

Acknowledgements

The authors wish to thank Drs. P. Petrusz and A. Rustioni (Department of Anatomy and Physiology, University of North Carolina at Chapel Hill) for the use of their glutamate antibody and J. Orefice for production of the illustrations. This research was supported by National Institutes of Health Grants HL 18974 and NS 22721.

References

Barman, S.M. and Gebber, G.L. (1985) Axonal projection patterns of ventrolateral medullospinal sympathoexcitatory neurons. *J. Neurophysiol.*, 53: 1551 – 1566.

Braitman, D.J. and Coyle, J.T. (1987) Inhibition of ³H-kainate acid receptor binding by divalent cations correlates with ion affinity for the calcium channel. *Neuropharmacology*, 26: 1247 – 1251.

Brown, D.L. and Guyenet, P.G. (1984) Cardiovascular neurons of brain stem with projections to spinal cord. *Am. J. Physiol.*, 247: R1009 – R1016.

Cohen, R.S., Carlin, R.K., Grab, D.J. and Sukevitz, P. (1982) Phosphoproteins in postsynaptic densities. In W.H. Gispen and A. Routtenberg (Eds.), *Brain Phosphoproteins, Progress in Brain Research, Vol. 56*, Elsevier, Amsterdam, pp. 49 – 76.

Cravo, S., Ruggiero, D.A., Anwar, M. and Reis, D.J. (1988) Quantitative-topographic analysis of adrenergic and non-adrenergic spinal projections of cardiovascular area of RVL. *Soc. Neurosci. Abstr.*, 14: 328.

Ernsberger, P., Arango, V. and Reis, D.J. (1988a) A high density of muscarinic receptors in the ventrolateral medulla of the rat is revealed by correction for autoradiographic efficiency. *Neurosci. Lett.*, 85: 179 – 186.

Ernsberger, P., Arneric, S.P., Arango, V. and Reis, D.J. (1988b) Quantitative distribution of muscarinic receptors and choline acetyltransferase in rat medulla: examination of transmitter-receptor mismatch. *Brain Res.*, 452: 336 – 344.

Ernsberger, P., Feinland, G., Meeley, M.P. and Reis, D.J. (1988c) Characterization and visualization of clonidine-sensitive imidazole sites in rat kidney which recognize clonidine-displacing substance. *Am. J. Hypertension* (in press).

Foster, A.C. and Fagg, G.E. (1984) Acidic amino acid binding sites in mammalian neuronal membranes: their characteristics and relationship to synaptic receptors. *Brain Res. Rev.*, 7: 103 – 164.

Foster, A.C., Mena, E.E., Monaghan, D.T. and Cotman, C.W. (1981) Synaptic localization of kainic acid binding sites. *Nature*, 289: 73 – 75.

Granata, A.R., Ruggiero, D.A., Park, D.H., Joh, T.H. and Reis, D.J. (1985) Brain stem area with C1 epinephrine neurons mediates baroreflex vasodepressor responses. *Am. J. Physiol.*, 248: H547 – H567.

Greenamyre, J.T., Young, A.B. and Penney, J.B. (1984) Quantitative autoradiographic distribution of L-^{3}H-glutamate binding sites in rat central nervous system. *J. Neurosci.*, 4: 2133 – 2144.

Guyenet, P.G. and Cabot, J.B. (1981) Inhibition of sympathetic preganglionic neurons by catecholamines and clonidine: mediation by an alpha-adrenergic receptor. *J. Neurosci.*, 1: 908 – 917.

Guyenet, P.G., Sun, M-K. and Les Brown, D. (1987) Role of GABA and excitatory amino acids in medullary baroreflex pathways. In J. Ciriello, F.R. Calaresu, L.P. Renaud and C. Polosa (Eds.), *Organization of the Autonomic Nervous System: Central and Peripheral Mechanisms*, Alan R. Liss, New York, pp. 215 – 225.

Hepler, J.R., Toomim, C.S., McCarthy, K.D., Conti, F., Battaglia, G., Rustioni, A. and Petrusz, P. (1988) Characterization of antisera to glutamate and aspartate. *J. Histochem. Cytochem.*, 36: 13 – 22.

Herkenham, M. (1987) Mismatches between neurotransmitter and receptor localizations in brain: observations and implications. *Neuroscience*, 23: 1 – 38.

Mayer, M.L. and Westbrook, G.L. (1987) The physiology of excitatory amino acids in the vertebrate central nervous system. *Prog. Neurobiol.*, 28: 197 – 276.

Milner, T.A., Morrison, S.F., Abate, C. and Reis, D.J. (1988) Phenylethanolamine *N*-methyltransferase-containing terminals synapse directly on sympathetic preganglionic neurons in the rat. *Brain Res.*, 448: 205 – 222.

Mo, N. and Dun, N.J. (1987) Excitatory postsynaptic potentials in neonatal rat sympathetic preganglionic neurons: possible mediation by NMDA receptors. *Neurosci. Lett.*, 77: 327 – 332.

Monaghan, D.T. and Cotman, C.W. (1982) The distribution of ^{3}H-kainic acid binding sites in rat CNS as determined by autoradiography. *Brain Res.*, 252: 91 – 100.

Monaghan, D.T. and Cotman, C.W. (1985) Distribution of *N*-methyl-D-aspartate-sensitive L-^{3}H-glutamate binding sites in rat brain. *J. Neurosci.*, 5: 2909 – 2919.

Morrison, S.F. and Reis, D.J. (1989) Reticulospinal vasomotor neurons in the RVL mediate the somatosympathetic reflex. *Am. J. Physiol.*, 256: R1084 – R1097.

Morrison, S.F., Milner, T.A. and Reis, D.J. (1988) Reticulospinal vasomotor neurons of the rat rostral ven-

trolateral medulla: relationship to sympathetic nerve activity and the C1 adrenergic cell group. *J. Neurosci.*, 8: 1286 – 1301.

Munson, P.J. and Rodbard, D. (1980) LIGAND: a versatile computerized approach for characterization of ligand binding systems. *Anal. Biochem.*, 107: 220 – 239.

Nishi, S., Yoshimura, M. and Polosa, C. (1987) Synaptic potentials and putative transmitter actions in sympathetic preganglionic neurons. In J. Ciriello, F.R. Calaresu, L.P. Renaud and C. Polosa (Eds.), *Organization of the Autonomic Nervous System: Central and Peripheral Mechanisms*, Alan R. Liss, New York, pp. 15 – 26.

Ottersen, O.P. and Storm-Mathisen, J. (1984) Glutamate- and GABA-containing neurons in the mouse and rat brain, as demonstrated with a new immunocytochemical technique. *J. Comp. Neurol.*, 229: 374 – 392.

Pickel, V.M. (1981) Immunocytochemical methods. In L. Heimer and M.J. Robards (Eds.), *Neuroanatomical Tract Tracing Methods*, Plenum Publ. Co., New York, pp. 483 – 509.

Riveros, N. and Orrego, F. (1982) A search in rat brain cortex synaptic vesicles for endogenous ligands for kainic acid receptors. *Brain Res.*, 236: 492 – 496.

Ross, C.A., Ruggiero, D.A., Park, D.H., Joh, T.H., Sved, A.F., Fernandez-Pardal, J., Savedra, J.M. and Reis, D.J. (1984) Tonic vasomotor control by the rostral ventrolateral medulla: effect of electrical or chemical stimulation of the area containing C1 adrenaline neurons on arterial pressure, heart rate, and plasma catecholamines and vasopressin. *J. Neurosci.*, 4: 474 – 494.

Seybold, V.S. and Elde, R.P. (1984) Receptor autoradiography in thoracic spinal cord: correlation of neurotransmitter binding sites with sympathoadrenal neurons. *J. Neurosci.*, 4: 2533 – 2542.

Sternberger, L.A. (1979) *Immunocytochemistry*, John Wiley, New York.

Sun, M.K. and Guyenet, P.G. (1986) Hypothalamic glutamatergic input to medullary sympathoexcitatory neurons in rats. *Am. J. Physiol.*, 251: R798 – R810.

Uchizono, K. (1965) Characterization of excitatory and inhibitory synapses in the CNS of the cat. *Nature*, 207: 642 – 643.

Unnerstall, J.R. and Wamsley, J.K. (1983) Autoradiographic localization of high-affinity ^{3}H-kainic acid binding sites in the rat forebrain. *Eur. J. Pharmacol.*, 86: 361 – 371.

Yoshimura, M., Polosa, C. and Nishi, S. (1987) Slow EPSP and the depolarizing action of noradrenaline on sympathetic preganglionic neurons. *Brain Res.*, 414: 138 – 142.

Young, W.S., III and Kuhar, M.J. (1980) Noradrenergic α_1- and α_2-receptors: light microscopic autoradiographic localization. *Proc. Natl. Acad. Sci. U.S.A.*, 77: 1696 – 1700.

J. Ciriello, M.M. Caverson and C. Polosa (Eds.)
Progress in Brain Research, Vol. 81
© 1989 Elsevier Science Publishers B.V. (Biomedical Division)

CHAPTER 12

Cholinergic mechanisms subserving cardiovascular function in the medulla and spinal cord

Hreday N. Sapru

Section of Neurosurgery and Department of Pharmacology, University of Medicine and Dentistry of New Jersey, New Jersey Medical School, Newark, NJ 07103, U.S.A.

Introduction

The importance of the nucleus tractus solitarius (NTS), ventrolateral medullary pressor area (VLPA), ventrolateral medullary depressor area (VLDA) and intermediolateral column (IML) of the spinal cord in cardiovascular regulation is well-established (Willette et al., 1983a; Blessing et al., 1984; Dampney et al., 1985; Ciriello et al., 1986; Guyenet et al., 1987; Reis et al., 1987). A schematic representation of these areas is shown in Fig. 1. Information regarding the neurotransmitters and neuromodulators in various projections connecting the NTS, VLPA, VLDA and IML is just beginning to be accumulated. A glutamate-like substance has been implicated as the excitatory transmitter of the primary baroreceptor afferent terminals (Talman et al., 1980), the projections from NTS to VLPA (Urbanski and Sapru, 1988a,b) and of the projections from NTS to VLDA (Gordon, 1987; Guyenet et al., 1987; Urbanski and Sapru, 1988, 1989). The inhibitory transmitter in the projection from the VLDA to VLPA is believed to be GABA (Willette et al., 1983b, 1984b; Blessing, 1988; Urbanski and Sapru, 1989).

Address for correspondence: Dr. H. Sapru, Neurosurgery, Medical Sciences Bldg., Room H592, New Jersey Medical School, 185 South Orange Ave., Newark, NJ 07103, U.S.A.

The presence of acetylcholine esterase, choline acetyltransferase and muscarinic receptors has been demonstrated in the various regions of the medulla and the spinal cord which are known to be involved in cardiovascular regulation (Navaratnam and Lewis, 1970; Butcher and Woolf, 1984; Kimura et al., 1984; Watson et al., 1987). These observations suggest that cholinergic mechanisms in these regions may be involved in cardiovascular regulation. Recently, subtypes of muscarinic receptors have been identified in the brains of experimental animals and humans (Cortes et al., 1986a,b). Specific agonists and antagonists are available for only two (M_1 and M_2) muscarinic receptor subtypes (Watson et al., 1987). Cloning

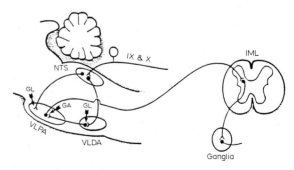

Fig. 1. Schematic diagram showing the relationships between the nucleus tractus solitarius (NTS), ventrolateral medullary pressor area (VLPA), ventrolateral medullary depressor area (VLDA) and the intermediolateral column of the spinal cord (IML). GA = GABA; GL = glutamate.

studies have revealed that M_1 and M_2 receptors represent distinct gene products and have different amino acid sequences (Kubo et al., 1986). In this chapter the cardiovascular actions of these subtype selective cholinergic agonists and antagonists microinjected in different regions of the medulla and the spinal cord are briefly reviewed.

Methods

Male Wistar rats, weighing 300 – 350 g, were used. The rats were anesthetized with pentobarbital sodium (45 – 50 mg/kg i.p.), immobilized with d-tubocurarine (0.1 – 0.2 mg/kg, i.v.) and artificially ventilated. Blood pressure (BP), mean arterial pressure (MAP), heart rate (HR), the rate of increase in the left ventricular pressure (dP/dt) and contractility index (CI) were monitored with standard techniques (Willette et al., 1983a; Lokhandwala et al., 1985). Rectal temperature was monitored and maintained at 37 ± 0.5°C.

In the experiments on the NTS the animals were placed prone in a stereotaxic instrument. The NTS was identified bilaterally (Sundaram et al., 1989b) with microinjections of L-glutamate (1.77 nmol/site in 20 – 50 nl of 0.9% sodium chloride solution, pH 7.4); the coordinates (expressed in mm) were 0.5 rostral, 0.5 lateral with reference to the calamus scriptorius and 0.5 deep from the dorsal surface of the brainstem.

For identification of the VLPA and the VLDA, the rats were placed supine in a stereotaxic instrument. The larynx, esophagus and underlying musculature were excised to expose the basal portion of the occipital bone. A window, approximately 6 mm wide and 7 mm long, was then created in this bone. The most caudal border of the occipital foramen served as a landmark. The VLPA was located 3.5 – 4.1 mm rostral to the landmark, 1.4 – 1.9 mm lateral to the midline and 0.5 – 1 mm deep from the ventral surface of the medulla. The VLDA was located 1.8 – 2.0 mm rostral to the landmark, 1.5 – 1.9 mm lateral to the midline and 0.5 – 1.0 mm deep from the ventral surface of the medulla (Willette et al., 1983a).

The IML was identified as follows. The rats were fixed prone in a stereotaxic instrument to which a spinal unit was attached. The dorsal surface of the spinal cord from C_7 to T_5 level was exposed by laminectomy. Microinjections of L-glutamate (1.77 nmol in 20 nl of 0.9% sodium chloride solution, pH 7.4) were used to locate neurons eliciting positive inotropic and chronotropic effects. The coordinates for these sites were 0.6 – 0.7 mm lateral to the midline and 0.7 – 0.9 mm deep from the dorsal surface of the spinal cord (Sundaram et al., 1989a).

The following muscarinic receptor subtype selective agonists and antagonists were used (Watson et al., 1987): AFDX-116 (a specific antagonist for M_2 muscarinic receptors); pirenzepine (PZ, a specific antagonist for M_1 muscarinic receptors); cis-methyldioxolane (CD; a specific agonist for M_2 muscarinic receptors); McN-A343 (a specific agonist for M_1 muscarinic receptors). AFDX-116 was dissolved in 0.05 N HCl. All other agents were dissolved in 0.9% sodium chloride solution. The pH of all microinjection solutions was adjusted to 7.4. The vehicle alone was injected in all cases. No effect of the vehicle was observed.

Results

Nucleus tractus solitarius

Bilateral microinjections (25 nl) of CD (0.2 – 2.0 nmol/site) into the previously identified cardiovascular sites in the NTS (Fig. 2A) decreased MAP and HR (Fig. 2B). Dose-response relationships [number of animals (n) = 28] for the maximum bradycardic and hypotensive effects which were obtained within 1 – 2 min of the microinjections are shown in Fig. 2C,D, respectively. The duration of these effects was from 3 to 6 min. Intravenous injections of the same doses of CD produced no response. Maximum hypotensive (-52 ± 1.2 mmHg) and bradycardic (-50 ± 2.7 bpm) responses were observed at 0.8 nmol/site. Control MAP and HR in these rats were 102 ± 4 mmHg and 346 ± 8 beats/min (bpm), respectively. At a higher dose (2 nmol/site), the depressor and bradycardic responses were significantly smaller ($P < 0.05$) than those observed at 0.8 nmol/site. Smaller responses to larger doses of CD may be due to the depolarization blockade property of this cholinergic agonist. Confirmation of this inference was obtained as follows. L-glutamate (1.77 nmol) was microinjected unilaterally into the NTS ($n = 5$); a decrease in MAP (-37 ± 1.2 mmHg) was observed. Five minutes later, CD (0.8 nmol) was microinjected at the same site; a decrease in MAP (-20 ± 3.2 mmHg) was observed as expected. When the BP had recovered to control levels (8 min), L-glutamate (1.77 nmol) was

again microinjected at the same site; the decrease in MAP (-35 ± 1.5 mmHg) remained unchanged. The same experiment was repeated using the higher dose of CD (2 nmol) in another group of rats ($n = 5$). The response to microinjections of glutamate was significantly ($P < 0.05$) reduced after the microinjections of 2 nmol CD; the decrease in MAP induced by glutamate was 38 ± 2.5 and 21 ± 1.8 mmHg before and after the microinjection of CD, respectively. The response to L-glutamate recovered after $40 - 50$ min indicating absence of permanent tissue damage. Bilateral vagotomy did not affect the hypotensive and bradycardic effects of CD ($n = 5$) in the NTS.

In another group of rats ($n = 6$), AFDX-116 (0.8 nmol/site) was microinjected into the NTS sites previously identified bilaterally with microinjections of L-glutamate; a slight increase ($+10 \pm 3.2$ mmHg) in BP was observed. Initially AFDX-116 induced a depression of neurons as indicated by the lack of responses to glutamate. The response to L-glutamate recovered within $15 - 20$ min after the microinjection of AFDX-116. At this time (i.e. 25 min after the microinjection of AFDX-116), microinjections of CD (0.8 nmol/site) at the same sites failed to evoke the usual depressor and bradycardic responses. On the other hand, the same dose of AFDX-116 did not alter the responses to a comparable dose (0.8 nmol/site) of glutamate. Bilateral microinjections of PZ (2 nmol/site) into the NTS did not alter the responses to CD or L-glutamate ($n = 4$).

McN-A343 (3 nmol/site) or PZ (1.5 nmol/site) failed to evoke any response (Fig. 3) in the NTS. Control MAP and HR in this group of rats ($n = 6$) were 98 ± 4 mmHg and 348 ± 12 bpm, respectively.

Ventrolateral medullary pressor area

An increase in MAP and HR was evoked by bilateral microinjections of CD (Fig. 4B). Dose-response relationships ($n = 30$) for the hypertensive and tachycardic effects of CD ($0.004 - 4$ nmol/site) are shown in Fig. 4C,D, respectively.

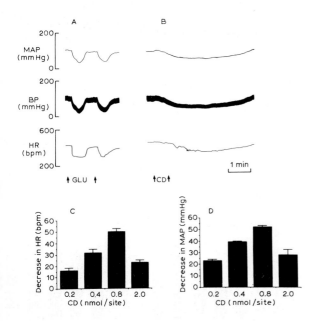

Fig. 2. M_2 agonist applied in NTS decreases arterial pressure and heart rate. In (A,B): top trace is mean femoral arterial pressure (MAP, mmHg); middle trace is pulsatile femoral arterial pressure (BP, mmHg); bottom trace is heart rate (HR, bpm). (A) NTS was identified bilaterally by the drop in MAP and HR produced by microinjecting L-glutamate monosodium 1.77 nmol/site (arrows). (B) Bilateral microinjections of *cis*-methyldioxolane (0.8 nmol/site) at the same sites induced a slow onset, long-lasting decrease in BP and HR. Dose-response relationships [number of animals (n) = 28] for the bradycardic and hypotensive effects are shown in (C,D), respectively. Each bar represents mean value $\pm$ S.E. (Reproduced with permission from Sundaram et al., 1989b.)

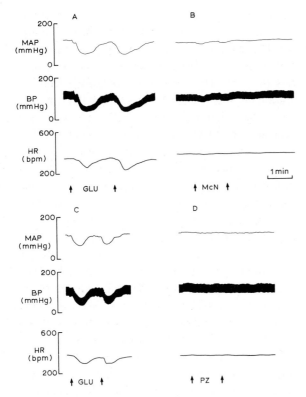

Fig. 3. Lack of effect on arterial pressure and heart rate of M_1 agonist and antagonist applied in NTS. Same traces as in Fig. 2. (A) Identification of cardiovascular sites in the NTS. (B) Bilateral microinjection of McN-A343 (3 nmol/site) at the same sites evoked no significant change in BP or HR. (C) NTS sites in a different rat. (D) Microinjections of pirenzepine (1.5 nmol/site) at the same sites evoked no response. (Reproduced with permission from Sundaram et al., 1989b.)

Control MAP and HR in these rats were 100 ± 10 mmHg and 350 ± 30 bpm, respectively. These effects had an onset delay of $2 - 5$ sec and a duration of $10 - 50$ min. Maximal hypertensive and tachycardic responses were observed at 0.4 nmol/site. At 4 nmol/site, the pressor and tachycardic responses were significantly smaller than those observed at 0.4 nmol/site ($P < 0.001$ and 0.05, respectively). These effects were mediated via the sympathetic nervous system because they were prevented by pretreatment with a ganglion blocker (chlorisondamine, 3 mg/kg, i.v., $n = 4$).

Microinjection of the M_2 antagonist AFDX-116 ($0.2 - 1.6$ nmol/site) produced a dose-dependent

decrease in BP ($5 - 20$ mmHg) lasting $60 - 150$ min. After microinjection of AFDX-116 the pressor response to CD was attenuated at the time when the response to glutamate had recovered from the depression produced by the antagonist. McN-A343 and PZ failed to evoke any response.

Intravenous injections of the anticholinesterase inhibitor physostigmine sulfate ($25 - 200$ μg/kg, $n = 4$) which crosses the blood-brain barrier and elevates endogenous acetylcholine (ACh) levels in the brain (Brezenoff and Giuliano, 1982) induced an increase in MAP (Punnen et al., 1986). This effect was mediated via M_2 receptors located in the VLPA because microinjections of AFDX, but not

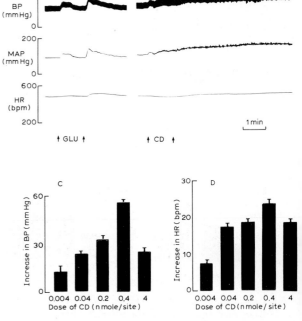

Fig. 4. M_2 agonist applied in VLPA increases arterial pressure and heart rate. Top trace: pulsatile femoral BP (mmHg); middle trace: mean arterial pressure (mmHg); bottom trace: heart rate (bpm). (A) VLPA was identified bilaterally by the increase in MAP and HR produced by microinjecting L-glutamate monosodium 1.77 nmol/site (arrows). (B) Bilateral microinjections of cis-methyldioxolane (0.4 nmol/site) at the same sites induced a slow onset, prolonged increase in BP and HR. The increase in BP (panel C) and HR (panel D) induced by CD was dose-dependent. Each bar represents mean value $\pm$ S.E. (Reproduced with permission from Sundaram et al., 1988.)

of PZ, into the VLPA prevented this effect of intravenous physostigmine.

The drug 3,4-diaminopyridine (DAP) releases transmitters, including ACh, from nerve terminals (Glover, 1982). Microinjection of DAP (0.1–2.0 nmol/site) into the VLPA produced an increase in BP and HR which lasted 20–40 min. Microinjection of scopolamine or AFDX-116 prevented these effects of DAP (Sundaram and Sapru, 1988).

Ventrolateral medullary depressor area

In the VLDA, bilateral microinjections of CD (0.2–1.6 nmol/site) decreased MAP and HR in a dose-dependent manner. Maximum hypotensive (−71 ± 2.4 mmHg) and bradycardic (−62 ± 6 bpm) responses were observed at 0.4 nmol/site. At 0.8 and 1.6 nmol/site, the depressor responses were significantly smaller ($P < 0.5$) than those observed at 0.4 nmol/site. Microinjections of AFDX-116 (1.2 nmol/site) into the VLDA blocked the effects of subsequent injections of CD at the same sites. Microinjections of McN-A343 (3 nmol/site) or PZ into the VLDA failed to evoke any response. Microinjection of DAP (0.1–2.0 nmol/site) decreased BP and HR. Microinjection of scopolamine or AFDX-116 prevented these effects.

Intermediolateral column of the spinal cord

Microinjections of L-glutamate were used to functionally identify the sympathoexcitatory cardiac sites in the right and left IML at T_1 to T_3 cord segment level (Sundaram et al., 1989a). The maximum increase in HR or contractility was elicited from the T_2 segment. The coordinates for this site were 0.6–0.7 mm lateral to the mid-line and 0.7–0.9 mm deep from the dorsal surface of the spinal cord. Microinjections of ACh (0.01–1.00 nmol) into this site on the right side produced a marked dose-dependent tachycardia (Fig. 5B). The dose-response relationship ($n = 12$), presented in Fig. 5C, is based on the maximum tachycardic response elicited by a given ACh dose from one site

in the T_2 segment of each rat. This effect has onset delay of 20–30 sec and duration of 4–8 min. The response at the dose of 1 nmol was significantly smaller than that at 0.1 nmol ($P < 0.05$). No changes in BP were observed at any of the doses of ACh or L-glutamate. Control MAP and HR in these rats were 102 ± 4 mmHg and 338 ± 32 bpm, respectively. The specificity of these effects was tested as follows ($n = 7$). The site eliciting maximum positive chronotropic response (52 ± 9 bpm) was identified by microinjections of glutamate (1.77 nmol). Atropine hemisulfate (0.2 nmol) was microinjected at the same site; no significant change in HR was observed (Fig. 5E). Fifteen min later, microinjections of ACh (0.1 nmol) at the same site failed to produce the usual increase in HR (Fig. 5G) while the positive chronotropic responses to glutamate persisted (Fig. 5F). Carbachol, a stable analogue of ACh, also produced

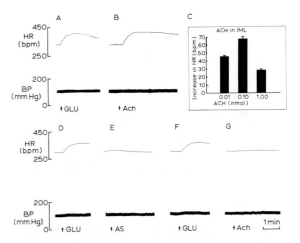

Fig. 5. Acetylcholine microinjected into the right IML at T_2 level increases heart rate. In each panel showing polygraph tracings the top trace is heart rate (bpm) and the bottom trace is femoral BP (mmHg). (A) Microinjection of L-glutamate (1.77 nmol) into the right IML produced an increase in HR. (B) Microinjection of acetylcholine (0.1 nmol) at the same site produced increase in HR. (C) The tachycardic response was dose-dependent. (D) Control tachycardic response to 1.77 nmol of glutamate microinjected into the right IML. (E) Atropine hemisulfate (0.2 nmol) was microinjected into the same site; no significant change in HR was observed. Atropine did not alter the effect of glutamate (1.77 nmol, panel F) but did block the effect of acetylcholine (0.1 nmol, panel G).

tachycardia when injected into the T_2 site. Intravenously administered chlorisondamine blocked the carbachol-induced tachycardia from the IML.

Spinal transection rostral (C_4 level; $n = 5$) or caudal (T_6 level; $n = 5$) to the site from which maximal tachycardic responses were induced by the microinjections of carbachol or glutamate (T_2 level) did not alter the responses.

Microinjection of CD (0.2 – 0.8 nmol) into the right IML at T_2 level elicited an increase in HR (20 – 70 bpm). The onset and duration of action were 20 – 40 sec and 45 – 60 min, respectively. Prior microinjections of AFDX-116 (0.8 nmol), but not of PZ (2 nmol), prevented the positive chronotropic action of CD. The responses to glutamate, tested 5 min prior to the injection of CD, were not altered by AFDX-116. McN-A343 and PZ elicited no response when microinjected into the previously identified right IML at T_2.

A functional asymmetry between the left and

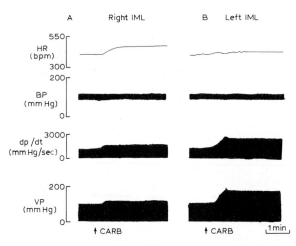

Fig. 6. Asymmetry in the tachycardic and positive inotropic responses to microinjections of carbachol into the right and left IML at T_2 level. Top trace is heart rate (bpm), second trace is femoral BP (mmHg), third trace is maximum rate of contraction of the left ventricle (dP/dt, mmHg/sec) and bottom trace is left ventricular pressure (mmHg). (A) Microinjection of carbachol (660 pmol) into the right IML produced a predominant increase in HR with a small increase in the left ventricular dP/dt or pressure and no change in BP. (B) Microinjection of the same dose of carbachol into the left IML produced a predominant increase in the left ventricular dP/dt and pressure with a small increase in HR and no change in BP.

right sides of IML at $T_1 - T_3$ level was observed. On the right side at T_2 level, microinjections of carbachol (660 pmol) into the IML produced a marked increase in HR and a minimal increase in left ventricular pressure and dP/dt (Fig. 6A) while on the left side the reverse was true (Fig. 6B).

Discussion

The results presented show that cholinergic agonists applied by microinjection produce cardiovascular responses from various regions of the medulla and the spinal cord. The use of specific agonists and antagonists at M_1 and M_2 receptors revealed that these responses were mediated by M_2 receptors. The M_2 receptor agonist CD evoked cardiovascular responses when microinjected into the areas of medulla and spinal cord under study while injections of the M_1 receptor agonist McN-A343 in the same sites had no effect. The specificity of these muscarinic responses was confirmed by the selective block of the response by an M_2, but not by an M_1, antagonist. Although microinjections of AFDX-116 rendered neurons unresponsive to L-glutamate, this effect was transient and the responses recovered to control levels within 20 – 150 min depending on the dose used. At the time when the responses to glutamate had recovered, AFDX-116 completely blocked the responses to CD and this effect lasted for 2 h suggesting that the muscarinic receptor blocking properties of AFDX-116 outlast its initial unspecific depressant effect on neurons. The results presented here are consistent with quantitative autoradiographic studies which demonstrate that muscarinic receptors in the hind brain are predominantly of the M_2 type (Cortes et al., 1986a,b). Although pharmacological studies have demonstrated the presence of nicotinic receptors in the VLPA and NTS (Kubo, 1987; Sapru, 1987) and the IML (unpublished observations), ACh and its analogues seem to mediate cardiovascular actions from these areas via muscarinic receptors (Sapru, 1987).

In the NTS (Sundaram et al., 1989b), depressor and bradycardic responses are elicited when an M_2

muscarinic agonist was microinjected. These observations are consistent with earlier studies in which non-selective muscarinic receptor agonists and antagonists were used (Criscione et al., 1983). Cholinergic agonists induced M_2-mediated depressor and bradycardic responses in the VLDA also.

In the VLPA these agents evoked pressor and tachycardic responses (Sundaram and Sapru, 1988; Sundaram et al., 1988). These results have been confirmed by Giuliano et al. (1989). Systemically administered physostigmine elicits a hypertensive response which appears to be mediated via the VLPA (Punnen et al., 1986; Sundaram et al., 1988) since the effect was blocked by microinjection of AFDX-116 into the VLPA. This effect was observed when responsiveness of the neurons in the VLPA to L-glutamate was normal, indicating that blockade of M_2 muscarinic receptors in the VLPA, rather than non-specific effects of AFDX-116, abolished the effects of systemically administered physostigmine.

Atropine sulfate or scopolamine hydrochloride, when microinjected alone into the VLPA, induced a dose-dependent fall in BP which lasted for 60 – 150 min. This effect was attributed to blockade of muscarinic receptors in the VLPA (Willette et al., 1984a; Sundaram et al., 1988). These observations suggest that the VLPA is under tonic excitatory cholinergic control. However, the source of this input remains to be established.

Positive chronotropic and inotropic effects were produced when ACh and its analogues were microinjected into the right and left IML at $T_1 - T_3$ level. These results have not been previously reported. In this study, we utilized the L-glutamate microinjection technique to identify neuronal pools regulating cardiac function in the IML. Using this technique it is possible to avoid the activation of ascending or descending fibers in the spinal cord which complicates the technique of intraspinal stimulation (Henry and Calaresu, 1974; Chung and Wurster, 1976; Cabot et al., 1979; Faden et al., 1979; Eberhart and Schramm, 1987). Electrical stimulation of such pathways may be responsible for some differences between our results and those of others. For example, tachycardic responses were elicited from T_1 to L_4 spinal segments (Henry and Calaresu, 1972; Faden et al., 1978a,b, 1979, 1980). In our studies (Sundaram et al., 1989a) these responses were restricted to the $T_1 - T_3$ spinal cord segments. Concomitant pressor responses have also been reported (Henry and Calaresu, 1972) while we observed no changes in BP. Inotropic responses have been reported to show right-sided preponderance (Faden and Jacobs, 1980) while in our studies increase in cardiac contractility was evoked by cholinergic agonists from the left IML at $T_1 - T_3$ level. Similar functional asymmetry was observed with microinjections of glutamate (Sundaram et al., 1989a) and is perhaps related to the different target sites of the right and left sympathetic nerves innervating the heart (Randall et al., 1957). Since scopolamine blocked these effects, muscarinic receptors must be mediating these responses. Chlorisondamine (a ganglion blocker) prevented the responses of carbachol indicating that sympathetic nervous system was involved in these actions. The implication of ascending or descending spinal pathways was excluded because the responses to carbachol remained unchanged after spinal transections rostral or caudal to the site of microinjection in the T_2 spinal segment. The effect of ACh, the natural transmitter, was similar to that of carbachol except that its action was of shorter duration. These results suggest that muscarinic receptors are located in the IML regulating sympathoexcitatory cardiac functions. Based on the techniques used in our study, it was not possible to ascertain if these receptors are located on the preganglionic sympathetic neurons (which are cholinergic but may or may not be cholinoreceptive), interneurons or nerve terminals. The physiological role played by these muscarinic receptors in the IML remains to be established.

Summary

This investigation was designed to study the role of muscarinic receptor subtypes in the cardiovascular responses elicited by microinjection of cholinergic agonists in the intermediate portion of the NTS, the VLPA and VLDA areas and the IML of the spinal cord. Microinjections of L-glutamate (1.77 nmol in $20-50$ nl in 0.9% sodium chloride solution) were used to identify these areas. Bilateral microinjections ($0.02-2$ nmol/site) of a potent M_2 muscarinic receptor agonist, CD, but not those of a relatively selective M_1 receptor agonist (McN-A343; 3 nmol/site), into the intermediate portion of NTS and the VLDA induced depressor and bradycardic responses. In the VLPA these agonists elicited pressor and tachycardic effects while in the IML at $T_1 - T_3$ only increase in HR was observed. Previous microinjections of a selective competitive M_2 receptor antagonist (AFDX-116; $0.8-1.6$ nmol/site), but not those of a potent selective M_1 receptor antagonist (PZ; $1.5-2.0$ nmol/site), into these areas blocked the effects of CD. These results indicate that the muscarinic receptors of M_2 type may play a part in the regulation of cardiovascular function in the above-mentioned cardiovascular areas in a yet unidentified manner.

Acknowledgements

The work presented here was done with my colleagues Drs. Kalyana Sundaram and Jaya Murugaian. This work was supported by grants from N.I.H. (HL24347) and American Heart Association (New Jersey affiliate). AFDX-116 and PZ were received as gifts from Boehringer Ingelheim Pharmaceuticals Inc., CT, U.S.A.

References

Blessing, W.W. (1988) Depressor neurons in the rabbit caudal medulla act via GABA receptors in rostral medulla. *Am. J. Physiol.*, 254: H686 – H693.

Blessing, W.W., Sved, A.F. and Reis, D.J. (1984) Arterial pressure and plasma vasopressin: regulation by neurons in the caudal ventrolateral medulla of the rabbit. In I.H. Slater (Ed.), *Clinical and Experimental Hypertension*, Marcel Dekker, New York, pp. 149 – 156.

Brezenoff, H.E. and Giuliano, R. (1982) Cardiovascular con-
trol by cholinergic mechanisms in the central nervous system. *Annu. Rev. Pharmacol. Toxicol.*, 22: 341 – 381.

Butcher, L.L. and Woolf, N.J. (1984) Histochemical distribution of acetylcholine esterase in the central nervous system: clues to the localization of cholinergic neurons. In A. Bjorklund, T. Hökfelt, and M.J. Kuhar (Eds.), *Handbook of Chemical Anatomy, Vol. 3*, Elsevier, New York, pp. 1 – 50.

Cabot, J.B., Wild, J.M. and Cohen, D.H. (1979) Raphe inhibition of sympathetic preganglionic neurons. *Science*, 203: 184 – 186.

Chung, J.M. and Wurster, R.D. (1976) Ascending pressor and depressor pathways in the cat spinal cord. *Am. J. Physiol.*, 231: 786 – 792.

Ciriello, J., Caverson, M.M. and Polosa, C. (1986) Function of the ventrolateral medulla in the control of the circulation, *Brain Res. Rev.*, 11: 359 – 391.

Cortes, R. and Palacios, J.M. (1986a) Muscarinic cholinergic receptor subtypes in the rat brain. I. Quantitative autoradiographic studies. *Brain Res.*, 362: 227 – 238.

Cortes, R. and Palacios, J.M. (1986b) Muscarinic cholinergic receptor subtypes in the human brain. II. Quantitative autoradiographic studies. *Brain Res.*, 362: 239 – 253.

Criscione, L., Reis, D.J. and Talman, W.T. (1983) Cholinergic mechanisms in the nucleus tractus solitarii and cardiovascular regulation in the rat. *Eur. J. Pharmacol.*, 88: 47 – 55.

Dampney, R.A.L., Goodchild, A.K. and Tan, E. (1985) Vasopressor neurons in the rostral ventrolateral medulla of the rabbit, *J. Auton. Nerv. Syst.*, 14: 239 – 254.

Eberhart, J.A. and Schramm, L.P. (1987) Projections from cervical spinal cord to lower thoracic cord in the rat. *Soc. Neurosci. Abst.*, 13: 270.

Faden, A.I. and Jacobs, T.P. (1980) Cardiac contractility and the spinal sympathetic neuron. *Neurol. Res.*, 1: 227 – 237.

Faden, A.I., Jacobs, T.P. and Woods, M. (1978a) Cardioacceleratory sites in the zona intermedia of the cat spinal cord. *Exp. Neurol.*, 61: 301 – 310.

Faden, A.I., Jacobs, T.P., Woods, M. and Tyner, C.F. (1978b) Zona intermedia pressor sites in the cat spinal cord: right-left asymmetry. *Exp. Neurol.*, 61: 571 – 581.

Faden, A.I., Jacobs, T.P. and Woods, M. (1979) An intraspinal sympathetic preganglionic pathway: physiological evidence in the cat. *Brain Res.*, 162: 13 – 20.

Giuliano, R., Ruggiero, D., Morrison, S., Ernsberger, P. and Reis, D.J. (1989) Cholinergic regulation of arterial pressure by the C_1 area of the rostral ventrolateral medulla. *J. Neurosci.*, 9: 923 – 942.

Glover, W.E. (1982) The aminopyridines. *Gen. Pharmacol.*, 13: 259 – 285.

Gordon, F.J. (1987) Aortic baroreceptor reflexes are mediated by NMDA receptors in caudal ventrolateral medulla. *Am. J. Physiol.*, 252: R628 – R633.

Guyenet, P.G., Sun, M. and Brown, D.L. (1987) Role of

GABA and excitatory amino acids in medullary baroreflex pathways. In J. Ciriello, L. Renaud and C. Polosa (Eds.), *Organization of the Autonomic Nervous System: Central and Peripheral Mechanisms*, Alan R. Liss, New York, pp. 215 – 225.

Henry, J.L. and Calaresu, F.R. (1972) Distribution of cardioacceleratory sites in intermediolateral nucleus of the cat. *Am. J. Physiol.*, 222: 700 – 704.

Henry, J.L. and Calaresu, F.R. (1974) Excitatory and inhibitory inputs from medullary nuclei projecting to spinal cardioacceleratory neurons in the cat. *Exp. Brain Res.*, 20: 485 – 504.

Kimura, H., McGeer, P.L. and Peng, J.H. (1984) Choline acetyltransferase containing neurons in the rat brain. In A. Bjorklund, T. Hökfelt, and M.J. Kuhar (Eds.), *Handbook of Chemical Anatomy, Vol. 3*, Elsevier, New York, pp. 51 – 67.

Kubo, T. (1987) Central nicotinic regulation of arterial blood pressure. In W.R. Martin, G.R. Van Loon, E.T. Iwamoto and L. Davis (Eds.), *Tobacco Smoking and Nicotine: A Neurobiologic Approach*, Plenum Press, New York, pp. 277 – 286.

Kubo, T., Fukuda, K., Mikami, A., Maeda, A., Takahashi, H., Mishina, M., Haga, T., Haga, K., Ichiyama, A., Kangawa, K., Kojima, M., Matsuo, H., Hirose, T. and Numa, S. (1986) Cloning, sequencing and expression of complementary DNA encoding the muscarinic acetylcholine receptor. *Nature*, 323: 411 – 416.

Lokhandwala, M.F., Sabouni, M.H. and Jandhyala, B.S. (1985) Cardiovascular actions of an experimental antitumor agent, homoharringtonine, in anesthetized dogs. *Drug Dev. Res.*, 5: 157 – 163.

Navaratnam, V. and Lewis, P.R. (1970) Cholinesterase-containing neurons in the spinal cord of the rat. *Brain Res.*, 18: 411 – 425.

Punnen, S., Willette, R.N., Krieger, A.J. and Sapru, H.N. (1986) Medullary pressor area: site of action of intravenous physostigmine. *Brain Res.*, 382: 178 – 184.

Randall, W.C., McNally, H., Cowan, J., Caliguiri, L. and Rohse, W.G. (1957) Functional analysis of the cardioaugmentor and cardioaccelerator pathways in the dog. *Am. J. Physiol.*, 191: 213 – 217.

Reis, D.J., Ross, C., Granata, A.R. and Ruggiero, D.A. (1987) Role of C1 area of rostroventrolateral medulla in cardiovascular control. In J.P. Buckley and C.M. Ferrario (Eds.), *Brain Peptides and Catecholamines in Cardiovascular Regulation*, Raven Press, New York, pp. 1 – 14.

Sapru, H.N. (1987) Control of blood pressure by nicotinic and muscarinic receptors in the ventrolateral medulla. In L. Davis (Ed.), *Tobacco Smoking and Nicotine: A Neurobiologic Approach*, Plenum Press, New York, pp. 287 – 300.

Sundaram, K. and Sapru, H.N. (1988) Cholinergic nerve terminals in the ventrolateral medullary pressor area: pharmacological evidence. *J. Auton. Nerv. Syst.*, 22: 221 – 228.

Sundaram, K., Krieger, A.J. and Sapru, H.N. (1988) M2 muscarinic receptors mediate pressor responses to cholinergic agonists in the ventrolateral medullary pressor area. *Brain Res.*, 449: 141 – 149.

Sundaram, K., Murugaian, J. and Sapru, H.N. (1989a) Cardiac responses to microinjections of excitatory amino acids into the intermediolateral cell column of the rat spinal cord. *Brain Res.*, 482: 12 – 22.

Sundaram, K., Murugaian, J., Watson, M. and Sapru, H.N. (1989b) M_2 muscarinic receptor agonists produce hypotension and bradycardia when injected into the nucleus tractus solitarius. *Brain Res.*, 477: 358 – 362.

Talman, W.T., Perrone, M.H. and Reis, D.J. (1980) Evidence for L-glutamate as the neurotransmitter of baroreceptor afferent nerve fibers. *Science*, 209: 813 – 814.

Urbanski, R.W. and Sapru, H.N. (1988a) Evidence for a sympathoexcitatory pathway from the nucleus tractus solitarius to the ventrolateral medullary pressor area. *J. Auton. Nerv. Syst.*, 23: 161 – 174.

Urbanski, R.W. and Sapru, H.N. (1988b) Putative neurotransmitters involved in medullary cardiovascular regulation. *J. Auton. Nerv. Syst.*, 25: 181 – 193.

Watson, M., Roeske, W.R. and Yamamura, H.I. (1987) Cholinergic receptor heterogeneity. In H.Y. Meltzer (Ed.), *Psychopharmacology: A Third Generation of Progress*, Raven Press, New York, pp. 241 – 248.

Willette, R.N., Barcas, P.P., Krieger, A.J. and Sapru, H.N. (1983a) Vasopressor and depressor areas in the rat medulla. *Neuropharmacology*, 22: 1071 – 1079.

Willette, R.N., Krieger, A.J., Barcas, P.P. and Sapru, H.N. (1983b) Medullary GABA receptors and the regulation of blood pressure in the rat. *J. Pharmacol. Exp. Ther.*, 226: 893 – 899.

Willette, R.N., Punnen, S., Krieger, A.J. and Sapru, H.N., (1984a) Cardiovascular control by cholinergic mechanisms in the rostral ventrolateral medulla. *J. Pharmacol. Exp. Ther.*, 231: 457 – 463.

Willette, R.N., Barcas, P.P., Krieger, A.J. and Sapru, H.N. (1984b) Endogenous GABAergic mechanisms in the medulla and the regulation of blood pressure. *J. Pharmacol. Exp. Ther.*, 230: 34 – 39.

J. Ciriello, M.M. Caverson and C. Polosa (Eds.)
Progress in Brain Research, Vol. 81
© 1989 Elsevier Science Publishers B.V. (Biomedical Division)

CHAPTER 13

Multiple actions of noradrenaline on sympathetic preganglionic neurons of the cat studied in the spinal cord slice

M. Yoshimura[1], C. Polosa[2] and S. Nishi[1]

[1]Department of Physiology, Kurume University School of Medicine, Kurume, Japan, and [2]Department of Physiology, McGill University, Montreal, Quebec, Canada

Introduction

Several lines of evidence suggest that catecholamines (CA) have a role as mediators, or modifiers, of synaptic actions on the sympathetic preganglionic neuron (SPN). The intermediolateral (IML) nucleus of the gray matter of the thoracic spinal cord is rich in CA-containing axons (Carlsson et al., 1964). This innervation is of supraspinal origin. Several CA-synthesizing neuron sets of brainstem and hypothalamus, some of which are located in the ventrolateral medulla, are considered the source of this dense CA innervation of the IML column (see reviews by Coote, 1988 and Laskey and Polosa, 1988). CA-containing axons form typical synapses with identified SPNs (Chiba and Masuko, 1986; Milner et al., 1988). Binding studies show that adrenoceptors are present in the IML nucleus (Cabot et al., 1984; Seybold and Elde, 1984; Dashwood et al., 1985). Iontophoresis of CA on SPNs produced depressant effects mediated by an α_2-adrenoreceptor (see reviews by Coote, 1988 and Laskey and Polosa, 1988). The influence of the CA-innervation on sympathetic activity is the subject of controversy.

Pharmacological studies suggested that CA mediate inhibitory (Dembowsky et al., 1980; Coote et al., 1981) or excitatory (Taylor and Brody, 1976; Franz et al., 1987) synaptic actions.

This chapter summarizes the results obtained in an analysis of CA actions on SPNs carried out by intracellular recording in the slice of the upper thoracic spinal cord of the cat (Yoshimura et al., 1986a, 1987a,b,c,d). These data describe what CA actually do to the SPN and therefore permit prediction of the effects CA are likely to mediate in the intact animal.

Methods

Details of the methods pertaining to specific experiments can be found in the original papers of Yoshimura et al. (1986a,b,c; 1987a,b,c,d). The general methodology only is summarized here. Cats were anesthetized with α-chloralose and Na pentobarbitone (60 and 10 mg/kg i.p., respectively). After laminectomy, thoracic spinal cord segments 2 – 3 were excised, desheathed and cut with a vibratome into 500 μM thick transverse sections. The slice was placed in a recording chamber and superfused with oxygenated Krebs solution at 37°C and pH 7.4. The Krebs solution contained, in mM, NaCl 117, KCl 3.6, NaH_2PO_4 1.2, $CaCl_2$ 2.5, $MgCl_2$ 1.2, glucose 11.0, $NaHCO_3$ 25.00. The

Address for correspondence: C. Polosa, Department of Physiology, McGill University, McIntyre Medical Sciences Bldg., 365, Drummond Street, Montreal, Quebec H3G 1Y6.

composition of the Krebs solution was modified when required in particular experiments. Under the dissecting microscope and with transillumination from below, the IML nucleus was clearly identifiable as described in anatomical studies (e.g. Réthelyi, 1972). Glass microelectrodes filled with 3 M KCl, 2 M K citrate or 2 M K acetate and of resistance from 40 to 120 MΩ were used. Intracellular recordings were made from SPNs that were identified by their antidromic response to stimulation of the segmental white ramus or ventral rootlets or of the axon path from the IML nucleus to the ventral root exit zone, along the lateral edge of the ventral horn. The antidromic latencies corresponded to axonal conduction velocities of 1 – 9 m/sec. Stability of impalement was demonstrated by membrane potential, input resistance and size of the after hyperpolarization that were stable over periods of recording lasting several hours.

Results

General properties of the neurons

Resting potential of the SPNs studied was around −60 mV at the extracellular K concentration of 3.6 mM. Neuron input resistance was 67.5 ± 3.7 MΩ and time constant was 11.5 ± 1.2 msec at the resting membrane potential. The action potential had peak amplitude of 70 – 80 mV and duration of 3 msec. It involves Na, Ca and K currents (Yoshimura et al., 1986c). The action potential was followed by a longlasting afterpotential of complex configuration that results from the combination of two outward K currents [fast and slow after hyperpolarization (AHP), Yoshimura et al., 1986b] and an inward Ca current (Yoshimura et al., 1987e). A transient K current (Yoshimura et al., 1987f) may also be part of the afterpotential. Focal stimulation of the slice produced excitatory and inhibitory synaptic potentials of the fast (time course of tens of msec) and slow (time course of sec) variety (Nishi et al., 1987).

Slow post-synaptic potentials and catecholamines

As mentioned above, focal stimulation of the slice produced in SPNs slow post-synaptic potentials (PSPs) with time course of seconds in addition to fast PSPs with time scale of tens of msec (Nishi et al., 1987). A fast excitatory post-synaptic potential (EPSP), which sometimes triggered a spike, consistently preceded the slow PSPs. Both fast EPSPs and slow PSPs were reversibly abolished by superfusion with tetrodotoxin (TTX 0.6 μM) or with low Ca (0.25 mM) Krebs, which proves that both were synaptically produced. Two sets of observations suggest a relation between slow PSPs and CA. One is that some slow PSPs are blocked by adrenoceptor antagonists (Yoshimura et al., 1987b,c), the other is that NA, applied by superfusion, produced in the majority of SPNs depolarizing or hyperpolarizing responses with properties similar to those of the slow EPSP or slow IPSP, respectively (Yoshimura et al., 1987b,c). The actual breakdown of the frequency of occurrence of these NA-evoked responses is 38% depolarization, 25% hyperpolarization and 19% mixed responses, the balance showing no response ($n = 50$).

The slow EPSP has rise time of 2 – 3 sec and decay time of 10 – 20 sec. It could be graded in amplitude and duration according to the stimulus strength, from barely detectable to large enough to reach firing threshold. When firing occurred it was characterized by long-duration spike trains of low frequency. The afterpotential of the spikes evoked by the slow EPSP had an appearance similar to that observed during superfusion with NA in the 10 – 50 μM concentration range. Namely, the afterpotential had a triphasic appearance, due to the fact that the early and late hyperpolarizing components (Yoshimura et al., 1986b) were separated by a transient phase of accelerated depolarization. In the presence of NA, the triphasic configuration is due to the addition of a depolarizing component of the afterpotential due to a Ca-dependent inward Na current (Yoshimura et al., 1987a). Neuron input resistance, measured at the plateau of the slow EPSP, while membrane potential was manually maintained at approximately control level, increased by $10-30\%$. Membrane hyperpolarization reduced the amplitude of the slow EPSP. At membrane potentials between -86 and -93 mV the slow EPSP was undectectable. This membrane potential is presumed to be Ek in 3.6 mM KCl Krebs solution, because in a previous study the fast component of the AHP reversed at around -90 mV (Yoshimura et al., 1986b).

Hyperpolarization beyond these values did not cause reversal of the slow EPSP. When the K concentration of the Krebs solution (control 3.6 mM) was changed at constant membrane potential, the amplitude of the slow EPSP increased in low K (0.36 mM) and decreased in high K (10.0 mM). These properties suggest that the slow EPSP is due to a decrease in K conductance of the SPN membrane. Failure to reverse the slow EPSP with membrane hyperpolarization was also observed in high K. The α-adrenoceptor antagonist phentolamine ($5-10$ μM) and the α_1-adrenoceptor antagonist prazosin (300 μM) blocked some of the slow EPSPs evoked by focal stimulation and the resulting repetitive discharge. In one of the cells prazosin unmasked a slow IPSP. Phentolamine or prazosin did not depress the fast EPSP evoked by focal stimulation. The α_2-adrenoceptor antagonist yohimbine (1 μM) had no appreciable effect on the slow EPSP.

NA ($10-50$ μM) produced a membrane depolarization, alone or preceded by hyperpolarization, in 57% of the cells tested. The depolarization could also be evoked during superfusion with TTX. In some cases the depolarization was large enough to produce repetitive firing. The NA-evoked depolarization, like the slow EPSP, was associated with a $10-40\%$ increase in neuron-input resistance. Like the slow EPSP, the NA-evoked depolarization decreased in amplitude during progressive membrane hyperpolarization and was nullified at membrane potentials between -87 and -95 mV. No response was observed when the membrane was hyperpolarized beyond these values.

When K in the Krebs solution (control 3.6 mM) was changed at constant membrane potential, the amplitude of the NA-evoked depolarization increased in low K (0.36 mM) and decreased in high K (10.0 mM). Thus, the NA-evoked depolarization, like the slow EPSP, seems due to a decrease in K conductance of the SPN membrane. Phentolamine and prazosin blocked the NA-evoked depolarization at the same doses at which they block the slow EPSP. In many cases prazosin unmasked a hyperpolarization. Yohimbine had no effect or enhanced the depolarization. The β-adrenoceptor antagonist propranolol ($1-4$ μM) had no effect. The analogies of the properties of the slow EPSP and of the NA-evoked depolarization suggest that NA, or another transmitter which activates α_1-adrenoceptors, mediates some slow EPSPs of the SPN. The observation of changes in the shape of the afterpotential of spikes evoked by the slow EPSP similar to those evoked by superfusion with NA (Yoshimura et al., 1987a) suggests that CA-releasing axon terminals evoke the slow EPSP monosynaptically rather than by excitation of segmental interneurons antecedent to the SPN.

The slow IPSP, evoked by focal stimulation, had rise time of $0.3-0.6$ sec and half-decay time of $3-6$ sec. The slow IPSP could be graded in amplitude and duration by varying stimulus strength. As mentioned above, this slow response was preceded, as a rule, by a fast EPSP which, in some cases, evoked a spike. In these cases, the slow IPSP was superimposed on the AHP which followed the spike. In these cases the slow IPSP could be distinguished from the AHP because (1) the slow IPSP is graded while the AHP is all-or-none; (2) the time-to-peak and duration are longer for the slow IPSP than for the AHP and (3) the α_2-adrenoceptor antagonist yohimbine attenuated the slow IPSP (see below) but had no effect on the AHP (Yoshimura et al., 1987c). In some of the cells the slow IPSP was followed by a slow EPSP. Neuronal input resistance decreased during the slow IPSP. The slow IPSP was recorded with electrodes filled with KCl, K acetate or K citrate. When a KCl-filled electrode was used, the slow

IPSP had stable amplitude and time course over the whole duration of recording, which was 30 – 60 min on average. Since over the same period leakage of Cl from the electrode tip would result in a progressive increase in internal Cl concentration until it exceeds external Cl concentration (as shown by the finding that fast IPSPs and the response is not due to a change in the Cl conducing) the fact that the slow IPSP remained hyperpolarizing and was stable suggests that this response is not due to a change in the Cl conductance of the SPN membrane. The slow IPSP amplitude increased when the membrane was depolarized and decreased when the membrane was hyperpolarized. In 3.6 mM KCl Krebs the response was nullified at a membrane potential of approximately – 90 mV. Hyperpolarization beyond this value resulted in a reversal of the response, from hyperpolarizing to depolarizing. The slow IPSP amplitude increased in low K Krebs (0.36 mM KCl) and decreased in high K Krebs (10.0 mM KCl). These properties suggest that the slow IPSP is due to an increase in K conductance of the SPN membrane. The slow IPSP was blocked by yohimbine (0.5 – 1.0 μM) or phentolamine (5 μM) but not by prazosin (1 μM) or propranolol (1 – 5 μM). In some cases yohimbine unmasked a slow EPSP. This suggests that slow EPSPs and IPSPs occur simultaneously in a number of SPNs and that the observed response is the algebraic sum of the two events.

NA (10 – 50 μM) produced membrane hyperpolarization, alone or followed by depolarization in 22 of 50 cells tested. This hyperpolarization is not mediated synaptically because it can be evoked during superfusion with TTX or with low Ca (0.25 mM) high Mg (5 mM) Krebs solution. During the NA-evoked hyperpolarization, like during the slow IPSP, the neuron-input resistance decreased. Like for the slow IPSP, the amplitude of the NA-evoked hyperpolarization decreased with membrane hyperpolarization or in high K and increased with membrane depolarization or in low K. In 3.6 mM Krebs the response reversed from hyperpolarizing to depolarizing at around – 90 mV.

This reversal potential, as well as the influence of membrane potential and of external K concentration, suggests that the NA-evoked hyperpolarization is due to an increase in K conductance of the SPN membrane. The hyperpolarizing response to NA was blocked by yohimbine but not by prazosin or propranolol. In all cases yohimbine unmasked a depolarization which was blocked by prazosin.

As in the case of the slow, prazosin-sensitive EPSP, it seems likely that CA-releasing axon terminals evoke the slow, yohimbine-sensitive, IPSP monosynaptically, rather than by excitation of segmental inhibitory interneurons antecedent to the SPN which could then release glycine or GABA on the SPN membrane. Various observations which suggest monosynaptic mediation of the yohimbine-sensitive IPSP are the fact that NA is the only putative transmitter studied so far which produces an increase in K conductance of the SPN membrane, whereas both glycine and GABA produce an increase in Cl conductance of the SPN membrane (Yoshimura and Nishi, 1982); the demonstration of CA-containing axon terminals forming axo-somatic and axo-dendritic synapses on the SPN (Chiba and Masuko, 1986); the presence of α_2-binding sites in the IML, presumably on the SPN membrane (Cabot et al., 1984; Seybold and Elde, 1984; Dashwood et al., 1985); the fact that the NA-evoked hyperpolarization is not blocked by the Ca-antagonist cobalt or by TTX and hence is due to a direct action of NA on the SPN membrane (Yoshimura et al., 1987c).

The rhythmic bursting induced in sympathetic preganglionic neurons by noradrenaline

The observations on the effects of NA on the SPN membrane potential, reported in the previous section, were made with brief (10 – 60 sec) exposure of the slice to the drug. When the exposure was prolonged beyond this duration, almost all neurons that were depolarized by NA showed a spontaneous, slow, relatively regular, oscillation in membrane potential. Bursts of spikes were superimposed on the depolarizing phase of the membrane potential oscillation. The oscillation, and the associated rhythmic bursting, persisted for as long as NA was present in the perfusate. The longest recorded stretch of bursting was 25 min duration. The mean frequency of the oscillation ranged from 0.2 to 1.0 Hz at membrane potentials of -45 to -65 mV. In the presence of NA, the oscillation disappeared when the membrane was hyperpolarized or depolarized by more than 10 mV from the resting potential level (-60 mV). The oscillation also disappeared when the NA was washed out. The bursting, and the underlying oscillation in membrane potential, are endogenous. This is demonstrated by three sets of observations. The first is that in TTX the bursting disappeared but the oscillation in membrane potential persisted, thus showing that the oscillation was not the result of synaptic input. The second is that the frequency of the oscillation was voltage-dependent, the frequency increasing with depolarization within the range of membrane potentials over which the oscillation occurs. This shows that the timing of the cellular events underlying the oscillation in membrane potential is set within the cell itself. Finally, the latter inference is supported by the observation that the rhythm of the oscillation is reset by firing the neuron with an intracellular current pulse: the duration of the oscillation cycle subsequent to the stimulated cycle was prolonged. The prolongation was phase-dependent, being less for stimulation in the first half than in the second half of the cycle. This spontaneous oscillation in membrane potential was associated with changes in neuron input resistance. During the depolarizing wave the neuron input resistance was markedly decreased. The oscillation was abolished by the Ca-channel blocker cobalt or by low Ca.

These findings show that this neuron is a conditional-pacemaker. The shift from the non-pacemaker to the pacemaker condition is produced in the presence of NA. Similar observations of transformation of the activity of neurons from non-rhythmic, exogenously driven, to a rhythmic endogenous bursting activity have been reported for other neurons (e.g. NTS neurons in the presence of TRH; Dekin et al., 1985).

Catecholamine effects on the spike and afterpotential of the sympathetic preganglionic neuron

The depolarizing phase of the SPN action potential results from influx of both sodium and calcium (Yoshimura et al., 1986c). Sodium influx accounts for the fast component of the normal action potential, while calcium influx accounts for a slower component which is responsible for the "shoulder" on the repolarization phase of the SPN spike. In the absence of NA, antidromic or current-induced spikes of the SPN are followed by a prominent AHP of 2.8 sec average duration and 16 mV average peak amplitude (Yoshimura et al., 1986b). In most cases two components can be distinguished, an initial faster and usually larger component (the fast AHP) which was not affected by cobalt or low Ca, followed by a slowly decaying component (the slow AHP) which was suppressed by cobalt or low Ca. Both components of the AHP are due to an increase in K conductance, but only the slow AHP is due to a Ca-activated K conductance.

NA abolished the shoulder on the repolarizing phase of the SPN spike (Yoshimura et al., 1986a). The spike therefore became narrower and its repolarization proceeded at an approximately constant rate. This effect is very similar to the effect of cobalt (Yoshimura et al., 1986a) and is due to a depressant action of NA on the Ca component of the spike. This is confirmed by the observation that in TTX the amplitude and rate of rise of the Ca spike decreased during NA administration (Yoshimura et al., 1986a). The depression by NA of the inward Ca current which generates the shoulder of the normal action potential may result from depression of the voltage-dependent Ca conductance which underlies the Ca spike and/or from enhancement of the voltage-dependent K conductance which underlies the repolarization of the spike (Yoshimura et al., 1986c). Regardless of the actual mechanism, reduction of the inward calcium current could result in reduced activation of the Ca-dependent outward K current which underlies the slow component of the AHP (Yoshimura et al., 1986b).

In the presence of NA the slow AHP was suppressed and an ADP, absent in the absence of NA, appeared (Yoshimura et al., 1986a). This ADP is a component of the afterpotential which was observed in almost all cells studied regardless of the effect of NA on membrane potential (depolarization or hyperpolarization). The amplitude of the ADP was dose-dependent. A typical NA-evoked ADP had time-to-peak of 50 msec (measured from the onset of the spike) and half-decay time of 60–120 msec. Small ADPs were preceded by an undershoot, presumably representing the fast component of the AHP. Large amplitude ADPs were preceded by small undershoots or by no undershoot at all. The NA-evoked ADP is associated with a decrease in neuron-input resistance and has a strong voltage-dependence, decreasing in amplitude non-linearly when the membrane was hyperpolarized. No reversal was observed. In order for the ADP to be produced by NA, Ca and Na ions must be present. Thus, the NA-evoked ADP is suppressed by the Ca-channel blocker cobalt, by low Ca or by intracellular injection of the Ca-chelator EGTA. It is also suppressed in Na-free medium. The data suggest that a slow inward cation current underlies the NA-evoked ADP and that this current is a Ca-activated Na current. This slow inward current can result in repetitive firing of the neuron in response to a single intracellular current pulse (Yoshimura et al., 1987a). Thus, responsiveness of the neuron to synaptic input can be markedly modulated by NA.

The disappearance of the slow AHP is not due to masking of the outward current of the slow AHP by the inward current of the NA-evoked ADP nor is the NA-ADP appearance due to unmasking of an inward current by the depression of the outward current of the slow AHP because the two currents are not simultaneous. Although the early part of the slow AHP overlaps the tail end of the NA-ADP, the late part of the slow AHP extends beyond the end of the NA-ADP. In some cases the slow AHP was suppressed even though the ADP must have been very small as judged by the fact that its presence was only detected as an upward displacement of the fast AHP trajectory.

Moreover, in other cases the ADP appeared and grew to near maximum amplitude while the slow AHP was still present (Yoshimura et al., 1987a). The depression of the slow AHP occurred after the ADP amplitude had reached a plateau. The depression of the slow AHP may be due to depression by NA of the Ca influx during the spike, already described, or of intermediate steps coupling the Ca influx to activation of the K conductance. Regardless of the generation mechanism, the suppression of the slow AHP will result in increased SPN responsiveness to excitatory input, since the AHP has a marked role in reducing the post-spike responsiveness of the SPN (Yoshimura et al., 1986b).

Discussion

The data presented describe the many different effects we have observed on SPNs by superfusing the spinal cord slice with NA. Some of these effects (depolarization, hyperpolarization, pacemaker activity) appear when NA is applied to the resting SPN membrane. The others (depression of the Ca spike and slow AHP, activation of the slow inward Na current that produces the ADP) are only observed when the neuron generates a spike. It is possible, but this has not been tested yet, that the inward current underlying the NA-ADP can be turned on by a subthreshold depolarization, e.g. by an EPSP. In this case this current would boost the EPSP and provide an additional push toward threshold (analogous to prepotentials observed in some neurons during steady-current injection, e.g. Lanthorn et al., 1984). Thus, this current, in addition to amplifying the response of the neuron to suprathreshold input by changing a single spike response into a burst of spikes, may also amplify subthreshold input by adding its depolarizing effect to that of the excitatory synaptic current.

The multiple actions of NA on the SPN are remarkable but not surprising in view of the multiple effects NA is known to have on different neurons and also on the same neuron. Conductances which have been reported to be increased or decreased by NA are the resting G_k (North and Yoshimura, 1984; Akasu et al., 1985), the G_{KCa} (Akasu et al., 1985; Schwindt et al., 1988) and the G_{Ca} (Minota and Koketsu, 1977; Dunlap and Fischbach, 1981; Gray and Johnston, 1987). Examples of modifications of conductances by NA in only one direction are the decrease in a transient G_K (Aghajanian, 1985) and the increase in G_{Cl} (Segal, 1981). Examples of multiple NA actions in a given neuron are provided, for instance, by the hippocampal pyramidal cell (Langmoen et al., 1981; Madison and Nicoll, 1986), the hippocampal granule cell (Gray and Johnston, 1987; Haas and Rose, 1987; Lacaille and Schwartzkroin, 1988) and the vesical parasympathetic cells (Akasu et al., 1985).

The inference from the observation that some slow EPSPs and IPSPs are suppressed by α_1- and α_2-adrenoceptor antagonists, respectively, is that some axons presynaptic to the SPN release CA. Thus, these observations provide a functional significance to the observations of CA-containing axons in the IML forming synaptic contacts on SPNs (Chiba and Masuko, 1986; Milner et al., 1988). Concerning the slow, CA-mediated, EPSP it is important to define its role relative to that of the fast EPSP in tonic and reflex excitation of SPNs. Intracellular recording in vivo (Dembowsky et al., 1985) shows that the background firing of SPNs, underlying the neurogenic tone of effector cells, is due to summating fast EPSPs. The fast EPSP is due to the action of a glutamate-like transmitter (Nishi et al., 1987). Thus, the slow EPSP produced by CA can only have the role of facilitatory mechanism by virtue of the longlasting depolarization and increase in neuron-input resistance it produces. The slow, Ca-dependent, inward Na current can also have an important role in the process of SPN excitation, as discussed above, if it turns out that this current can be activated by subthreshold depolarizations, in particular by the fast EPSP. A similar reasoning applies to the SPN firing evoked by afferent or CNS stimulation. For the firing evoked by somatic or visceral afferents there is intracellular evidence in vivo (Dembowsky et al.,

1985) that the firing is generated by summating fast EPSPs. For other inputs, for which intracellular data are not available, extracellular spike recording shows latencies and durations of evoked firing only compatible with generation by fast EPSPs (see review by Laskey and Polosa, 1988). Thus, it is likely that the slow EPSP produced by NA, together with the slow, Ca-dependent, inward Na current, performs only a facilitatory role in the generation of the background or reflex SPN firing. These considerations are relevant in connection with previously suggested hypotheses concerning the role of medullary adrenergic neurons in the control of SPNs (e.g. Milner et al., 1988). All the same considerations, with the appropriate modifications, may apply to the hypothesis that NA mediates reflex or centrally evoked SPN inhibition. However, much less is known about synaptic inhibition than synaptic excitation of SPNs, and hence for inhibition several possibilities for a NA role cannot be ruled out as yet.

The fact that NA applied by superfusion produced both depolarization and hyperpolarization may seem confusing. However, these two effects are mediated by different adrenoreceptors and it seems possible that these two receptor types are controlled by different subsets of adrenergic presynaptic axons. Indirect support for this view is provided by previous observations on the effect of adrenergic blockers on the background activity and on reflex responses of SPNs. Both excitatory and inhibitory effects have been described (see review by Laskey and Polosa, 1988). The observation that with iontophoresis only inhibitory α_2 effects were produced can be explained if α_2-receptor distribution was dominantly somatic, because this would be the most likely location of receptors which are exposed to iontophoretic NA, since the electrode tip is likely to be near the neuron soma. In the in vitro slice preparation the dose-response relationships for the two NA effects, depolarizing and hyperpolarizing, are similar (Yoshimura et al., unpublished observations), therefore the possibility that the two receptor types have different sensitivity to NA can be disregarded. This problem is not unique to the SPN, since other neurons [e.g. hippocampal pyramidal cells (Langmoen et al., 1981; Madison and Nicoll, 1986), hippocampal granule cells (Gray and Johnston, 1987; Haas and Rose, 1987; Lacaille and Schwartzkroin, 1988) and vesical parasympathetic cells (Akasu et al., 1985)] show multiple responses to NA applied by superfusion.

Two of the effects of NA, the depression of the slow AHP and the production of a slow inward Na current, are likely to result in a marked increase in the excitability of the neuron. The suppression of the slow AHP is likely to enhance the bursting produced by the NA-ADP. The additional property of conditional pacemaker will have the consequence that once the membrane is depolarized, as a result of NA released by presynaptic axons, activity will continue for a long time, i.e. prolonged afterdischarge. In this context recent data in α-motoneurons (Conway et al., 1988) show that L-DOPA, a CA precursor, produces the appearance of spontaneous rhythmic depolarizing potentials associated with burst firing, reminiscent of those described in the SPN.

Consider the importance of SPN bursting in ganglionic transmission. On the assumption that firing of sympathetic ganglion cells, in response to input from preganglionic neurons, is the result of spatio-temporal summation of unitary subthreshold fast nicotinic EPSPs, bursting of the input, as produced by CA, may improve transmission, by comparison with a non-bursting input pattern of the same mean frequency, by virtue of pre- and post-synaptic mechanisms. Presynaptically, increased ACh stores (Birks, 1978) and release of ACh (Birks, 1982) have been described. It is possible that increased release of non-cholinergic excitatory transmitter(s) also occurs. Postsynaptically, larger fast EPSPs and activation of muscarinic receptors as well as of receptors for a hypothetical non-cholinergic excitatory transmitter are possible mechanisms by which bursting may facilitate ganglionic transmission.

Acknowledgements

This work was supported by grants to S. Nishi and M. Yoshimura by the Ministry of Education, Science and Culture of Japan, and to C. Polosa by the Medical Research Council of Canada and the Quebec Heart Foundation.

References

Aghajanian, G.K. (1985) Modulation of a transient outward current in serotonergic neurones by α_1-adrenoceptors. Nature, 315: 501–503.

Akasu, T., Gallagher, J.P., Nakamura, I., Shinnick-Gallagher, P. and Yoshimura, M. (1985) Noradrenaline hyperpolarization and depolarization in cat vesical parasympathetic neurones. J. Physiol., 361: 165–184.

Birks, R.I. (1978) Regulation by patterned preganglionic neural activity of transmitter stores in a sympathetic ganglion. J. Physiol., 280: 539–572.

Birks, R.I. (1982) Acetylcholine release during burst-patterned stimulation of a sympathetic ganglion: its relation to transmission efficacy. J. Physiol. (Paris), 78: 417–419.

Cabot, J.B., Edwards, E., Bogan, N. and Schechter, N. (1984) Alpha-2-adrenergic receptors in avian spinal cord: increases in apparent density associated with the sympathetic preganglionic cell column. J. Auton. Nerv. Syst., 11: 77–89.

Carlsson, A., Falck, B., Fuxe, K. and Hillarp, N.A. (1964) Cellular localization of monoamines in the spinal cord. Acta Physiol. Scand., 60: 112–119.

Chiba, T. and Masuko, S. (1986) Direct synaptic contacts of catecholamine axons on the preganglionic sympathetic neurons in the rat thoracic spinal cord. Brain Res., 380: 405–408.

Conway, B.A., Hultborn, H., Kiehn, O. and Mintz, I. (1988) Plateau potentials in α-motoneurones induced by intravenous injection of L-DOPA and clonidine in the spinal cat. J. Physiol., 405: 369–384.

Coote, J.H. (1988) The organization of cardiovascular neurons in the spinal cord. Rev. Physiol. Biochem. Pharmacol., 110: 147–285.

Coote, J.H., MacLeod, V.H., Fleetwood-Walker, S.M. and Gilbey, M.P. (1981) Baroreceptor inhibition of sympathetic activity at a spinal site. Brain Res., 220: 81–93.

Dashwood, M.R., Gilbey, M.P. and Spyer, K.M. (1985) The localization of adrenoceptors and the opiate receptors in regions of the cat central nervous system involved in cardiovascular control. *Neuroscience*, 15: 537 – 551.

Dekin, M.S., Richerson, G.B. and Getting, P.A. (1985) Thyrotropin-releasing hormone induces rhythmic bursting in neurons of the nucleus tractus solitarius. *Science*, 229: 67 – 69.

Dembowsky, K., Czachurski, J., Amendt, K. and Seller, H. (1980) Tonic descending inhibition of the spinal somato-sympathetic reflex from the lower brain stem. *J. Auton. Nerv. Syst.*, 2: 157 – 182.

Dembowsky, K., Czachurski, J. and Seller, H. (1985) An intracellular study of the synaptic input to sympathetic preganglionic neurons of the third thoracic segment of the cat. *J. Auton. Nerv. Syst.*, 13: 201 – 244.

Dunlap, K. and Fischbach, G.D. (1981) Neurotransmitters decrease the calcium conductance activated by depolarization of embryonic chick sensory neurones. *J. Physiol.*, 317: 519 – 535.

Franz, D.N., Steffensen, S.C., Miner, L.C. and Sangdee, C. (1987) Neurotransmitter regulation of excitability in sympathetic preganglionic neurons through interactions with adenylate cyclase. In J. Ciriello, F.R. Calaresu, L.P. Renaud and C. Polosa (Eds.), *Organization of the Autonomic Nervous System: Central and Peripheral Mechanisms*, Alan Liss, New York, pp. 121 – 130.

Gray, R. and Johnston, D. (1987) Noradrenaline and β-adrenoceptor agonists increase activity of voltage-dependent calcium channels in hippocampal neurons. *Nature*, 327: 620 – 622.

Haas, H.L. and Rose, G.M. (1987) Noreadrenaline blocks potassium conductance in rat dentate granule cells in vitro. *Neurosci. Lett.*, 78: 171 – 174.

Lacaille, J-C. and Schwartzkroin, P.A. (1988) Intracellular responses of rat hippocampal granule cells in vivo to discrete applications of norepinephrine. *Neurosci. Lett.*, 89: 176 – 181.

Langmoen, I.A., Segal, M. and Andersen, P. (1981) Mechanisms of norepinephrine actions on hippocampal pyramidal cells in vitro. *Brain Res.*, 208: 349 – 362.

Lanthorn, T., Storm, J. and Andersen, P. (1984) Current-to-frequency transduction in CAI hippocampal pyramidal cells: slow prepotentials dominate the primary range firing. *Exp. Brain Res.*, 53: 431 – 443.

Laskey, W. and Polosa, C. (1988) Characteristics of the sympathetic preganglionic neuron and its synaptic input. *Progr. Neurobiol.*, 31: 47 – 84.

Madison, D.V. and Nicoll, R.A. (1986) Actions of noradrenaline recorded intracellularly in rat hippocampal CA1 pyramidal neurones, in vitro. *J. Physiol.*, 372: 221 – 244.

Milner, T.A., Morrison, S.F., Abate, C. and Reis, D.J. (1988) Phenylethanolamine *N*-methyltransferase-containing terminals synapse directly on sympathetic preganglionic neurons in the rat. *Brain Res.*, 448: 205 – 222.

Minota, S. and Koketsu, K. (1977) Effects of adrenaline on the action potential of sympathetic ganglion cells in bullfrogs. *Jpn. J. Physiol.*, 27: 353 – 366.

Nishi, S., Yoshimura, M. and Polosa, C. (1987) Synaptic potentials and putative transmitter actions in sympathetic preganglionic neurons. In J. Ciriello, F.R. Calaresu, L.P. Renaud and C. Polosa (Eds.). *Organization of the Autonomic Nervous System: Central and Peripheral Mechanisms,* Alan Liss, New York, pp. 15 – 26.

North, R.A. and Yoshimura, M. (1984) The actions of noradrenaline on neurones of the rat substantia gelatinosa in vitro. *J. Physiol.*, 349: 43 – 55.

Réthelyi, M. (1972) Cell and neuropil architecture of the intermediolateral (sympathetic) nucleus of cat spinal cord. *Brain Res.*, 46: 203 – 213.

Schwindt, P.C., Spain, W.J., Foehring, R.C., Chubb, M.C. and Crill, W.E. (1988) Slow conductances in neurons from cat sensory motor cortex in vitro and their role in slow excitability changes. *J. Neurophysiol.*, 59: 450 – 467.

Segal, M. (1981) The action of norepinephrine in the rat hippocampus: intracellular studies in the slice preparation. *Brain Res.*, 206: 107 – 128.

Seybold, V.S. and Elde, R.P. (1984) Receptor autoradiography in thoracic spinal cord: correlation of neurotransmitter binding sites with sympathoadrenal neurons. *J. Neurosci.*, 4: 2533 – 2542.

Taylor, D.G. and Brody, M.J. (1976) Spinal adrenergic mechanisms regulating sympathetic outflow to blood vessels. *Circ. Res. 38, Suppl.* II: 10 – 20.

Yoshimura, M. and Nishi, S. (1982) Intracellular recordings from lateral horn cells of the spinal cord in vitro. *J. Auton. Nerv. Syst.*, 6: 5 – 11.

Yoshimura, M., Polosa, C. and Nishi, S. (1986a) Noradrenaline modifies sympathetic preganglionic neuron spike and afterpotential. *Brain Res.*, 362: 370 – 374.

Yoshimura, M., Polosa, C. and Nishi, S. (1986b) Afterhyperpolarization mechanisms in cat sympathetic preganglionic neuron in vitro. *J. Neurophysiol.*, 55: 1234 – 1246.

Yoshimura, M., Polosa, C. and Nishi, S. (1986c) Electrophysiological properties of sympathetic preganglionic neurons in the cat spinal cord in vitro. *Pflügers Arch.*, 406: 91 – 98.

Yoshimura, M., Polosa, C. and Nishi, S. (1987a) Noradrenaline-induced afterdepolarization in cat sympathetic preganglionic neurons in vitro. *J. Neurophysiol.*, 57: 1314 – 1324.

Yoshimura, M. Polosa, C. and Nishi, S. (1987b) Slow EPSP and the depolarizing action of noradrenaline on sympathetic preganglionic neurons. *Brain Res.*, 414: 138 – 142.

Yoshimura, M., Polosa, C. and Nishi, S. (1987c) Slow IPSP and noradrenaline-induced inhibition of the cat sympathetic preganglionic neuron in vitro. *Brain Res.*, 419: 383 – 386.

Yoshimura, M., Polosa, C. and Nishi, S. (1987d) Noradrenaline induces rhythmic bursting in sympathetic preganglionic neurons. *Brain Res.*, 420: 147 – 151.

Yoshimura, M., Polosa, C. and Nishi, S. (1987e) After-depolarization mechanism in the in vitro, caesium-loaded, sympathetic preganglionic neuron of the cat. *J. Neurophysiol.*, 57: 1325 – 1337.

Yoshimura, M., Polosa, C. and Nishi, S. (1987f) A transient outward rectification in the cat sympathetic preganglionic neuron. *Pflügers Arch.*, 408: 207 – 208.

SECTION IV

Cardiovascular and Respiratory Integration by Ventrolateral Medullary Neurons

J. Ciriello, M.M. Caverson and C. Polosa (Eds.)
Progress in Brain Research, Vol. 81
© 1989 Elsevier Science Publishers B.V. (Biomedical Division)

CHAPTER 14

Specific areas of the ventral medulla controlling sympathetic and respiratory activities and their functional synchronization in the rat

Stanislaw Baradziej and Andrzej Trzebski

Department of Physiology, Medical Academy, 00 325 Warsaw, Poland

Introduction

A role for the rostral ventrolateral medulla (RVLM) in the generation of centrally or reflexly induced sympathetic activity and of pressor responses has been demonstrated in several different species (Trzebski et al., 1971; Guertzenstein and Silver, 1974; Dampney et al., 1982, 1985, 1986; McAllen, 1982; Hilton et al., 1983; Willette et al., 1983; Ross et al., 1984; Brown and Guyenet, 1985; Gatti et al., 1985; McAllen, 1986; Sun and Guyenet, 1986; Guyenet and Brown, 1986; for a review see Ciriello et al., 1986; Morrison et al., 1988). The ventrolateral medulla has also been extensively investigated for its role in generating the central respiratory drive (for review see Schlaefke, 1981; Loeschcke, 1982; Millhorn and Eldridge, 1986). Little, however, is known on the role of the ventrolateral medulla in the synchronization of the sympathetic activity with the central respiratory generator (CRG), an interaction known to exist (for a review see Koepchen et al., 1980; Bachoo and Polosa, 1987). Within the cat nucleus subretrofacialis of the RVLM separate sites have been identified where electrical stimulation produces activation only of the phrenic nerve, only of sympathetic neurons or of both of them (Dampney and McAllen, 1988). Glutamate microinjection in lateral regions of the RVLM produces depression of phrenic nerve activity and pressor response, presumably due to sympathoexcitation (Lawing et al., 1987).

The purpose of this chapter is to map out systematically the ventral medullary surface of the rat with microinjections of glutamate for effects on sympathetic and respiratory motoneuron activity. Another aim of our study is a search for some neuronal population within the ventral medulla which relays the input from different respiratory medullary neurons onto sympathetic premotoneurons. In our previous studies (Czyzyk et al., 1987) we have shown that the pattern of respiratory synchronization of sympathetic discharge in the rat of the normotensive Wistar-Kyoto strain is characterized by a peak of discharge in the early expiratory phase, while in inspiration, depression of activity occurs. In spontaneously hypertensive rats (SHRs) of the Okamoto-Aoki strain, depression of sympathetic activity in inspiration is absent, or limited only to early inspiration, and there is a peak of activity in late inspiration.

Methods

The experiments were carried out on adult Wistar rats (290 – 340 g), anesthetized with pentobarbital (Nembutal, 100 mg/kg, i.p.) followed by α-chloralose (50 mg/kg, i.v.). All animals were paralyzed with Pancuronium bromide (Pavulon 1 mg/kg, i.v.) and artificially ventilated with tidal volume of 1.5–2.0 ml and frequency of 60–80 strokes · min^{-1}. An expiratory load of 1–2 cm H_2O was imposed. End-tidal CO_2 was monitored with a Beckman gas analyzer and maintained at about 4.0%. Arterial blood pressure was recorded with a cannula in the femoral artery connected to a Statham pressure transducer. Another cannula was inserted into the femoral vein for intravenous infusions. Body temperature was monitored and maintained at 37–38°C with a heating pad.

All animals were placed in a stereotaxic instrument (David Kopf Instruments) in a supine position. Both vagus and aortic nerves were isolated and cut in the neck. The right phrenic nerve root, cervical sympathetic trunk, sympathetic lumbar chain between L4 and L5 and renal sympathetic nerve were isolated and put on a bipolar platinum electrode in a paraffin oil pool for recording. The electrical activity was amplified (30–3000 Hz band pass) and integrated after full-wave rectification (time constant 0.2–1.0 sec).

For determining the timing of sympathetic discharge within the respiratory cycle, the integrated sympathetic activity was averaged by Anops 105 signal averaging and histogram analyzer (Warsaw Institute of Technology Research). The onset of the integrated phrenic burst triggered the averager for 16 respiratory cycles.

The nerve activity was monitored on a 4-channel Tektronix oscilloscope and stored on a Racall Type ST 706 tape recorder for subsequent off-line analysis. An Elema Scholander pen recorder was used for continuous recording. In most of the animals phrenic nerve activity was recorded simultaneously with the activities of two of the three sympathetic nerves.

The ventral medulla was exposed after drilling through the occipital bone. The exposed area was approximately 8 mm long from the trapezoid bodies and about 6 mm wide, 3 mm on each side of the basilar artery.

Microinjections of 1 M L-glutamate monosodium dissolved in 0.9% buffered NaCl were performed through glass micropipettes with an outside tip diameter of 16 μm. A PV 830 Pneumatic Pico-Pump microinjector was used for the microinjection. Volumes injected ranged between 20 and 40 nl over 2 sec. Microinjections of the same volume of vehicle (buffered saline) into each area were used as control.

Microinjections were performed into different points of the exposed ventral medulla ipsilaterally or contralaterally to the nerves whose activity was recorded. Microinjections were either superficial, 100–400 μm beneath the ventral surface of the medulla, or deep, down to 1200 μm. Sites of microinjections were marked with Evans blue added to the glutamate solution. The brains were subsequently frozen and thin sections were cut. The area of dye deposit was approximately equal to twice the diameter of the micropipette tip. Microinjection sites were compared with the atlas of Paxinos and Watson (1986) and with the anatomical data of Newman (1984). Superficial microinjections into the RVLA corresponded to the ventral, superficial part of the lateral paragigantocellular nucleus (PGL). Microinjections into medial regions corresponded to the gigantocellular reticular ventral nucleus (GRV). Deep microinjections into the RVLA corresponded to the dorsal part of the PGL and those into the medial region corresponded to the rostroventrolateral reticular nucleus according to Paxinos and Watson (1986). No dye deposit was found in the nucleus ambiguus (Bieger and Hopkins, 1987). Some dye deposits were found within the reticular formation close to the ventral and ventromedial boundaries of the subcompact subdivision of the nucleus ambiguus. This region has been called the para-ambigual area (PA; Baradziej and Trzebski, 1989).

Results

Rostral ventrolateral medulla

Glutamate microinjections produced different effects on phrenic and sympathetic nerves depending

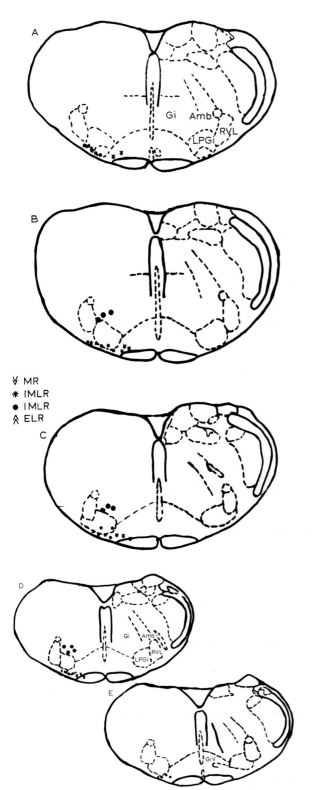

♦ MR
* IMLR
● IMLR
⋀ ELR

on the site of injection. For facilitating description the rostral medullary area, extending from 1.4 to 2.2 mm caudally to the trapezoid bodies (Fig. 1), is subdivided into: (1) a medial region (MR) 0.8 – 1.4 mm laterally to the midline; (2) an intermediate lateral region (IMLR) 1.4 – 1.8 mm from the midline; and (3) an extreme lateral region (ELR) 1.8 – 2.2 mm from the midline. Within the IMLR a superficial and a deep portion were distinguished. Within the deep portion a region ventral and medial to the nucleus ambiguus, defined as the PA (Fig. 2), was the only region where microinjections modified the timing of the synchronization of the sympathetic discharge to the respiratory cycle.

Medial region

Glutamate microinjections, ipsilateral or contralateral to the recorded nerves, 100 – 400 μm below the ventral medullary surface into GRV (Paxinos and Watson, 1986) produced an increase in the amplitude and duration of phrenic bursts (T1, Fig. 3) or shortening of the intervals between them (T_E). No significant sympathetic or blood pressure response was noted (Fig. 3). Microinjections into deeper structures were less effective and usually no effect was obtained at 400 – 500 μm beneath the ventral surface. The timing of the respiratory synchronization of sympathetic discharge remained unchanged, i.e. a clear inspiratory depression and early expiratory facilitation was observed in the normotensive Wistar rat.

Intermediate lateral region

Superficial, ipsilateral or contralateral microinjections into the IMLR, 100 – 400 μm beneath the

Fig. 1. Cross sections of the rostral medulla in rostrocaudal direction (A – E). ♦ MR = medial region; * IMLR = superficial intermediate lateral region; ⊛ IMLR = deep intermediate lateral region; ⋀ ELR = extreme lateral region. Only selected sites of glutamate microinjections are presented for clarity of the picture. Gi = gigantocellular reticular nucleus; LPGi = lateral paragigantocellular nucleus; Amb = nucleus ambiguus; RVL = rostroventrolateral reticular nucleus.

196

ventral medullary surface, at sites corresponding to the ventral part of PGL, produced an increase in amplitude, and often in duration of phrenic bursts, as well as in the level of activity recorded in all three sympathetic nerves. At times an initial transient inhibition of phrenic nerve activity was observed. A blood pressure rise always accompanied the sympathoexcitatory effect (Fig. 4).

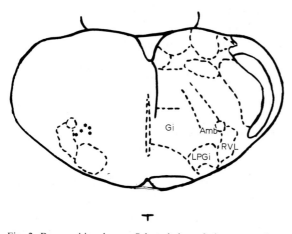

Fig. 2. Para-ambigual area. Selected sites of glutamate micro-injections are marked. Abbreviations as in Fig. 1.

Glutamate microinjections into deeper regions of PGL, 800 – 1200 μm beneath the ventral surface, produced greater sympathoexcitatory response in all three nerves than superficial injections (Fig. 5). Both sympathoexcitatory and pressor responses to a single glutamate microinjection lasted for up to 10 min. In contrast, the phrenic nerve excitatory response diminished gradually with application of glutamate into deeper structures of the IMLR and the inhibition of phrenic nerve activity was more prominent (Fig. 6). No shift in the timing of the respiration-synchronous sympathetic discharge within the respiratory cycle was observed.

Para-ambigual area

Glutamate microinjections into this area (Fig. 2) altered the timing of the respiratory synchronization of the sympathetic discharge. The depression of sympathetic activity during inspiration, typical for normotensive Wistar rats, could be changed into a facilitation of discharge while the early expiratory facilitation was changed into depression (Fig. 7D). Such a pattern of respiratory syn-

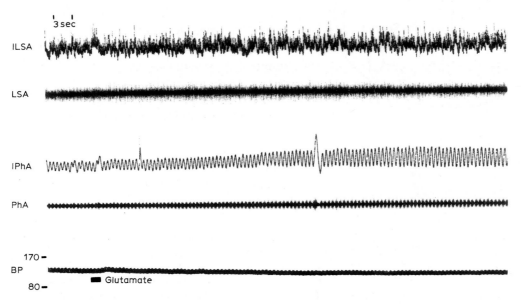

Fig. 3. Effect of glutamate microinjection into the medial region of rostroventral medulla. From top: ILSA = integrated lumbar trunk activity; LSA = lumbar trunk activity; IPhA = integrated phrenic nerve activity; PhA = phrenic nerve activity; BP = blood pressure. Note that the increase in amplitude of phrenic nerve discharge is not accompanied by changes in sympathetic activity.

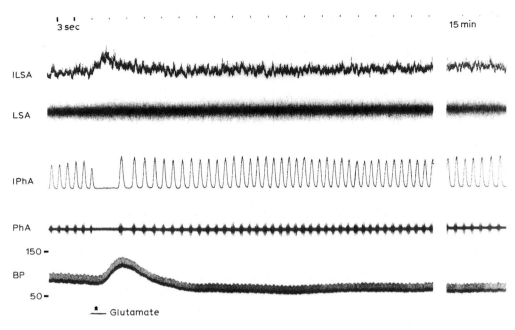

Fig. 4. Effect of glutamate microinjection into the superficial intermediate lateral region (IMLR). Abbreviations as in Fig. 3. Sympathoexcitatory and pressor effects are accompanied by augmented phrenic nerve discharge. Transient inhibition of phrenic nerve activity at the onset of microinjection is also observed.

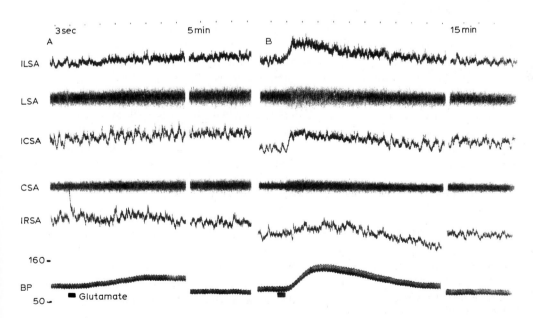

Fig. 5. Comparison of the sympathoexcitatory effects in three sympathetic nerves produced by superficial (A) and deep (B) glutamate microinjections into the intermediate lateral region (IMLR) in the same rat. From top: ILSA = integrated lumbar trunk activity; LSA = lumbar trunk sympathetic activity; ICSA = integrated cervical nerve sympathetic activity; CSA = cervical nerve sympathetic activity; IRSA = integrated renal nerve sympathetic activity; BP = arterial blood pressure.

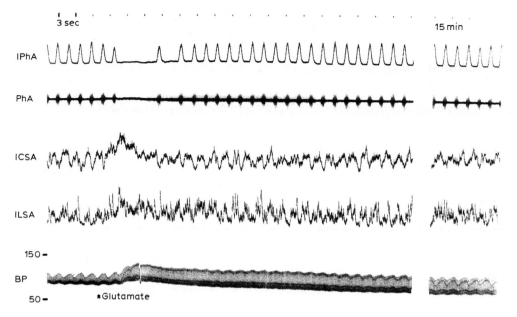

Fig. 6. Effect of glutamate microinjection into the deep intermediate lateral region (IMLR) 1.2 mm beneath ventral surface of the medulla. Abbreviations as in Fig. 5. Note that the strong sympathoexcitatory effect was not accompanied by increase in the phrenic nerve discharge.

chronization of sympathetic discharge produced by glutamate microstimulation of PA mimicked that found in the spontaneously hypertensive rat (Czyzyk-Krzeska and Trzebski, 1987). Sym-

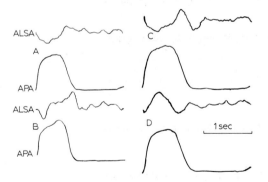

Fig. 7. Averaged lumbar sympathetic activity (ALSA) triggered by the onset of the phrenic nerve burst. (A) Control; (B) after glutamate microinjection into a site within the para-ambigual area; (C,D) after glutamate microinjections into other sites within the para-ambigual area. All records are from the same experiment. The pattern shown in (D) is similar to the timing of sympathetic discharge within the respiratory cycle in spontaneously hypertensive rats (i.e. facilitation in inspiration and depression in early expiration).

pathoexcitatory and pressor effects accompanied this modification of the pattern of synchronization of phrenic and sympathetic discharge.

The extent of the changes in synchronization varied with the site of injection (Fig. 7B – D). Similar changes in the pattern of respiratory synchronization were observed in all sympathetic nerves studied. Diffusion of glutamate into the nucleus ambiguus, which contains part of the ventral group of respiratory neurons (Saether et al., 1987; Ezure et al., 1988) can not be excluded although dye deposits were not found within this nucleus (Fig. 2).

Usually the frequency, amplitude and duration of the phrenic bursts increased following glutamate microinjection into the PA. However, in a few cases microinjections produced significant phase-shifts of the respiratory sympathetic discharge without changes of amplitude and/or frequency of phrenic nerve bursts. The functional properties of the PA have been reported elsewhere (Baradziej and Trzebski, 1989).

Extreme lateral region

Glutamate microinjections into the ELR, 100 – 400 μm beneath the medullary surface, were into the PGL. The most striking effect was a longlasting inhibition of phrenic nerve activity. In contrast, the activity of three sympathetic nerves increased significantly and arterial blood pressure increased (Fig. 8A). Glutamate microinjections into the most lateral part of this area produced only inhibition of phrenic nerve discharge with no

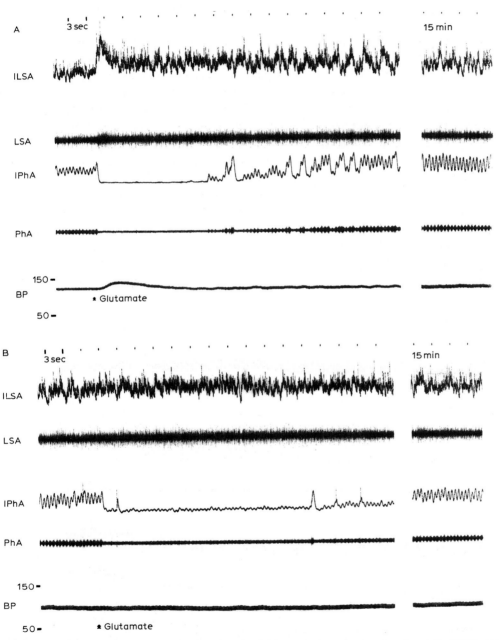

Fig. 8. Effect of glutamate microinjection into the superficial extreme lateral rostroventral medulla (ELR). Abbreviations as in Fig. 3. (A) Prolonged apnoea with accompanying sympathoexcitatory effect; (B) glutamate microinjection applied more laterally produces prolonged inhibition of phrenic nerve activity and no changes of sympathetic activity or arterial blood pressure.

change in blood pressure and sympathetic activity (Fig. 8B). Thus, this most lateral region appears to contain mainly the neuron population responsible for inhibition of inspiratory activity.

Caudal ventrolateral medulla

Glutamate microinjections, either ipsilateral or contralateral, into an area situated 5.0 – 5.5 mm caudal to the trapezoid bodies and 1.9 – 2.1 mm lateral to the midline, about 1 mm beneath the ventral medullary surface, a region corresponding to the A1 area (Granata et al., 1985), produced a depression of activity in all three sympathetic nerves and a fall of arterial blood pressure. This sympathoinhibitory effect was always accompanied by prolonged depression of phrenic nerve discharge (Fig. 9). The timing of the respiratory sympathetic discharge remained unchanged. The inhibitory area was found to be restricted. Frequently, microinjections applied into neighboring regions were followed by sympathoexcitatory and

pressor effects as well as apneustic phrenic nerve discharge.

Discussion and conclusions

The results of the present study indicate that distinct subpopulations of neurons exist in the rat ventral medulla that drive inspiratory or sympathetic nerve activities. The finding of spatial separation between respiratory and sympathetic-related neurons in the cat is in general agreement with the findings of McAllen (1986). However, the sites where selective respiratory stimulation was obtained were located more medially than the area described in cats by Lawing et al. (1987).

The medial region of RVLM (MR), from which selective excitatory effects on phrenic nerve activity were obtained, corresponds to the intermediate area described in cats (for a review see Schlaefke, 1981), which receives excitatory inputs from numerous sources maintaining the central respiratory drive (Millhorn and Eldridge, 1987).

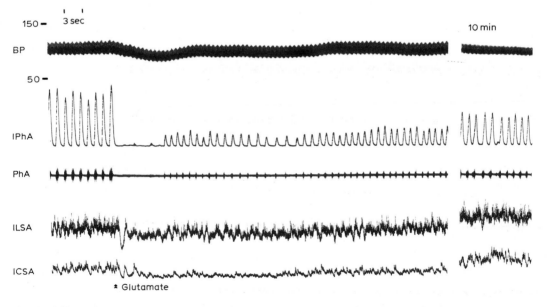

Fig. 9. Effect of glutamate microinjection into the caudal ventrolateral medulla. From top: BP = blood pressure; IPhA = integrated phrenic nerve activity; ILSA = integrated lumbar trunk activity; ICSA = integrated cervical trunk activity. Prolonged depression of phrenic nerve burst activity with parallel decreases of sympathetic activity and of arterial blood pressure are observed.

There is no evidence of bulbospinal respiratory neurons in close proximity to the surface of the ventral medulla. Therefore, the excitation of phrenic nerve activity from the MR must be mediated by known projections from the ventral medulla to bulbospinal respiratory neurons of the dorsal and ventral group, in deeper regions. No change in sympathetic discharge accompanied the excitation of respiratory activity from the superficial medial region, showing that in this region the respiratory network may be activated independently of sympathetic activity. Another striking example of dissociation was the simultaneous sympathetic excitation and inspiratory inhibition occurring after injection of glutamate within the lateral division of the PGL. Similar inspiration-inhibitory effects with accompanying pressor response have been observed after glutamate microinjections into the ventrolateral medulla in the cat (Lawing et al., 1987). This area may overlap with the caudal extension of the nucleus retrofacialis, the area known as Boetzinger complex or rostral group of expiratory neurons. These neurons inhibit monosynaptically the contralateral bulbospinal inspiratory neurons and phrenic motoneurons (Lipski and Merrill, 1980; Merrill et al., 1983; Merrill and Fedorko, 1984; for review see Long and Duffin, 1986). Recently, similar rostral expiratory neurons, presumably corresponding to the Boetzinger neurons in cats, have been identified in the rat (Ezure et al., 1988). It must be mentioned, however, that knowledge of the synaptic organization of respiratory neurons in the rat is still scanty. A systematic study by Seather et al. (1987) showed similarities between the rat and cat respiratory neurons as far as localization and classification according to firing pattern is concerned. On the other hand, in the rat only a few respiratory-related neurons are found in the dorsal group, most of them being concentrated in the ventrolateral group (Ezure et al., 1988).

A spatial separation between neuron sets driving respiratory and sympathetic activity was also evident within the IMLR. Here phrenic nerve responses were maximal close to the surface, while sympathoexcitatory effects were prominent at greater depths.

At all sites, sympathetic and phrenic nerve responses were produced by both ipsi- and contralateral glutamate injections. This result agrees with the findings of Dampney and McAllen (1988) in cats and with anatomical evidence that descending spinal projections from PGL and from other nuclei, in which microinjections were performed in the present study, cross the midline in the rat (Newman, 1985). Also the projections from bulbospinal respiratory neurons to phrenic motoneurons cross the midline of the rat medulla (Gauthier et al., 1986).

No site produced effects selectively on any of the three sympathetic nerves studied. This result contrasts with the finding of McAllen (1986b), and Dampney and McAllen (1988) who described in the cat discrete regions within the ventral medulla driving selectively skin or muscle vasoconstrictor fibers. Possible reasons for the discrepancy are the use in the present study of whole nerve recording, with the associated averaging of effects on fibers with different targets, and of larger injection volumes [20–40 nl compared with 2–20 nl in Dampney and McAllen's (1988) study].

Generalized inhibitory effects were produced by glutamate application to sites of the caudal ventrolateral medulla corresponding to the A1 area (Granata et al., 1985) and to the caudal vasodepressor area in the rat (Willette et al., 1983, 1984). This study provides the first evidence that the caudal sympathoinhibitory area of the ventrolateral medulla inhibits also inspiratory drive. This inhibitory area overlaps the retroambigual area where expiratory neurons are located in the cat. However, in this species caudal expiratory neurons do not inhibit premotor bulbospinal inspiratory neurons (Merrill, 1979) nor phrenic motoneurons (for review see Long and Duffin, 1986) in contrast to rostral expiratory neurons (Merrill and Fedorko, 1984). Therefore, an inhibitory pathway involving neurons other than caudal expiratory neurons may be considered, possibly one involving propriobulbar inhibitory neurons as described in the cat (Ballantyne and Richter, 1985).

Our study has also provided evidence that a specific area, the PA, controls the sympathorespiratory synchronization. Saether et al. (1987) described in the rat propriobulbar inspiratory or expiratory neurons within the reticular formation surrounding the nucleus ambiguus. These neurons could be excited by the glutamate microinjections applied to the para-ambigual area in the present study. Perhaps these neurons receive input from different categories of respiratory neurons (Saether et al., 1987) and project it to the sympathetic premotoneurons in the rostroventrolateral medulla in the rat (Guyenet and Brown, 1986). Respiration-related activity of some sympathetic premotoneurons has been reported by Haselton and Guyenet (1988) and McAllen (1987) in the cat. The respiratory modulated neurons within the rostroventrolateral medulla project to spinal preganglionic neurons. The patterns of respiration-related firing of preganglionic sympathetic neurons in the rat (Gilbey et al., 1986) are consistent with the firing patterns reported by Haselton and Guyenet (1988) in medullary sympathetic premotoneurons. We suggest therefore that the para-ambigual neuronal population identified in the present study is antecedent to the more superficial medullary sympathetic premotoneurons exhibiting respiratory related activity described by Haselton and Guyenet (1988). Further research is needed to test this hypothesis.

An additional hypothesis that can be made is that if the timing of the sympathorespiratory synchronization in the rat is controlled by a set of neurons in the PA, it is conceivable that the same neurons may be responsible for the differences in the pattern of sympathetic activity during the respiratory cycle between various strains of rats, e.g. Sprague-Dawley (Numao et al., 1987) versus Wistar rats (Czyzyk et al., 1987) or normotensive Wistar Kyoto rats versus SHRs (Czyzyk-Krzeska and Trzebski, 1987).

Our final conclusion is that the nature of the mechanism of interaction or coordination between the central respiratory rhythm generator and central sympathetic neurons cannot be solved until the neuronal wiring between these two neuron systems has been established. Further study of the synaptic connections and functional characteristics of the para-ambigual reticular neurons and perhaps other neuronal subpopulations within the ventrolateral medulla, may provide an answer to the question of how the circulatory and respiratory central control systems are mutually synchronized.

Acknowledgement

This study was supported by the Polish Academy of Sciences, grant no. 06-02 III.1.4.

References

Bachoo, M. and Polosa, C. (1987) Properties of the inspiratory related activity of sympathetic preganglionic neurones of the cervical trunk in the cat. *J. Physiol. (Lond.)*, 385: 545–564.

Baradziej, S. and Trzebski, A. (1989) Para-ambigual area neurons in the ventrolateral medulla oblongata control the pattern of respiratory-related synchronization of the sympathetic discharge in the rat. *Neurosci. Lett.*, (in press).

Bieger, D. and Hopkins, D.A. (1987) Viscerotopic representation of the upper alimentary tract in the medulla oblongata in the rat: the nucleus ambiguus. *J. Comp. Neurol.*, 262: 546–562.

Blessing, W.W. and Reis, D.J. (1982) Inhibitory cardiovascular function of neurons in the caudal ventrolateral medulla of the rabbit. Relationship to the area containing A_1 NE neurons. *Brain Res.*, 253: 161–172.

Brown, D.L. and Guyenet, P.G. (1985) Electrophysiological study of cardiovascular neurons in the rostral ventrolateral medulla in rats. *Circ. Res.*, 56: 359–369.

Christensen, K., Lewis, E. and Kuntz, A. (1979) Innervation of the renal blood vessels in the cat. *J. Comp. Neurol.*, 185: 23–29.

Ciriello, J., Caverson, M.M. and Polosa, C. (1986) Function of the ventrolateral medulla in the control of the circulation. *Brain Res. Rev.*, 11: 359–391.

Czyzyk, M.F., Fedorko, L. and Trzebski, A. (1987) Pattern of the respiratory modulation of the sympathetic activity is species dependent: synchronization of the sympathetic outflow over the respiratory cycle in the rat. In J. Ciriello, F.R. Calaresu, L.P. Renaud and C. Polosa (Eds.), *Organization of the Autonomic Nervous System: Central and Peripheral Mechanisms, Vol. 31*, Alan R. Liss, New York, pp. 143–152.

Czyzyk-Krzeska, M.F. and Trzebski, A. (1987) Respiratory synchronization of the sympathetic activity (SA) in spontaneously hypertensive rats (SHRs). *Neurosci., Suppl.* 22: 981P (*Abstr.*), p. S327.

Dampney, R.A.L. and McAllen, R.M. (1988) Differential control of sympathetic fibers supplying hindlimb skin and muscle by subretrofacial neurones in the cat. *J. Physiol. (Lond.),* 395: 41 – 56.

Dampney, R.A.L., Goodchild, A.K., Robertson, L.G. and Montgomery, W. (1982) Role of ventrolateral medulla in vasomotor regulation: a correlative anatomical and physiological study. *Brain Res.,* 249: 223 – 235.

Dampney, R.A.L., Goodchild, A.K. and Tan, E. (1985) Vasopressor neurons in the rostral ventrolateral medulla of the rabbit. *J. Auton. Nerv. Syst.,* 14: 239 – 254.

Ezure, K., Manaba, M. and Yamada, H. (1988) Distribution of medullary respiratory neurons in the rat. *Brain Res.,* 455: 262 – 270.

Gatti, P.J., Taveria DaSilva, A.M., Hamosh, P. and Gillis, R.A. (1985) Cardiorespiratory effects produced by application of L-glutamic acid and kainic acid to the ventral surface of the cat hindbrain. *Brain Res.,* 330: 21 – 29.

Gatti, P.J., Norman, W.P., Taveria DaSilva, A.M. and Gillis, R.A. (1986) Cardiorespiratory effects produced by microinjecting L-glutamic acid into medullary nuclei associated with the ventral surface of the feline medulla. *Brain Res.,* 381: 281 – 288.

Gauthier, P., Saether, K. and Monteau, R. (1986) Respiratory activity in the rat and the cat after sagittal splitting of the medulla. *Neurosci. Lett. Suppl.,* 26: S577.

Gilbey, M.P., Numao, Y. and Spyer, K.M. (1986) Discharge patterns of cervical sympathetic preganglionic neurones related to central respiratory drive in the rat. *J. Physiol. (Lond.),* 378: 253 – 265.

Granata, A.R., Kumada, M. and Reis, D.J. (1985) Sympathoinhibition by A_1-noradrenergic neurons is mediated by neurons in the C_1 area of the rostral medulla. *J. Auton. Nerv. Syst.,* 14: 387 – 395.

Guertzenstein, P.G. and Silver, A. (1974) Fall in blood pressure produced from discrete regions of the ventral surface of the medulla by glycine and lesions. *J. Physiol. (Lond.),* 242: 489 – 503.

Guyenet, P.G. and Brown, D.L. (1986) Nucleus paragigantocellularis lateralis and lumbar sympathetic discharge in the rat. *Am. J. Physiol.,* 250: R1081 – R1094.

Haselton, J.R. and Guyenet, P.G. (1988) Central respiratory generator-related activity of sympathetic premotoneurons in the rat rostral ventrolateral medulla (Abstr.). *Proc. 18th Annual Meeting Society for Neuroscience, Toronto,* 14.1.

Hilton, S.M., Marshall, J.M. and Timms, R.J. (1983) Ventral medullary relay neurons in the pathway from the defense areas of the cat and their effect on blood pressure. *J. Physiol. (Lond.),* 345: 149 – 166.

Koepchen, H.P., Hilton, S.M. and Trzebski, A. (Eds.) (1980) *Central Interaction between Respiratory and Cardiovascular Control Systems,* Springer-Verlag, Berlin – Heidelberg – New York.

Lawing, W.L., Millhorn, D.E., Bayliss, D.A., Dean, J.B. and Trzebski, A. (1987) Excitatory and inhibitory effects on respiration of L-glutamate microinjected superficially into the ventral aspects of the medulla oblongata in cat. *Brain Res.,* 435, 322 – 326.

Lipski, J. and Merrill, E.G. (1980) Electrophysiological demonstration of the projection from expiratory neurones in rostral medulla to contralateral dorsal respiratory group. *Brain Res.,* 197: 321 – 329.

Loeschcke, H.H. (1982) Central chemosensitivity and the reaction theory. *J. Physiol (Lond.),* 332: 1 – 24.

Long, S. and Duffin, J. (1986) The neuronal determinants of respiratory rhythm. *Prog. Neurobiol.,* 22: 101 – 182.

McAllen, R.M. (1986a) Action and specificity of ventral medullary vasopressor neurones in the cat. *Neuroscience,* 18: 51 – 59.

McAllen, R.M. (1986b) Location of neurones with cardiovascular and respiratory function at the ventral surface of the cat's medulla. *Neuroscience,* 18: 43 – 49.

McAllen, R.M. (1987) Central respiratory modulation of subretrofacial bulbospinal neurones in the cat. *J. Physiol. (Lond.),* 388: 533 – 545.

McAllen, R.M., Neil, J.J. and Loewy, A.D. (1982) Effects of Kainic acid applied to the ventral medullary surface on vasomotor tone, the baroreceptor reflex and hypothalamic autonomic responses. *Brain Res.,* 238: 65 – 76.

Merrill, E.G. (1979) In C. Von Euler and H. Lagercrantz (Eds.). *Central Nervous Control Mechanisms of Breathing,* Pergamon Press, Oxford, pp. 239 – 254.

Merrill, E.G. and Fedorko, L. (1984) Monosynaptic inhibition of phrenic motoneurons: a long descending projection from Botzinger neurons. *J. Neurosci.,* 4: 2350 – 2353.

Merrill, E.G., Lipski, J., Kubin, L. and Fedorko, L. (1983) Origin of the expiratory inhibition of nucleus tractus solitarius inspiratory neurons. *Brain Res.,* 263: 43 – 50.

Millhorn, D.E. and Eldridge, F.L. (1986) Role of ventrolateral medulla in regulation of respiratory and cardiovascular systems. *J. Appl. Physiol.,* 61: 1249 – 1263.

Morrison, S.F., Milner, T.A. and Reis, D.J. (1988) Reticulospinal vasomotor neurons of the rat rostral ventrolateral medulla: relationship to sympathetic nerve activity and the C_1 adrenergic cell group. *J. Neurosci.,* 8: 1286 – 1301.

Newman, D.B. (1985) Distinguishing rat brainstem reticulospinal nuclei by their neuronal morphology. I. Medullary nuclei. *J. Hirnforschung,* 26: 187 – 226.

Numao, Y., Koshiya, N., Gilbey, M.P. and Spyer, K.M. (1987) Central respiratory drive-related activity in sympathetic nerves of the rat: the regional differences. *Neurosci. Lett.,* 81: 279 – 284.

Paxinos, G. and Watson, C. (1986) *The Rat Brain in Stereotax-*

204

ic Coordinates, 2nd. edn., Academic Press, Sydney.

Richter, D.W., Ballantyne, D. and Remmer, J.E. (1986) How is the respiratory generated? A model. *News Physiol. Sci.*, 1: 109–112.

Ross, C.A., Ruggiero, D.A., Park, P.H., Joh, T.H., Sved, A.F., Fernandez-Pardal, J., Saavedra, J.M. and Reis, D.J. (1984a) Tonic vasomotor control by the rostral ventrolateral medulla, effect of electrical and chemical stimulation of the area containing C_1 adrenaline neurons on arterial pressure, heart rate and plasma catecholamines and vasopressin. *J. Neurosci.*, 4: 474–494.

Ross, C.A., Ruggiero, D.A., Joh, T.H., Park, D.H. and Reis, D.J. (1984b) Rostral ventrolateral medulla: selective projections to the thoracic autonomic cell column from the region containing C_1 adrenaline neurones. *J. Comp. Neurol.*, 228: 168–185.

Saether, K., Hilaire, G. and Monteau, R. (1987) Dorsal and ventral respiratory groups of neurons in the medulla of the rat. *Brain Res.*, 419: 87–96.

Schlaefke, M.E. (1981) Central chemosensitivity: a respiratory drive. *Rev. Physiol. Biochem. Pharmacol.*, 90: 171–244.

Sun, N.K. and Guyenet, P.G. (1986) Medullospinal sympathoexcitatory neurons in normotensive and spontaneously hypertensive rats. *Am. J. Physiol.*, 250: R910–R917.

Trzebski, A., Zielinski, A., Lipski, J. and Majcherczyk, S. (1971) Increase of the sympathetic preganglionic discharges and of the peripheral vascular resistance following stimulation by H^+ ions of the superficial chemosensitive areas of the medulla oblongata in cats. *Proceed. Sci., Vol. 9, XXV Int. Congress, Munich*, 1971, p. 571. (Abstr. 1701).

Willette, R.N., Barcas, P.P., Krieger, A.J. and Sapru, H.N. (1983) Vasopressor and depressor areas in the rat medulla. Identification by microinjection of L-glutamate. *Neuropharmacology*, 22: 1071–1080.

Willette, R.N., Krieger, A.J., Barcas, P.P. and Sapru, H.N. (1984) Interdependence of rostral and caudal ventrolateral medullary areas in the control of blood pressure. *Brain Res.*, 321: 169–174.

J. Ciriello, M.M. Caverson and C. Polosa (Eds.)
Progress in Brain Research, Vol. 81
© 1989 Elsevier Science Publishers B.V. (Biomedical Division)

CHAPTER 15

Role of the ventrolateral medulla in the cardiovascular responses to changes in the carbon dioxide tension in the arterial blood

Franco Lioy

Department of Physiology, University of British Columbia, Vancouver, B.C., Canada, V5T 1W5

Introduction

During the past few years the role of the ventrolateral medulla (VLM) in the regulation of the respiratory and cardiovascular systems has been the object of numerous investigations which have been discussed in depth in some excellent reviews (e.g. see Koepchen et al., 1981; Ciriello et al., 1986; Millhorn and Eldridge, 1986). This chapter will focus on the role of structures located on the surface of the VLM in mediating the cardiovascular responses to changes in the concentration of CO_2 in the arterial blood.

Three chemosensitive regions, a cranial area M (Mitchell et al., 1963), an intermediate area S (Schlaefke and Loeschcke, 1967) and a caudal area L (Loeschcke et al., 1970), have been identified whose stimulation by solutions with high PCO_2/low pH induce hyperventilation while superfusion with low PCO_2 alkaline solutions induces the opposite effect. It also became apparent the some cardiovascular effects could be induced by stimulation or inhibition of neurons located on the surface of the VLM and/or in regions immediately below it. After the initial demonstration by Loeschcke and Koepchen (1958) that application of procaine to the VLM surface induced a large fall in systemic arterial pressure (SAP), other investigators showed that electrical or chemical

stimulation or cold blockade of various sites on the VLM surface could have profound effects on SAP (Schlaefke and Loeschcke, 1967; Loeschcke et al., 1970; Schlaefke et al., 1970).

Feldberg and Guertzenstein (1972) identified two areas on the VLM surface which exert important cardiovascular effects: a rostral area located immediately below the inferior border of the trapezoid bodies and roughly overlapping with area M and the rostral part of intermediate area S of the pH sensitive areas (Schlaefke, 1981), and a caudal area, located laterally to the pyramids and 6 – 9 mm caudal to the trapezoid bodies (Feldberg and Guertzenstein, 1976; Guertzenstein and Lopes, 1984). Electrical stimulation of the rostral area (the "glycine area") induces a pressor response, while application of pentobarbitone or of inhibitory agents such as glycine or GABA causes a fall in blood pressure. McAllen (1986a) showed that microinjections in this area of amino acids which selectively activate cell bodies induce large increases in SAP and renal nerve activity. Since bilateral electrolytic lesions within this area decrease SAP to levels seen after high spinal section (Guertzenstein and Silver, 1974; Bousquet et al., 1975) it seems that this region is an important source of the supraspinal component of vascular tone. Electrical stimulation or application of nicotine or of excitatory amino acids to the caudal area (the "nicotine area") induce a large fall in SAP (and also secretion of vasopressin by hypothalamic neurons) (Bisset et al., 1975; Feldberg and Guertzenstein, 1976; Guertzenstein and Lopes, 1984). An interaction between these two areas has been postulated (Willette et al., 1984): the nicotine area appears to exert its depressor effect by inhibiting, possibly via noradrenergic fibers, the sympathoexcitatory neurons located in the "glycine area" (Granata et al., 1985).

The VLM surface and the neurogenic cardiovascular responses to CO_2

CO_2 produces conflicting effects on the cardiovascular system: while it causes bradycardia and vasodilatation by its direct action on the cardiac pacemaker and the vascular smooth muscle (Suutarinen, 1966) it also induces sympathetic excitation which results in vasoconstriction, tachycardia and an increase in myocardial contractility. The involvement of CNS structures in these effects was suggested by Downing and Siegel (1963) who found that administration of hypercapnic gas mixtures to anesthetized dogs increased the discharge rate of the inferior cardiac nerve even after sino-aortic denervation. Lioy et al. (1978) perfused at constant flow the innervated, vascularly isolated hindlimbs of the cat with normocapnic normoxic blood, while the $PaCO_2$ in the rest of the body was changed from hypocapnic to hypercapnic levels (Fig. 1). A direct relationship between $PaCO_2$ and hindlimb vascular resistance was observed and it was calculated that $25-30\%$ of the neurogenic vascular tone, i.e. of that fraction which was lost after administration of phentholamine, was dependent on the presence of normocapnic levels of CO_2. Deafferentation of the peripheral chemoreceptors (PCh) did not affect this relationship. Experiments which more directly pointed to an intracranial mechanism for this relationship between CO_2 and sympathetic tone were performed by perfusing the cephalic circulation with hypercapnic and/or hypoxic blood: this resulted in increases in SAP, heart rate, total

peripheral resistance and myocardial contractility (Kao et al., 1962; Downing et al., 1963; De Geest et al., 1965; Hainsworth et al., 1984).

Small inconstant changes in SAP had been observed upon application of solutions of different pH to the chemosensitive areas of the VLM (Schlaefke et al., 1970). However, in these experiments the animals were breathing spontaneously and the cardiovascular effects could have been masked by the simultaneous changes in intrapleural pressure, arterial blood gases and lung volume induced by the changes in ventilation. Szulczyk and Trzebski (1976) injected acid solutions (pH 6.6 – 6.8) over the surface of the VLM of

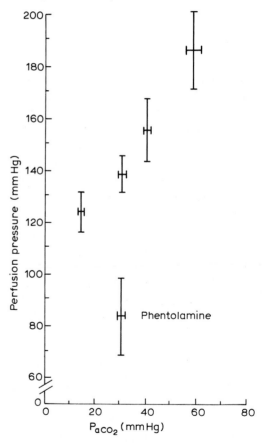

Fig. 1. Effect of changes of $PaCO_2$ in six cats on the perfusion pressure (PP) of the isolated hindlimb perfused at constant flow. The lowest point indicates the PP after phentolamine injection into the perfusion system. Horizontal and vertical bars illustrate the standard errors of the mean. (Courtesy of Lioy et al., 1978.)

anesthetized, artificially ventilated, vagotomized and sino-aortic deafferented cats and observed, besides the expected increase in phrenic nerve activity, an increase in SAP, hindlimb vascular resistance and sympathetic nerve firing. Superfusion of the exposed VLM surface with hypercapnic acidic solutions in similarly prepared normocapnic cats induced an increase in phrenic activity and SAP, a small but significant increase in heart rate and a reduction of the hindlimb blood flow. Opposite effects were obtained by VLM superfusion with hypocapnic, alkaline solutions (Lioy et al., 1981). The increase in vascular resistance induced by systemic hypercapnia in anesthetized vagotomized, sino-aortic denervated rats is not uniformly distributed (Lioy et al., 1985), the larger vasoconstrictor effects being seen in the skin, skeletal muscle, intestine, kidneys and pancreas. Cardiac output and heart rate were not significantly affected. Different responses of different sympathetic nerves to changes in CO_2 were also observed by Koepchen et al. (1981). Recently,

Gatti and Massari (1988) observed that stimulation of area S with L-glutamate induced an increase in femoral artery resistance which was larger than that seen in the renal vascular bed.

The intermediate area S of the VLM surface appears to be of particular importance in mediating the CO_2 sensitivity of sympathetic vasoconstrictor tone. Cold blockade (12°) of this area in vagotomized, sino-aortic denervated cats significantly reduces the slope of the relationship between $PaCO_2$ and hindlimb vascular resistance (Hanna et al., 1979). It is interesting to note that during hypocapnia cold blockade of area S has practically no effect on hindlimb resistance (Fig. 2A). This is in agreement with the observation that sympathetic preganglionic neurons (SPNs) have a very low sensitivity to CO_2 in the hypocapnic range (Hanna et al., 1981): therefore, cold blockade of area S, by removing an input mediating CO_2 sensitivity, cannot be expected to have a significant effect on sympathetic vasoconstrictor tone. Cooling the whole of the VLM sur-

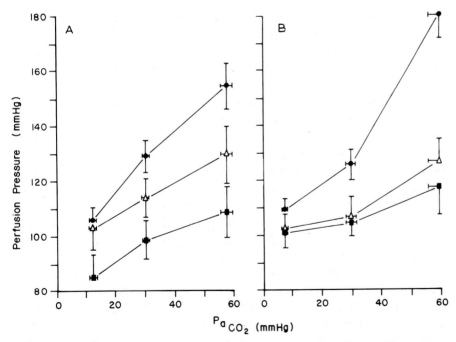

Fig. 2. Relationship between $PaCO_2$ and hindlimb perfusion pressure. ●, Control (medullary surface temperature 37°); △, selective cooling of area S (12°); ■, cooling of the whole ventral surface (12°). (A) Control group ($n = 12$); (B) adrenalectomized group ($n = 5$). Horizontal and vertical bars illustrate the standard errors of the mean. (Courtesy of Hanna et al., 1979.)

face to 12° decreased vascular resistance but did not further decrease the sensitivity to CO_2: it seems therefore that area S mediates the whole of the supraspinal component of the CO_2 sensitivity of the SPNs. This is confirmed by the fact that the hindlimb vascular resistance to CO_2 after area S blockade was of the same magnitude as that observed in spinal animals (Rohlicek and Polosa, 1986; Accili et al., 1988). The effect of area S blockade persisted after adrenalectomy and therefore the decrease in the vascular resistance sensitivity to CO_2 was not due to a decrease in catecholamine release. Superficial cells in the VLM have been shown to stimulate catecholamine release (McAllen, 1986b): these cells must not play a significant role in the CO_2 sensitivity of the vascular resistance. However, they may be important in the maintenance of the basal sympathetic vascular tone since the further decrease in vascular resistance observed when the whole VLM surface was cooled to 12° was no longer seen after adrenalectomy (Fig. 2B).

These results were recently verified by Millhorn (1986) who found that the integrated activity of the cervical sympathetic trunk increased during hypercapnia and that cooling of area S to 20° abolished this increase. Moreover, stepwise cooling of area S in normocapnia induced stepwise reductions in SAP and sympathetic activity confirming the importance of this area in the maintenance of basal sympathetic tone.

The VLM and the peripheral chemoreceptors

The interaction between the central chemosensitive areas and the PCh has also been extensively studied. Millhorn et al. (1982) found that the respiratory response to PCh stimulation was clearly decreased by cooling area S. Hanna et al. (1981) observed an increase of the activity of single SPN fibers in the cervical sympathetic trunk of vagotomized cats during progressive changes of $PaCO_2$ from 20 to 90 mmHg, both before and after PCh deafferentation. They estimated that between $PaCO_2$ values of 40 – 60 mmHg the cen-

tral and peripheral chemoreceptor inputs were responsible for a similar proportion of the overall SPN response. Above 60 mmHg there appeared to be occlusion between the two inputs because, after carotid sinus nerve section, the SPN response was greater than 50% of that seen before the section. Superficial cells in and around the lateral reticular nucleus of the VLM, which is in close proximity to area S, project to the SPNs in the intermediate lateral column of the spinal cord (see Ciriello, 1986) and are excited by activation of the carotid bodies (Caverson et al., 1984). Moreover, electrolytic lesions of this nucleus reduce the PCh-induced pressor response (Ciriello and Calaresu, 1977).

It appears therefore that area S plays an important role in mediating the CO_2 sensitivity of the SPNs also by modulating the effectiveness of the PCh input.

Effects of CO_2 on the respiratory and sympathetic outputs

There are remarkable similarities between the CO_2 response of SPNs and respiratory neurons. The average response of a population of SPNs to changes in $PaCO_2$ describes a sigmoid curve which is very similar to that of the simultaneously recorded phrenic-nerve response (Hanna et al., 1981). The only significant difference is that in hypocapnia rhythmic phrenic activity disappears while the SPN activity reaches a plateau at 20% of the maximal response and becomes CO_2-independent.

The question arises if the chemosensitive areas of the VLM affect the respiratory and sympathetic outputs independently or if the changes in sympathetic activity are secondary to those of the respiratory centres.

It is well known that some sympathetic neurons show activity which is phase locked to the central inspiratory activity (Preiss et al., 1975; Polosa et al., 1980; Bainton et al., 1985). A number of experiments have shown that maneuvers that modify the respiratory drive also alter in a similar way the respiration-synchronous sympathetic activity

(Bachoo and Polosa, 1985, 1986, 1987). In PCh deafferented cats there was a fixed delay between the onset of the inspiratory burst of sympathetic nerve activity and that of the phrenic nerve burst. This delay remained constant up to respiratory frequencies of 300 per min (Bachoo and Polosa, 1987). In other experiments Bachoo and Polosa (1985) found that both the phrenic activity and the inspiratory-synchronous sympathetic activity were suppressed by stimulation of low threshold afferent fibers in the superior laryngeal nerve. This inspiratory component of the SPN discharge was responsible for 24% of the neurogenic vascular resistance present in normocapnia. This is very similar to the 25–30% of hindlimb neurogenic vascular tone which is lost when the animals are exposed to hypocapnia (Lioy et al., 1978). This similarity suggests that in normocapnia the CO_2 sensitive component of neurogenic vascular resistance is due only to the inspiration-synchronous component of the sympathetic activity.

An experimental approach which could clarify this problem would be one that modifies the sympathetic output without affecting the respiratory one. Millhorn (1986) found that if rhythmic phrenic activity was not present an increase in $PaCO_2$ did not increase sympathetic activity. He concluded that only chemoreceptor information which was first filtered through the respiratory neuron network reached the sympathetic neurons.

However, he kept the phrenic motor neurons below the apneic threshold by cooling area S: this would be expected to affect also those chemoreceptive mechanisms which could directly influence the sympathetic system, thus invalidating his conclusion.

On the other hand, Koepchen et al. (1981) found that when phrenic activity was suppressed in hypocapnic cats considerable activity persisted in the cervical sympathetic trunk and that, once the $PaCO_2$ was raised, an increase in sympathetic activity sometimes could be detected before phrenic bursts reappeared. Similar results were obtained by Trzebski and Kubin (1981) who found that when $PaCO_2$ was progressively increased in hypocapnic apneic cats the SAP and the sympathetic activity started increasing at $PaCO_2$ levels that were lower than those which induced resumption of rhythmic phrenic activity. These different CO_2 thresholds for the pressor and respiratory effects were confirmed by Lioy and Trzebski (1984) in vagotomized, sino-aortic denervated rats which were made apneic by hypocapnia. A step increase of $PaCO_2$ from 15 to 22 mmHg induced an immediate sustained increase in SAP which could persist for up to 45 min in the absence of any rhythmic phrenic activity. A further increase of $PaCO_2$ to 25 mmHg induced an immediate larger increase in SAP and then, when rhythmic phrenic activity resumed, an additional step increase in SAP was observed (Fig.

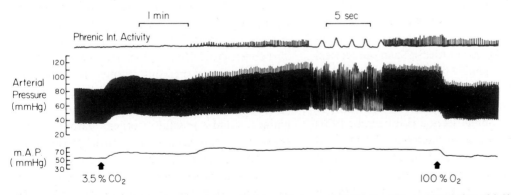

Fig. 3. Vagotomized, sino-aortic deafferented rat. Hyperventilation with 100% O_2. Effect of inhalation of 3.5% CO_2 in O_2 on the arterial pressure and the integrated electrical activity of the phrenic nerve (Phrenic Int. Activity). m.A.P. = mean arterial pressure. (Courtesy of Lioy and Trzebski, 1984.)

3). It can be noticed that this second increase in SAP was also characterized by rhythmic oscillations, with the pressure increasing after each phrenic burst. It appears therefore that, although CO_2 stimulation of the central chemosensitive areas can induce a pressor effect in the absence of rhythmic respiratory activity, the central sympathetic mechanisms involved also receive excitatory inputs from the respiratory oscillator, which are then transmitted to the cardiovascular effectors by respiratory-modulated sympathetic neurons (Preiss et al., 1975; Preiss and Polosa, 1977). The simplest explanation for these conflicting experimental results is that there were differences in the preparations which altered the percentage of spontaneously active preganglionic neurons with afferent "CO_2 connections". The effect of an inspiratory synchronous, CO_2-dependent input on the generation of the sympathetic response to CO_2 is probably quite significant but more investigation will be necessary before definite conclusions can be made.

Cardiovascular effects of CO_2 in spinal animals

The spinal cord may represent an additional source of CO_2-dependent neurogenic vascular tone. After section of the cervical spinal cord systemic hypercapnia can induce an increase in SAP in rats (Lioy and Trzebski, 1984) and cats (Johnson et al., 1968). Szulczyk and Trzebski (1976) observed an increase in SAP and sympathetic nerve firing in spinal cats in response to superfusion of the first thoracic spinal segment with acidic solutions. Increases in the firing rate of the SPNs in the cervical trunk during systemic hypercapnia in spinal animals were also observed (Zhang et al., 1982). CO_2-mediated vasoconstriction was not present immediately after spinal section (Lioy et al., 1978) but a direct relationship between $PaCO_2$ and hindlimb vascular resistance, both in the hypocapnic and hypercapnic range, was observed 3 – 4 h after the transection (Rohlicek and Polosa, 1986). The role of the sympathetic nervous system in this CO_2-induced vasoconstriction was demonstrated by the abolition of the vasoconstriction after ganglionic blockade. However, no change in postganglionic nerve activity in response to hypercapnia was observed in spinal dogs (Alexander, 1945) and cats (Meckler and Weaver, 1985).

Accili et al. (1988) perfused separately the vascularly isolated hindlimbs of the spinal (C2) cat. One leg was sympathetically denervated by sectioning the lumbar chain. An increase in $PaCO_2$ induced an immediate vasoconstriction in the innervated leg, followed by a delayed, sustained vasoconstriction which was present also in the denervated leg. This late vasoconstriction was drastically reduced, but not abolished, after bilateral adrenalectomy. It appears therefore that in the spinal animal the CO_2-mediated vasoconstriction is due not only to the activation of sympathetic neurons but also to the release of adrenal catecholamines. Since some vasoconstriction was still present in the denervated leg after adrenalectomy, it is possible that also other vasoconstrictor substances may have been released during hypercapnia.

Hypercapnia has been shown to induce release of adrenal catecholamines in spinal animals (Millar, 1960; Cantu et al., 1966), probably by direct stimulation of the medullary cells (Nahas et al., 1967). Hypercapnia also induces an increase of the circulating levels of renin, angiotensin and vasopressin (Anderson et al., 1980; Wang et al., 1984) which can affect blood pressure (Staszewska-Barczak, 1978; Walker, 1987). In previous experiments (Hanna et al., 1979) we observed that adrenalectomy did not significantly change the vasoconstrictor effect of hypercapnia in cats with an intact central nervous system. It is possible, however, that in the spinal animal, in which the sympathetic tone is decreased, circulating catecholamines, and possibly other vasoconstrictor substances, may assume a much more important role both in the maintenance of the basal vascular tone and in its sensitivity to CO_2. From the experimental evidence reviewed it is apparent that CO_2, both in the hypocapnic and hypercapnic range, is an important factor in the regulation of vascular resistance and arterial pressure.

The direct relaxing effect of CO_2 on the vascular smooth muscle is counteracted in most vascular territories by the increase in vasoconstrictor sympathetic activity mediated through the VLM chemosensitive areas, the PCh and the spinal cord. It is likely that CO_2 influences vascular resistance not only by this action on the neurogenic tone but also by affecting the release of vasoconstrictor substances such as adrenal catecholamines and possibly angiotensin and vasopressin. However, the importance of these humoral factors, as well as that of the spinal cord, in the CO_2-mediated regulation of the vascular resistance in the intact animal is not clear and should be the object of more detailed investigations.

Acknowledgements

The support of the Medical Research Council of Canada and of the British Columbia Heart Foundation is gratefully acknowledged.

References

Accili, E.A., Puttaswamaiah, S. and Lioy, F. (1988) Effects of carbon dioxide on hindlimb vascular resistance in the acute spinal cat. *J. Auton. Nerv. Syst.*, 23: 87 – 94.

Alexander, R.S. (1945) The effects of blood flow and anoxia on spinal cardiovascular centres. *Am. J. Physiol.*, 143: 689 – 708.

Anderson, R.J., Rose, Jr., C.E., Berns, A.S., Erickson, A.L. and Arnold, P.E. (1980) Mechanism of effect of hypercapnic acidosis on renin secretion in the dog. *Am. J. Physiol.*, 238: F119 – F125.

Bachoo, M. and Polosa, C. (1985) Properties of a sympatho-inhibitory and vasodilator reflex evoked by superior laryngeal nerve afferents in the cat. *J. Physiol. (Lond.)*, 364: 183 – 198.

Bachoo, M. and Polosa, C. (1986) The pattern of sympathetic neurone activity during expiration in cat. *J. Physiol. (Lond.)*, 378: 375 – 390.

Bachoo, M. and Polosa, C. (1987) Properties of the inspiration-related activity of sympathetic preganglionic neurones of the cervical trunk in the cat. *J. Physiol. (Lond.)*, 385: 545 – 564.

Bainton, C.R., Richter, D.W., Seller, H., Ballantyne, D. and Klein, J.P. (1985) Respiratory modulation of sympathetic activity. *J. Auton. Nerv. Syst.*, 12: 77 – 90.

Bisset, G.W., Feldberg, W., Guertzenstein, P.G. and Rocha e

Silva, M., Jr. (1975) Vasopressin release by nicotine: the site of action. *Br. J. Pharmacol.*, 54: 463 – 474.

Bousquet, W.W., Feldman, J., Kelly, J. and Block, R. (1975) Role of the ventral surface of the brainstem in the hypotensive action of clonidine. *Eur. J. Pharmacol.*, 34: 151 – 156.

Cantu, R.C., Nahas, G.G. and Manger, W.C. (1966) Effect of hypercapnic acidosis and of hypoxia on adrenal catecholamine output of the spinal dog. *Proc. Soc. Exp. Biol. Med.*, 122: 434 – 437.

Caverson, M.M., Ciriello, J. and Calaresu, F.R. (1984) Chemoreceptor and baroreceptor inputs to ventrolateral medullary neurons. *Am. J. Physiol.*, 247: R872 – R879.

Ciriello, J. and Calaresu, F.R. (1977) Lateral reticular nucleus: a site of somatic and cardiovascular integration in the cat. *Am. J. Physiol.*, 233: R100 – R109.

Ciriello, J., Caverson, M.M. and Polosa, C. (1986) Function of the ventrolateral medulla in the control of the circulation. *Brain Res. Rev.*, 11: 359 – 391.

De Geest, H., Levy, M.N. and Zieske, H. (1965) Reflex effects of cephalic hypoxia, hypercapnia and ischemia upon ventricular contractility. *Circ. Res.*, 17: 349 – 358.

Downing, S.E. and Siegel, J.H. (1963) Baroreceptors and chemoreceptors influence on sympathetic discharge to the heart. *Am. J. Physiol.*, 20: 471 – 479.

Downing, S.E., Mitchell, J.H. and Wallace, A.G. (1963) Cardiovascular responses to ischemia, hypoxia and hypercapnia of the central nervous system. *Am. J. Physiol.*, 204: 881 – 887.

Feldberg, W. and Guertzenstein, P.G. (1972) A vasodepressor effect of pentobarbitone sodium. *J. Physiol. (Lond.)*, 224: 83 – 103.

Feldberg, W. and Guertzenstein, P.G. (1976) Vasodepressor effects obtained by drugs acting on the ventral surface of the brainstem. *J. Physiol. (Lond.)*, 258: 337 – 355.

Gatti, P.J. and Massari, V.J. (1988) Regional hemodynamic effects produced following medullary ventral surface application of L-glutamic acid in the cat. *Physiologist*, 31: A52.

Granata, A.R., Ruggiero, D.A., Park, D.H., Joh, T.H. and Reis, D.J. (1985) Brainstem area with C_1 epinephrine neurons mediates baroreceptor vasodepressor responses. *Am. J. Physiol.*, 248: H547 – H567.

Guertzenstein, P.G. and Lopes, O.U. (1984) Cardiovascular responses evoked from the nicotine-sensitive area on the ventral surface of the medulla oblongata in the cat. *J. Physiol. (Lond.)*, 347: 345 – 360.

Guertzenstein, P.G. and Silver, A. (1974) Fall in blood pressure produced from discrete regions of the ventral surface of the medulla by glycine and lesions. *J. Physiol. (Lond.)*, 242: 489 – 503.

Hainsworth, R., McGregor, K.H., Rankin, A.J. and Soladoye, A.O. (1984) Cardiac inotropic responses from changes in carbon dioxide tension in the cephalic circulation of anaesthetized dogs. *J. Physiol. (Lond.)*, 357: 23 – 35.

Hanna, B.D., Lioy, F. and Polosa, C. (1979) The effect of cold

212

blockade of the medullary chemoreceptors on the CO_2 modulation of the vascular tone and heart rate. *Can. J. Physiol. Pharmacol.*, 57: 461–468.

Hanna, B.D., Lioy, F. and Polosa, C. (1981) Role of carotid and central chemoreceptors in the CO_2 response of sympathetic preganglionic neurons. *J. Auton. Nerv. Syst.*, 3: 421–435.

Johnson, R.H., Crampton Smith, A. and Walker, J.M. (1968) Heart rate and blood pressure of spinal cats inspiring CO_2 before and after injection of hexamethonium. *Clin. Sci.*, 36: 257–265.

Kao, F.F., Suntay, R.G. and Li, W.K. (1962) Respiratory sensitivity to CO_2 in cross-circulated dogs. *Am. J. Physiol.*, 202: 1024–1028.

Koepchen, H.P., Klüssendorf, D. and Sommer, D. (1981) Neurophysiological background of central neural cardiovascular-respiratory coordination: basic remarks and experimental approach. *J. Auton. Nerv. Syst.*, 3: 335–368.

Lioy, F. and Trzebski, A. (1984) Pressor effect of CO_2 in the rat: different thresholds of the central cardiovascular and respiratory responses to CO_2. *J. Auton. Nerv. Syst.*, 10: 43–54.

Lioy, F., Hanna, B.D. and Polosa, C. (1978) CO_2-dependent component of the neurogenic vascular tone in the cat. *Pflügers Arch.*, 374: 187–191.

Lioy, F., Hanna, B.D. and Polosa, C. (1981) Cardiovascular control by medullary surface chemoreceptors. *J. Auton. Nerv. Syst.*, 3: 1–7.

Lioy, F., Blinkhorn, M.T. and Garneau, C. (1985) Regional hemodynamic effects of changes in $PaCO_2$ in the vagotomized, sino-aortic deafferented rat. *J. Auton. Nerv. Syst.*, 12: 301–314.

Loeschcke, H.H. and Koepchen, H.P. (1958) Versuch zur Lokalisation des Angriffsortes des Atmungs – und Kreislauf-wirkung von Novocain in Liquor Cerebrospinalis. *Pflügers Arch.*, 266: 628–664.

Loeschcke, H.H., Delattre, J., Schlaefke, M.E. and Trouth, C.O. (1970) Effects on respiration and circulation of electrically stimulating the ventral surface of the medulla oblongata. *Respir. Physiol.*, 10: 184–197.

McAllen, R.M. (1986a) Location of neurones with cardiovascular and respiratory function at the ventral surface of the cat's medulla. *Neuroscience*, 18: 43–49.

McAllen, R.M. (1986b) Action and specificity of ventral medullary vasopressor neurones in the cat. *Neuroscience*, 18: 51–59.

Meckler, R.L. and Weaver, L.C. (1985) Splenic, renal and cardiac nerves have unequal dependence upon tonic supraspinal inputs. *Brain Res.*, 338: 123–135.

Millar, R.A. (1960) Plasma adrenaline and noradrenaline during diffusion respiration. *J. Physiol. (Lond.)*, 150: 79–90.

Millhorn, D.E. (1986) Neural respiratory and circulatory interaction during chemoreceptor stimulation and cooling of ventral medulla in cats. *J. Physiol. (Lond.)*, 370: 217–231.

Millhorn, D.E. and Eldridge, F.L. (1986) Role of ventrolateral medulla in regulation of respiratory and cardiovascular systems. *J. Appl. Physiol.*, 61: 1249–1263.

Millhorn, D.E., Eldridge, F.L. and Waldrop, T.G. (1982) Effects of medullary area $I_{(s)}$ cooling on respiratory response to chemoreceptor inputs. *Respir. Physiol.*, 49: 23–39.

Nahas, G.G., Zagury, D., Milhaud, A., Manger, W.M. and Pappas, G.D. (1967) Acidemia and catecholamine output of the isolated canine adrenal gland. *Am. J. Physiol.*, 213: 1186–1192.

Polosa, C., Gerber, U. and Schondorf, R. (1980) Central mechanism of interaction between sympathetic preganglionic neurons and the respiratory oscillator. In H.P. Koepchen, S.M. Hilton and A. Trzebski (Eds.), *Central Interactions Between Respiratory and Cardiovascular Control Systems*, Springer-Verlag, Berlin, pp. 137–143.

Preiss, G. and Polosa, C. (1977) The relation between end-tidal CO_2 and discharge patterns of sympathetic preganglionic neurons. *Brain Res.*, 112: 255–267.

Preiss, G., Kirchner, F. and Polosa, C. (1975) Patterning of sympathetic preganglionic neuron firing by the central respiratory drive. *Brain Res.*, 87: 363–374.

Rohlicek, C.V. and Polosa, C. (1986) Neural effects of systemic hypoxia and hypercapnia on hindlimb vascular resistance in acute spinal cats. *Pflügers Arch.*, 406: 392–396.

Schlaefke, M.E. (1981) Central chemosensitivity: a respiratory drive. *Res. Physiol. Biochem. Pharmacol.*, 90: 171–244.

Schlaefke, M.E. and Loeschcke, H.H. (1967) Lokalisation eines an der Regulation von Atmung und Kreislauf beteiligten Gebietes an der ventralen Oberflache der Medulla Oblongata durch Kalteblockade. *Pflügers Arch.*, 297: 201–220.

Schlaefke, M.E., See, W.R. and Loeschcke, H.H. (1970) Ventilatory response to alteration in H^+ ion concentration in small areas of the ventral medullary surface. *Respir. Physiol.*, 10: 198–212.

Staszewska-Barczak, J. (1978) Participation of the sympathetic and the renin-angiotensin systems in blood pressure control during hypercapnia in the anaesthetized dog. *Eur. J. Pharmacol.*, 49: 441–444.

Suutarinen, T. (1966) Cardiovascular response to changes in arterial carbon dioxide tension. *Acta Physiol. Scand. Suppl.*, 226: 1–75.

Szulczyk, P. and Trzebski, A. (1976) The local effect of pH changes in the cerebrospinal fluid on the ventrolateral areas of medulla oblongata and on the spinal cord surface on the activity of cardiac and vertebral sympathetic nerves. *Acta Physiol. Pol.*, 27: 9–17.

Trzebski, A. and Kubin, L. (1981) Is the central inspiratory activity responsible for pCO_2 dependent drive of the sympathetic discharge? *J. Auton. Nerv. Syst.*, 3: 401–420.

Walker, B.R. (1987) Cardiovascular effect of V_1 vasopressinergic blockade during acute hypercapnia in conscious rats. *Am. J. Physiol.*, 252: R127–R133.

Wang, B.C., Sundet, W.D. and Goetz, K.L. (1984) Vasopressin in plasma and cerebrospinal fluid of dogs during hypoxia or acidosis. *Am. J. Physiol.*, 247: E449–E455.

Willette, R.N., Punnen, S., Krieger, A.J. and Sapru, H.N. (1984) Interdependence of rostral and caudal ventrolateral medullary areas in the control of blood pressure. *Brain Res.*, 321: 169–174.

Zhang, T.-X., Rohlicek, C.V. and Polosa, C. (1982) Responses of sympathetic preganglionic neurons to systemic hypercapnia in the acute spinal cat. *J. Auton. Nerv. Syst.*, 6: 381–389.

J. Ciriello, M.M. Caverson and C. Polosa (Eds.)
Progress in Brain Research, Vol. 81
© 1989 Elsevier Science Publishers B.V. (Biomedical Division)

CHAPTER 16

Integration of cardiorespiratory responses in the ventrolateral medulla

N.S. Cherniack, E.M. Adams, N.R. Prabhakar, M. Haxhiu and J. Mitra

Case Western Reserve University, School of Medicine, 2119 Abington Road, Cleveland, OH 44106, U.S.A.

The circulatory and respiratory systems act together to extract oxygen from the air and deliver it to the tissues, and to preserve cellular pH homeostasis by removing the CO_2 produced by metabolic processes. Both the peripheral chemoreceptors and the baroreceptors evoke respiratory and circulatory responses and are mechanisms by which integration of cardiorespiratory actions can occur. There are, in addition, a number of sites in the brain stem and in higher brain centers which can produce effects both on breathing and on the circulation. These include the nucleus tractus solitarius in the medulla, the nucleus parabrachialis medialis and Kölliker-Fuse in the pons, sites in the hypothalamus and in the amygdala. Attention has been directed to the ventrolateral medulla as another such site (Schlaefke, 1981).

Interactive groups of pressor and depressor vasomotor neurons have been described in the rostral and caudal medulla, respectively (Brody et al., 1986; Ciriello et al., 1986). At approximately the same locations there are neurons which can dramatically alter respiratory activity. In a number of species including the rat, cat and rabbit, abrupt changes in the pattern of breathing can be produced by cooling the ventrolateral surface of the medulla to temperatures which block synaptic transmission as well as by neuroactive substances applied to the surface or microinjected within 1 ml of the surface of the ventral medulla (Cherniack et

al., 1979; Haxhiu et al., 1984; Gatti et al., 1986; McAllen, 1986). A small area of the ventral medullary surface (VMS) in the region of the nucleus paragigantocellularis lateralis from which apnea can be produced, even by unilateral cooling, has been described in the cat (Budzinska et al., 1985). A similar area has been described in dogs (Adams et al., 1987). It has been proposed that the VMS contains the central chemoreceptors responsible for the changes in ventilation produced by alterations in arterial PCO_2, but this issue remains controversial. It has also been proposed that there is a common set of neurons for respiratory and vasomotor control, which act together to provide an excitatory input needed to elicit respiratory, as well as vasomotor changes.

This chapter reviews some of our own investigations on the circulatory and respiratory effects which can be elicited by experimental interventions near the surface of the ventrolateral medulla. These studies suggest that the neurons evoking respiratory and circulatory changes may not be the same even though they may be tightly coupled since respiratory and circulatory changes of unequal magnitude or even in opposite direction may occur. In addition, we will demonstrate a possible role of angiotensin II (AII) in mediating the pressor effects from the ventrolateral medulla.

A number of observations demonstrate that neurons near the ventral surface of the medulla can simultaneously depress or excite respiration and vasomotor activity. Surface cooling in cats depresses breathing, lowers blood pressure frequently and reduces the respiratory oscillations in sympathetic activity (VanLunteren et al., 1987) (Fig. 1). The application of NMDA (a glutamate agonist) to the ventrolateral surface of cats raises blood pressure and increases sympathetic activity. When NMDA is applied to the medullary surface of cats made apneic by hyperventilation, respiratory activity reappears and at times oscillations in blood pressure (Mayer waves) appear at the same time. Similar changes can occur when

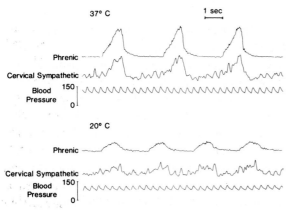

Fig. 1. Moving-average electrical activity recorded from phrenic and cervical sympathetic nerves in a cat ventilated with 7% CO_2 in O_2. Activity is shown with ventral medullary surface warm (37°C, top) and after cooling the intermediate area of the ventral medulla to 20°C (bottom). Blood pressure (Torr) is also shown before and after medullary cooling. Increased respiratory rate was not a consistent finding with medullary cooling. (From vanLunteren et al., 1987.)

apneic animals are given CO_2 to inhale (Fig. 2). Some instances of simultaneously occurring respiratory and circulatory changes may be overlooked if the appropriate variable has not been recorded. For instance, even when ventral surface manipulation produces undetectable or barely detectable alterations in tidal volume or phrenic nerve activity, changes can easily be discerned in the respiratory activity of the cranial nerves which innervate the muscles of the upper airways (Haxhiu et al., 1984b). Similarly, changes in vasomotor activity may be overlooked if blood pressure is measured rather than sympathetic activity.

On the other hand, there are clear instances in which the respiratory and circulatory effects of VMS manipulations can be dissociated. For example, microamounts of glutamate analogues can evoke only respiratory or only circulatory responses depending on the site of injection (McAllen, 1986). Nicotine applied to the caudal areas of the VMS in cats lowers blood pressure but increases respiratory activity (Janu et al., unpublished). Among glutamate analogues, kainate is more effective than NMDA in elevating blood pressure, while the converse is true for stimulating respiration, when the drugs are applied topically on the intermediate area of the VMS (Fig. 3). The same group has also shown that unilateral topical application of NMDA to the intermediate area evokes a maximal stimulation of respiration which cannot be further enhanced by NMDA application contralaterally (Mitra et al., 1987). In contrast,

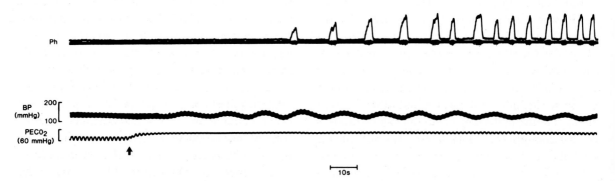

Fig. 2. Administration of 7% CO_2 in O_2 to a hyperoxic, hypocapnic, artificially ventilated, paralyzed, cat causes the appearance of phrenic nerve activity (upper trace) and of a regular oscillation in blood pressure (lower trace).

bilateral application of NMDA can produce a much greater rise of blood pressure than does unilateral application.

Systemically administered AII is known to produce some of its hypertensive effects by acting on structures in the anteroventral wall of the third ventricle (Catelli and Sved, 1988; Ferguson, 1988). In addition, it is believed that AII formed within the brain can modulate blood-pressure responses (Phillips, 1984). Recently, studies in humans and rabbits have demonstrated immunoreactive angiotensin in the rostral and caudal ventrolateral medulla (Allen et al., 1988; Mendelsohn et al., 1988). We have undertaken a series of experiments to assess the role of AII in the ventrolateral medulla on blood pressure and phrenic nerve activity. The experiments, although preliminary, suggest that the AII response is mediated in part through the ventral portion of the medulla. Experiments were performed in male Sprague-Dawley rats anesthetized with urethane (1.3 g/kg, i.p.) and tracheotomized. The femoral artery and vein were cannulated to monitor blood pressure and administer supplemental doses of anesthesia, respectively. The phrenic nerve (usually on the

right side) was isolated and cut. The animal's head was fixed in a stereotaxic apparatus. Dorsal craniotomy was performed to expose the medulla. At the end of surgery the animal was paralyzed (Pancuronium bromide, 0.6 mg/kg, i.v.) and artificially ventilated. The body temperature of the animal was maintained at 37°C with a servocontrolled heating blanket. The electrical activity of the phrenic nerve was recorded with a pair of stainless steel hook electrodes. The phrenic nerve signal was amplified with an AC-coupled amplifier (Grass Instruments, Quincy, MA, Model PG 511) having band pass filter settings of 0.1 to 3.0 KHz, full-wave rectified and processed by a moving averager (Charles Ward Enterprises, Philadelphia, PA) using a time constant of 100 msec. Drug microinjections into the ventrolateral medulla were made with a three barrel micropipette assembly having a total tip diameter of 50 μ. The barrels contained an AII antagonist ([sar^1 III^8] AII), lidocaine HCl and a NaCl solution. The first two barrels were connected to a pneumatic pressure system (Picospritzer, General Valve Corp., NJ) and the third barrel to a high input impedance AC amplifier for recording local neuronal activity. It is known that the rostroventrolateral (RVL) and the caudoventrolateral (CVL) medulla are situated below the nuclei ambiguus and retroambiguus, respectively. It is also known that these nuclei contain neurons having respiration-related activity. Since in our experiments the stereotaxic approach to the RVL and CVL were made from the dorsal medullary surface, our sites for injection were always below the nuclei ambiguus and retroambiguus as assessed by disappearance of respiration-related activity. We also used the effects of the injection of lidocaine as a second criterion for assessing the function of the target regions. Depressor effects produced by lidocaine were used to identify the RVL. It has been shown by Ross et al. (1984) that microinjection of GABA or tetrodotoxin in the RVL lowers blood pressure. The paraventricular hypothalamic nucleus (PVH) was electrically stimulated with an implanted concentric bipolar electrode (usually on the left side). We used

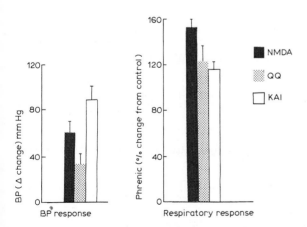

Fig. 3. Comparison of blood pressure and respiratory responses to the ventrolateral medullary surface (intermediate area) application of glutamate analogues at an end tidal PCO_2 level of 50 mmHg in cats. N-methyl-D-aspartate (NMDA) had a strong respiratory and kainate (KAI), a strong vasomotor effect. Quisqualate (QQ) was least effective in stimulating blood pressure and was as effective as KAI in stimulating respiration.

stereotaxic coordinates from Paxinos and Watson's atlas (Paxinos and Watson, 1986). Integrated phrenic nerve activity was analyzed with respect to the changes in peak activity occurring during inspiration measured from baseline levels during expiration. At least 10 breaths were measured during a control period to obtain an average value.

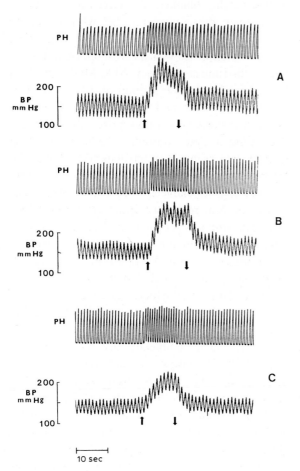

Fig. 4. The effect of paraventricular hypothalamic nucleus (PVH) stimulation on systemic blood pressure before and after microinjection of AII antagonist in the CVL and RVL in the rat. The animal was pretreated with a vasopressin antagonist (i.v.). (A) Control response to PVH stimulation. Integrated phrenic nerve activity (PH) at the top and systemic blood pressure (BP) at the bottom. Stimulus on and off are marked by arrows (100 μA, 0.2 msec, 50 Hz). (B) Stimulation of the PVH in the same animal after the microinjection (10 ng in 10 nl) of AII antagonist in the CVL. No change in BP response. (C) Stimulation of the PVH after the microinjection of AII antagonist in the RVL. BP response was attenuated.

Changes in blood pressure and phrenic nerve activity were either expressed in absolute values or as percent of control. All rats were given i.v. the vasopressin antagonist ([d(CH$_2$)$_5$^{1}, O-Me-Tyr^2, Arg8]-Vasopressin) to eliminate the effects of vasopressin released into the systemic circulation. Stimulation of the PVH (100 μA, 0.2 msec, 50 Hz) raised blood pressure. After injection of the AII agonist the effect of the PVH stimulus was attenuated (Fig. 4). This suggests that release of AII into the RVL may partially account for the rise in blood pressure seen with hypothalamic excitation. As shown in Fig. 5, injections of AII (10 ng in 10 nl) in the rostral ventrolateral medulla increased blood pressure and respiration while injection into the CVL decreased blood pressure and breathing. Moreover, injection of the AII antagonist (10 ng in 10 nl) into the RVL lowered blood pressure and caused apnea while injection into the CVL raised blood pressure and tended to reduce breathing. This finding indicates the possibility that AII has a tonic action on vasomotor activity in ventrolateral medullary regions. Also, although the effects of the AII antagonist in the two regions (rostral versus caudal) on blood pressure were opposite in direction, the effects on respiration were

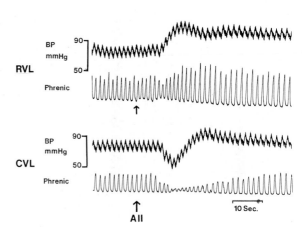

Fig. 5. Effects of AII microinjection on blood pressure and phrenic nerve activity in a rat. Upper panel shows the effects of microinjection of AII (10 ng in 10 nl) in the RVL. Both BP and phrenic nerve activity increased. Lower panel shows the effects of AII microinjection in the CVL. BP and phrenic nerve activity decreased.

qualitatively similar, supporting the idea obtained in the experiment described earlier that respiratory and vasomotor neurons in the ventral medulla are not identical. The blood pressure elevation caused by systemic administration of AII (in doses of 500 ng/kg and 5 µg/kg) was reduced by antagonist injection in the RVL but not by antagonist injection into the CVL (Fig. 6). Injection of the AII antagonist in either area failed to modify the blood pressure rise produced by doses of 10 µg/kg of AII nor did it alter the response to systemic norepinephrine. By contrast, lidocaine (20 ng in 10 nl) injection into either the RVL or CVL decreased blood pressure and greatly diminished the response to AII at all doses tried but failed to alter the response to intravenously administered norepinephrine. These studies suggest that a component of the hypertensive response to systemic AII arises from the rostral ventrolateral medulla. One possibility is that fiber tracts which use AII as synaptic transmitter or modulator descend to the medulla from structures on the anterior wall of the third ventricle.

It is not known on what cells AII acts in the ventrolateral medulla and in particular whether these cells contain epinephrine. It is possible that the attenuation of responses to systemic AII after injection of the antagonist into the RVL is the result of a change in the baroreceptor input since this input was intact.

Summary

Interventions confined to the region adjacent to the VMS can produce both respiratory and circulatory effects. Although it has been suggested that both breathing and vasomotor changes arise from the same neural elements near the VMS, our own investigations indicate that the neurons involved are closely linked but not identical. This belief is supported by recent studies which show that AII and angiotensin antagonists microinjected into the rostral portion of the VMS can significantly modify blood pressure and respiration but can produce effects of different sign. These observations, coupled with previous studies of the VMS, indicate the possibility that regions near the VMS may contribute to integration of circulatory and respiratory responses.

References

Adams, E.M., Chonan, T., von Euler, C. and Cherniack, N.S. (1987) Respiratory effect of focal cooling in the ventrolateral medulla of the dog. *Fed. Proc.*, 46: 826.

Allen, A.M., Chai, S.Y., Clevers, J., McKinley, M.J., Paxinos, G. and Mendelsohn, F.A.O. (1988) Localization and characterization of angiotensin II receptor binding and angiotensin converting enzyme in the human medulla oblongata. *J. Comp. Neurol.*, 269: 249–264.

Brody, M.J., Alper, R.H., O'Neill, T.P. and Porter, J.P. (1986) Central neural control of the cardiovascular system. In A. Zanchetti and R.C. Tarazi (Eds.), *Handbook of Hypertension, Vol. 8, Pathophysiology of Hypertension – Regulatory Mechanisms*, Elsevier, Amsterdam, pp. 1–25.

Budzinska, K., von Euler, C., Kao, F.F., Pantaleo, T. and Yamamoto, Y. (1985) Effects of graded focal cold block in rostral areas of the medulla. *Acta Physiol. Scand.*, 124: 329–340.

Catelli, J.M. and Sved, A.F. (1988) Lesions of the AV3V region attenuate sympathetic activation but not the hypertension

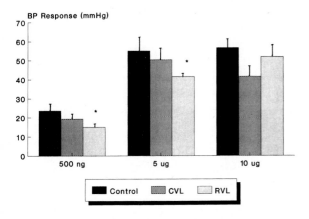

Fig. 6. Blood pressure response to systemic injection of AII (500 ng, 5 µg and 10 µg/kg) before and after the injection of AII antagonist (10 ng in 10 nl) in the CVL and RVL. BP increase from the control level has been plotted along the ordinals and different doses of AII along the abscissa. Lower (500 ng and 5 µg) but not the higher (10 µg) dose of AII effect on BP was attenuated by RVL injection of AII antagonist. Injection of AII antagonist in the CVL did not significantly attenuate the response.

elicited by destruction of the nucleus tractus solitarius. *Brain Res.*, 439: 330–336.

Cherniack, N.S., von Euler, C., Homma, I. and Kao, F.F. (1979) Graded changes in central chemoreceptor input by local temperature changes on the ventral surface of the medulla. *J. Physiol. (Lond.)*, 287: 191–211.

Ciriello, J., Caverson, M.M. and Polosa, C. (1986) Function of the ventrolateral medulla in the control of the circulation. *Brain Res. Rev.*, 11: 359–391.

Ferguson, A.V. (1988) Systemic angiotensin acts at the subformical organ to control the activity of paraventricular nucleus neurons with identified projections to the median eminena. *Neuroendocrinology*, 47: 489–497.

Gatti, P.J., Norman, W.P., Taveira Da Silva, A.M. and Gillis, R.A. (1986) Cardiorespiratory effects produced by microinjecting L-glutamic acid into medullary nuclei associated with the ventral surface of the feline medulla. *Brain Res.*, 381: 281–288.

Haxhiu, M.A., Mitra, J., vanLunteren, E., Bruce, E.N. and Cherniack, N.S. (1984a) Hypoglossal and phrenic responses to cholinergic agents to ventral medullary surface. *Am. J. Physiol.*, 247: R939–944.

Haxhiu, M.A., vanLunteren, E., Van De Graff, W.B., Strohl, K.P., Bruce, E.N., Mitra, J. and Cherniack, N.S. (1984b) Action of nicotine on respiratory activity of the diaphragm and genioglossus muscles and the nerves that innervate them. *Respir. Physiol.*, 57: 153–169.

McAllen, R.M. (1986) Location of neurones with cardiovascular and respiratory function, at the ventral surface of the cat's medulla. *Neuroscience*, 18: 43–49.

Mendelsohn, F.A.O., Allen, A.M., Clevers, J., Denton, D.A., Tarjan, E. and McKinley, M.J. (1988) Localization of angiotensin II receptor binding in rabbit brain by in vitro autoradiography. *J. Comp. Neurol.*, 270: 372–384.

Mitra, J., Prabhakar, N.R., Overholt, J.L. and Cherniack, N.S. (1987) Respiratory and vasomotor effects of excitatory amino acid on ventral medullary surface. *Brain Res. Bull.*, 18: 681–684.

Mitra, J., Prabhakar, N.R., Overholt, J.L. and Cherniack, N.S. (1988) The respiratory effects of *N*-methyl-D-aspartate on ventrolateral medullary surface (VMS) application. (in preparation)

Paxinos, G. and Watson, C. (1986) *The Rat Brain in Stereotaxic Coordinates, 2nd edn.*, Academic Press, New York.

Phillips, M.I. (1984) Brain renin – angiotensin and hypertension. In G.P. Guthrie, Jr. and T.A. Kotchen (Eds.), *Hypertension and the Brain*, Futura Publishing Co., New York, pp. 63–81.

Ross, C.A., Ruggiero, D.A., Park, D.H., Joh, T.H., Sved, A.F., Fernandez-Pardal, J., Saavedra, J.M. and Reis, D.J. (1984) Tonic vasomotor control by the rostral ventrolateral medulla: effect of electrical or chemical stimulation of the area containing C_1 adrenaline neurons on arterial pressure, heart rate and plasma catecholamines and vasopressin. *J. Neurosci.*, 4: 474–494.

Schlaefke, M. (1981) Central chemosensitivity: a respiratory drive. *Rev. Physiol. Biochem. Pharmacol.*, 90: 171–244.

VanLunteren, E., Mitra, J., Prabhakar, N.R., Haxhiu, M.A. and Cherniack, N.S. (1987) Ventral medullary surface inputs to cervical sympathetic respiratory oscillations. *Am. J. Physiol.*, 252: R1032–R1038.

SECTION V

Neuronal Circuitry in the Ventrolateral Medulla Involved in Integrative Function

J. Ciriello, M.M. Caverson and C. Polosa (Eds.)
Progress in Brain Research, Vol. 81
© 1989 Elsevier Science Publishers B.V. (Biomedical Division)

CHAPTER 17

Integrated function of neurones in the rostral ventrolateral medulla

T.A. Lovick[1] and P. Li[2]

[1]Department of Physiology, University of Birmingham, Birmingham B15 2TJ, U.K., and [2]Department of Physiology, Shanghai Medical University, Shanghai 200032, People's Republic of China

Introduction

Over the past decade the functioning of the neurones in the ventrolateral medullary reticular formation has attracted the interest of neuroscientists from many disciplines. It is now well-established that neurones in this region play a key role in setting the resting level of vasomotor tone by sending a tonic excitatory drive to the spinal sympathetic outflow. Moreover, it is becoming clear that there is a degree of viscerotopic organisation within the sympathoexcitatory neurones (Lovick, 1987a; Dampney and McAllen, 1988). This functional specificity allows them to generate different patterns of sympathetic discharge and hence to effect fine adjustments in response to the continuously changing needs of the cardiovascular system under different behavioural and environmental conditions.

Sympathoexcitation from the ventrolateral medulla is mediated by spinally-projecting neurones with terminations in the intermediolateral cell column. Electrophysiological studies in the rat, cat and rabbit have shown that the sympathoexcitatory cells have slowly conducting axons (< 10 m/sec) and perikarya which are localised in the subretrofacial portion of nucleus paragigantocellularis lateralis (PGL) (Brown and Guyenet, 1984, 1985; McAllen, 1986; Terui et al., 1986, 1987). However, these cells are only a part of the

heterogeneous population of spinally-projecting neurones in the ventrolateral medulla, many of which have conduction velocities outside the range measured for "cardiovascular" cells (Lebedev et al., 1984; Lovick, 1985a; Huangfu and Li, 1986). Indeed, the intense interest which has been focused on the "cardiovascular" neurones in PGL has meant that the role of the significant population of non-cardiovascular neurones in this area has been largely overlooked. Nevertheless, there is mounting evidence to suggest that these spinally-projecting neurones constitute a sensorimotor control system which shows many features in parallel with the sympathoexcitatory neurones. Furthermore, the two systems often appear to act in concert to produce an integrated response which may form part of a specific behavioural pattern.

Sensorimotor functions of ventrolateral medullary neurones

A potential role for ventrolateral medullary neurones in the control of sensorimotor activity is inferred from anatomical studies on the terminations of the spinally-projecting cells in this region. Dense terminal labelling in the ventral horn of the spinal cord has been described following injections of tritiated amino acids into the ventrolateral medulla (Loewy and McKellar, 1981; Martin et al., 1981). Furthermore, when the injection extended

224

into the area adjacent to the facial nucleus, labelling was also seen in the dorsal horn (laminae III and V), particularly in the cervical and lumbar cord.

Descending control of sensorimotor activity

Microinjection of an excitatory amino acid into PGL in lightly anaesthetised rats produced a pressor response and profound inhibition of the tail-flick response to noxious heat (Fig. 1) (Lòvick, 1986). In the cat too, electrical stimulation in this region inhibited responses of neurones in the dorsal horn of the spinal cord (Gray and Dostrovsky, 1985). In this study the fastest conduction in the descending pathway to the dorsal horn was

estimated at 13 m/sec. Furthermore, the inhibition evoked from PGL was found to be more potent than the inhibitory effects evoked by stimulation more medially in nucleus raphe magnus. Thus neurones in PGL appear to be an important source of descending modulation of spinal somasthetic information.

Tonic descending inhibition of noxious input

It has long been recognised that input to the spinal cord from peripheral nociceptors is subject to a tonic descending inhibitory influence of supraspinal origin. Somatosympathetic reflexes too appear to be under similar central inhibitory control. The tonic descending inhibition (TDI) is still present in decerebrate preparations (Wall, 1967; Dem-

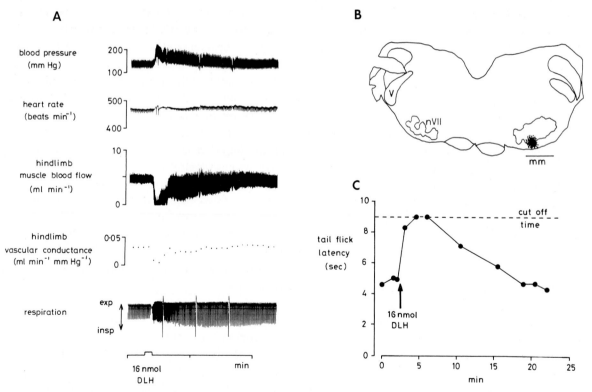

Fig. 1. (A) Cardiovascular and respiratory changes evoked by microinjection of D,L-homocysteic acid (DLH) into the ventrolateral medulla in the region ventral to the facial nucleus in a rat anaesthetised with Saffan. (B) Outline tracing of histological section through the injection site. The spread of dye which was coinjected with DLH is indicated by the stippled area. (C) Graph to show the time course of the inhibition of the tail-flick response which accompanied the autonomic changes. Abbreviations: nVII = facial nucleus; V = trigeminal tract. (Reproduced with permission from Lovick, 1986.)

bowsky et al., 1980) which suggests that the cells of origin lie somewhere in the brainstem. Recently, the active region has been localised to the ventrolateral medulla. Dembowsky and coworkers (Dembowsky et al., 1981) were the first to show that bilateral cooling of the ventrolateral medulla in the cat abolished tonic inhibitory control on the somato-sympathetic reflex evoked in the white ramus at T3 by stimulation of the corresponding intercostal nerves. Subsequently, Hall et al. (1982) made extensive electrolytic lesions in the medulla of the cat and found that TDI of noxious input from peripheral nerves was abolished only when the area of damage included the ventrolateral medulla. Effective lesions were always accompanied by a dramatic fall in blood pressure. Subsequent experiments have further localised the origin of TDI to the rostral part of PGL (Foong and Duggan, 1986) and it appears that TDI, like the tonic sympathoexcitatory drive, is subject to a tonic GABA-mediated inhibitory control (Lovick, 1987b).

Changes in motoneuronal activity

The spinal projection from the rostral ventrolateral medulla which terminates in the ventral horn appears to be largely excitatory. Electrical stimulation in PGL in the rat produced an increase in the amplitude of antidromic field potentials evoked in the ventral horn by stimulation of the sciatic nerve (Fig. 2). Recordings from single units in lamina IX also showed that motoneurones and other unidentified cells were facilitated by this stimulus (Lovick, 1987c). The excitatory responses with the shortest latency represented activation via a descending pathway conducting at 35 m/sec. In the cat too, Barman and Gebber (1985) noted that rapidly conducting spinally-projecting neurones in the ventrolateral medulla terminated in the ventral

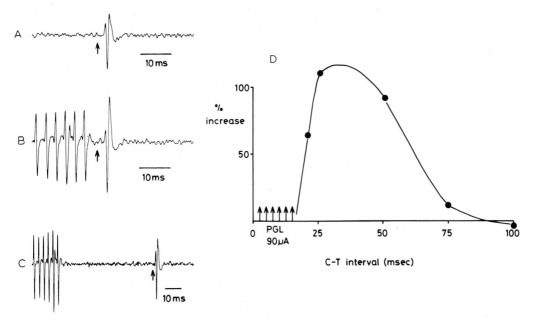

Fig. 2. (A) Antidromic field potential recorded in lamina IX in response to submaximal stimulation of the ipsilateral sciatic nerve (0.21V). Onset of stimulus is marked by the arrow. (B) Amplitude of the field potential is increased when the stimulus to the sciatic nerve is preceded by stimulation in PGL (90 μA). (C) Diminution of facilitating effect of stimulating in PGL at longer conditioning-testing interval. (D) Graph to show time course of the increase in amplitude of the sciatic field potential after conditioning stimulus to PGL.

grey matter. Thus a population of PGL neurones with fast-conducting axons may facilitate movement via the excitatory projection to the ventral horn. However, it remains to be seen whether this pathway is tonically active like its counterparts which terminate in the dorsal and lateral horns.

From the available evidence three major populations of spinally-projecting cells in PGL can be distinguished on the basis of their conduction velocity and site of termination in the cord (Fig. 3). The slowest fibres (< 10 m/sec) facilitate activity in the spinal sympathetic outflow whilst cells with axons that conduct in the middle range (up to 13 m/sec) exert an inhibitory influence on sensory input to the dorsal horn from nociceptors. The fastest-conducting cell group (up to 35 m/sec) appears to facilitate motoneuronal activity.

Activation of ventrolateral medullary control systems

Cardiovascular neurones

The presence of functionally distinct neuronal pools, each dedicated to controlling a specific sympathetic outflow (Lovick, 1987a; Dampney and McAllen, 1988) endows the ventrolateral cardiovascular control neurones with the potential for generating different patterns of cardiac and vasomotor nerve discharge by selectively adjusting the level of activity of the subpopulations of cells which control individual spinal sympathetic outflows. Indeed, the sympathoexcitatory neurones appear to form a common efferent limb in a number of cardiovascular reflex pathways, each of which can generate quite different patterns of cardiac and haemodynamic response. The most extensively studied of these has been the baroreceptor reflex pathway and it is now clear that second order barosensitive neurones in nucleus tractus solitarius exert an inhibitory influence on spinally-projecting sympathoexcitatory neurones in the ventrolateral medulla (Brown and Guyenet, 1984, 1985; McAllen, 1986; Terui et al., 1987). Interestingly, these same neurones receive excitatory inputs from "cardiovascular" areas within the hypothalamus (Brown and Guyenet, 1985; Terui et al., 1987). Indeed, cardiovascular responses to stimulating baroreceptors, the hypothalamus and midbrain were all severely attenuated when transmission through the ventrolateral medulla was blocked (McAllen et al., 1982; Hilton et al., 1983; Lovick, 1985b; Dean and Coote, 1986). Thus, the ventrolateral medullary neurones appear to form a common efferent pathway to the cord which is shared by a number of cardiovascular reflexes. Several studies have been made to ascertain the degree of convergence of afferent inputs onto individual neurones in the

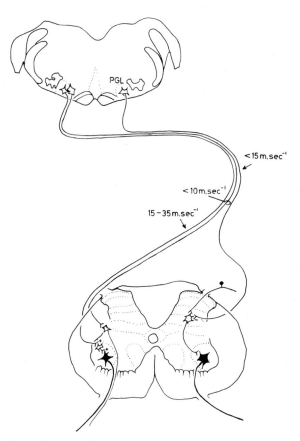

Fig. 3. Schematic diagram to show the spinal projections from nucleus paragigantocellularis (PGL). Neurones with slowly conducting axons (< 10 m/sec) project to the lateral horn whilst those with medium (up to 13 m/sec) and fast (up to 35 m/sec) conduction velocities project respectively to the dorsal and ventral horns.

ventrolateral medulla (Lovick et al., 1984; Li and Lovick, 1985; Terui et al., 1986; Huangfu and Li, 1988b; Lovick, 1988). In these experiments more than 60% of the cells tested responded to stimulation of two or more of the central nervous system regions which project directly to PGL. Inputs from the hypothalamus, dorsal periaqueductal grey (PAG) and parabrachial region were predominantly excitatory whilst afferent inputs from nucleus tractus solitarius and the medullary raphe were largely inhibitory (Fig. 4). Thus, individual ventrolateral medullary neurones do indeed appear

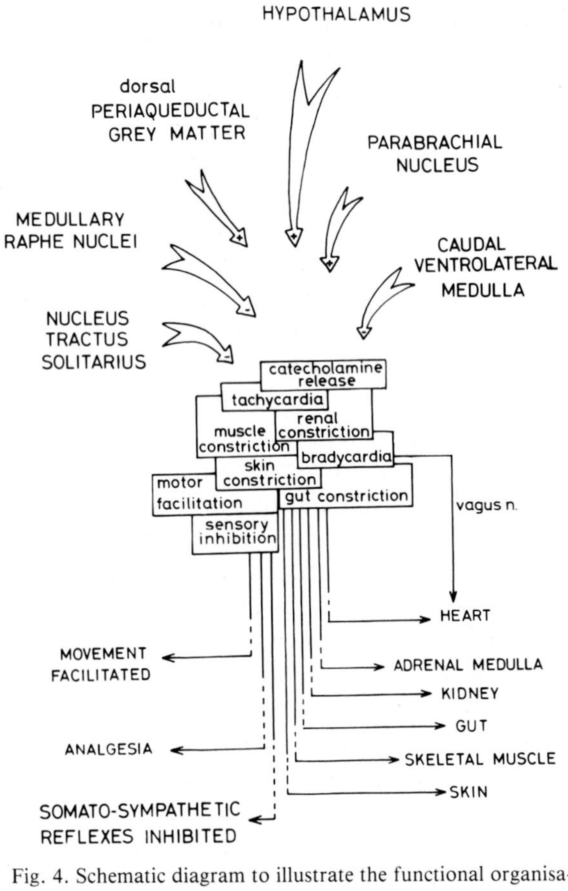

to be common to a number of cardiovascular reflex pathways and to integrate afferent information arriving simultaneously from different cardiovascular centres. The combination of viscerotopic organisation and convergence of cardiovascular reflex pathways on individual neurones endows a great deal of flexibility on the ventrolateral medullary control system and enables it to superimpose fine adjustments to individual sympathetic outflows onto the prevailing background level of vasomotor activity. The system is therefore able to integrate and respond efficiently to the numerous and often conflicting demands made by moment-to-moment changes in the cardiovascular status of the animal.

Pain control neurones

An increasing number of reports emphasise the association between cardiovascular control and reduced responsiveness to pain when sources of direct afferent input to the ventrolateral medulla are stimulated. For example, stimulation in the lateral hypothalamus, dorsal PAG, parabrachial complex and nucleus tractus solitarius all produce analgesia as well as evoking well-known patterns of cardiovascular adjustment (Mraovitch et al., 1982; Duggan and Morton, 1983; Katayama et al., 1984; Lovick, 1985b; Giradot et al., 1987; Lewis et al., 1987; Aimone and Gebhart, 1988; Ward, 1988). The fact that the efferent pathways to the spinal cord from all these sites converge on individual ventrolateral medullary neurones (see above) suggests that the anatomical association between the cardiovascular and pain control neurones in the ventrolateral medulla is more than fortuitous. Indeed, the close association between cardiovascular responses and analgesia has been a consistent feature in studies of the response evoked by stimulation in the PAG. Stimulation in the dorsal PAG has been shown to excite spinally-projecting neurones in PGL which have conduction velocities in the ranges expected for "cardiovascular", "somatosensory" and "motor" control neurones (Lovick et al., 1984 and un-

Fig. 4. Schematic diagram to illustrate the functional organisation of neurones in the ventrolateral medulla. Subpopulations of spinally-projecting neurones selectively control activity in individual spinal sympathetic outflows, as well as sensorimotor activity in the dorsal and ventral horns. Excitatory and inhibitory afferent inputs from diverse regions of the neuroaxis converge onto indidivual cells in the medulla.

published data). Responses of neurones in the dorsal horn to noxious sensory input are also attenuated by stimulation of the dorsal PAG (e.g. Duggan and Morton, 1983) whilst the responses of neurones in lamina IX are facilitated (Cale and Lovick, unpublished results). In conscious or decerebrate animals stimulation in the dorsal part of the PAG evokes aggressive or aversive behaviour which is accompanied by a characteristic pattern of autonomic changes and a reduction in responsiveness to painful stimuli (Abrahams et al., 1961; Fardin et al., 1984; Carrive et al., 1987). The autonomic changes include an increase in blood pressure, tachycardia, redistribution of the cardiac output to skeletal muscle at the expense of the circulation to the skin and viscera and an increase in the rate and depth of ventilation. Both the cardiorespiratory changes and the analgesia persist under light anaesthesia and both appear simultaneously as the intensity of stimulation in the dorsal PAG is increased (Duggan and Morton, 1983; Lovick, 1985b). Furthermore, both components of the response are severely attenuated following bilateral lesions in the ventrolateral medulla (Duggan and Morton, 1983; Lovick 1985b).

Simultaneous activation of cardiovascular and pain control systems under circumstances which evoke aggressive or defensive behaviour is a well-known phenomenon in man. Common examples include the analgesia experienced by soldiers in battle or sportsmen during competition: both situations in which there is a high level of aggression and sympathoexcitatory drive. The excitatory projection from the dorsal PAG onto cardiovascular and pain control neurones in the ventrolateral medulla appears to provide the major efferent pathway to the spinal cord by which these responses are mediated.

Inhibitory modulation of ventrolateral medullary neurones by the raphe nuclei

Recent evidence suggests that the activity of ventrolateral medullary neurones is subject to inhibitory modulation from the medullary raphe nuclei. In contrast to the pulse modulated phasic inhibition which is initiated by baroreceptor input to nucleus tractus solitarius (Brown and Guyenet, 1984, 1985; McAllen, 1986; Terui et al., 1986), inhibitory modulation from the raphe produces more subtle and long-lasting changes in the level of excitability of the ventrolateral descending control system.

Electrical stimulation in nucleus raphe magnus (NRM) and raphe obscurus (NRO) evokes predominantly inhibitory responses in neurones in PGL (Huangfu and Li, 1988b; Lovick, 1988). Furthermore, selective activation of nerve cell bodies, by microinjection of an excitatory amino acid into NRO, caused a reduction in the pressor response evoked by stimulation in the dorsal PAG (Huangfu and Li, 1988a). Interestingly, a similar attenuation of the pressor response evoked from the dorsal PAG could be produced by stimulation of the deep peroneal nerve, particularly the group II and III fibres (Huangfu and Li, 1985). This inhibitory effect was abolished by electrolytic lesions of or injection of local anaesthetic into NRO (Huangfu and Li, 1988a). These findings suggest that the inhibitory effects of peripheral nerve stimulation on transmission through the ventrolateral medulla are due to activation of the direct projection to PGL from the medullary raphe nuclei (Andrezik et al., 1981; Lovick, 1986; Huangfu et al., 1987). Indeed, neurones in the raphe are known to be excited by electrical stimulation of muscle (Liu et al., 1986). Furthermore, stimulation of muscle nerves has been shown to exert a sustained inhibitory influence on spinally-projecting neurones in PGL (Huangfu and Li, 1986; Terui et al., 1987). In these experiments prolonged (5 – 20 min) low frequency (10 Hz) stimulation of the deep peroneal nerve attenuated the responses of ventrolateral medullary neurones to stimulation of the dorsal PAG (Huangfu and Li, 1986). During the stimulation period there was also a gradual increase in the antidromic latency of spinally-projecting neurones in PGL, culminating in some cases in complete failure of the antidromic action potential to invade the soma (Fig. 5). The inhibitory effects lasted for 30 – 120 min. Thus, the reduction in the responses to stimulation in the dorsal PAG must be at least partly due to a postsynaptic inhibitory action in the ventrolateral medulla.

The inhibitory synapse in the ventrolateral medulla may also be an important site for the central sympathoinhibitory action of 5-HT. The ventrolateral medulla is rich in 5-HT-immunoreactive nerve terminals (Steinbusch, 1981), many of which are probably derived from the serotonin-containing perikarya of the medullary raphe. Microinjection of 5-HT (10 – 100 nmol) bilaterally into the ventrolateral medulla in rats produced a long-lasting depressor response. The fall in mean blood pressure (5 – 57 mmHg, mean 15.1) lasted up to 69 min (1 – 69 min, mean 33) and was usually accompanied by bradycardia. Furthermore, injection of 5-HT into the rostral part of the ventrolateral medulla, at the level of the facial nucleus, attenuated the pressor response and tachycardia evoked by stimulation in the dorsal periaqueductal grey (Fig. 6). These findings suggest that 5-HT is involved in the inhibitory pathway from the medullary raphe to the ventrolateral medulla and also indicate that this region could be a major site of action for the central antihypertensive action of 5-HT.

The physiological role of the inhibitory modulation of ventrolateral medullary neurones by the

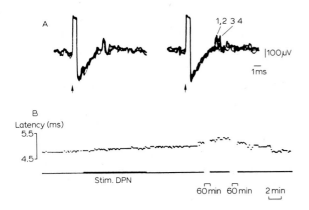

Fig. 5. Effect of stimulation of deep peroneal nerve on the response of an antidromically-activated spinally-projecting neurone in PGL. (A) Left side: Superimposed oscilloscope sweeps show constant latency of the response recorded during the control period. Right: Superimposed records show increased latency of the antidromic spike after stimulation of deep peroneal nerve (DPN, 0.5 msec pulses at 10 Hz, 400 µA for 10 min). Sweeps 1 and 2 were recorded at the start of the stimulation period and sweeps 3 and 4 at the end. Arrow marks stimulus artifact. (B) Time course of the increase in antidromic latency produced by stimulating the deep peroneal nerve. (Reproduced with permission from Huangfu and Li, 1986.)

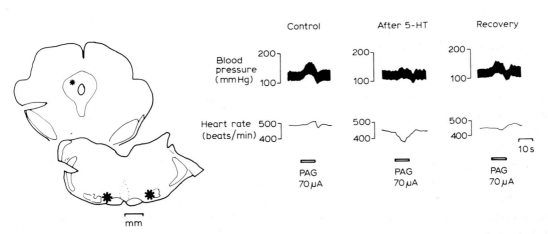

Fig. 6. Effect of microinjection of 50 nmol 5-HT bilaterally into PGL on the cardiovascular response to electrical stimulation in the dorsal PAG (70 µA, 1.0 msec pulses, 80 Hz for 10 sec). Asterisks on outline drawings of sections through the midbrain and medulla mark respectively the stimulation and injection sites in the dorsal PAG and ventrolateral medulla.

medullary raphe is intriguing. It is possible that the system is activated by the increased activity in muscle afferents produced during exercise. Indeed, low frequency stimulation of somatic afferents from muscle has been shown to produce a long-lasting fall in blood pressure in hypertensive rats (Yao et al., 1982; Hoffmann and Thoren, 1988). A reduction in blood pressure and sympathetic tone has also been reported to occur following exercise both in patients with essential hypertension and in spontaneously hypertensive strains of rat (Jennings et al., 1984; Shyu and Thoren, 1986). In Chinese medicine, the sympathoinhibitory effects of stimulating muscle afferents have already been exploited for several millennia in the form of acupuncture. The application of modern research methods to the study of this ancient form of therapy has revealed that effective needling requires the activation of group II afferents from muscle (Lu et al., 1981; Lu, 1983). Furthermore, there is abundant evidence that the raphe nuclei of the brainstem are essential both for the full expression of the autonomic changes evoked by acupuncture-like stimulation and for the production of acupuncture analgesia (e.g. Du and Chao, 1976; Chiang et al., 1979; Huangfu and Li, 1988a). The inhibitory projection from NRO to the ventrolateral medulla appears to be engaged during acupuncture for the suppression of descending sympathoexcitatory influences. In contrast, the direct inhibitory raphe-spinal pathway to the dorsal horn from NRM may be more important during acupuncture analgesia (Du and Chao, 1976; Chiang et al., 1979; Liu et al., 1986).

The midline raphe system is also thought to be concerned with initiating some of the physiological changes associated with sleep. For example, stimulation in NRO has been shown to elicit the pattern of sympathoinhibition that occurs during periods of desynchronised sleep (Futuro-Neto and Coote, 1982). The inhibitory projection from NRO to the "cardiovascular" cells in PGL may contribute to this effect.

Many facets of the functioning of the spinal projection from the ventrolateral medulla remain to be probed. However, it is already clear that this region is of central importance to both sympathetic and somatosensory function. It appears to fulfill many of the functions once ascribed to the "vasomotor centre" and to be the source of "tonic descending inhibition" of input from somatic and visceral nociceptors. The sympathoexcitatory neurones and sensory control neurones form the efferent limbs of many of the cardiovascular and somatosensory control systems which emanate from the brainstem. The integrated output from these cells to the spinal cord constitutes a major command signal which determines the level of activity in the sympathetic neurones as well as setting the level of responsiveness to noxious afferent input.

Acknowledgements

This work was supported by the Medical Research Council, the Science Fund of the Chinese Academy of Sciences and an IBRO/MacArthur Foundation Network Grant.

References

Abrahams, V.C., Hilton, S.M. and Zbrozyna, A.W. (1960) Active muscle vasodilatation produced by stimulation of the brainstem: its significance in the defence reaction. *J. Physiol. (Lond.)*, 154: 491 – 513.

Aimone, L.D. and Gebhart, G.F. (1988) Serotonin and/or an excitatory amino acid mediates stimulation-produced antinoception from the lateral hypothalamus in the rat. *Brain Res.*, 450: 170 – 180.

Andrezik, J.A., Chan-Palay, V. and Palay, S.L. (1981) The nucleus paragigantocellularis lateralis in the rat: demonstration of afferents by retrograde transport of horseradish peroxidase. *Anat. Embryol.*, 161: 373 – 390.

Barman, S. and Gebber, G. (1985) Axonal projection patterns of ventrolateral medullospinal sympathoexcitatory neurons. *J. Neurophysiol.*, 53: 1551 – 1566.

Brown, D.L. and Guyenet, P.G. (1984) Cardiovascular neurons of brain stem with projections to spinal cord. *Am. J. Physiol.*, 247: R1009 – R1016.

Brown, D.L. and Guyenet, P.G. (1985) Electrophysiological study of cardiovascular neurons in the rostral ventrolateral medulla in rats. *Circ. Res.*, 56: 359 – 369.

Carrive, P., Dampney, R.A.L. and Bandler, R. (1987) Excitation of neurones in a restricted portion of the periaqueductal grey elicits both behavioural and cardiovascular components of the defence reaction in the unanaesthetised decerebrate cat. *Neurosci. Lett.,* 81: 273 – 278.

Chiang, C.Y., Tu, H.C., Chao, Y.F., Pay, H., Ku, H.K., Cheng, J.K., Shan, H.Y. and Yang, F.Y. (1979) Effects of electrolytic lesions or intracerebral injections of 5,6-dihydroxytryptamine in raphe nuclei on acupuncture analgesia in rats. *Chin. Med. J.,* 92: 129 – 136.

Dampney, R.A.L. and McAllen, R.M. (1988) Differential control of sympathetic fibres supplying hindlimb skin and muscle by subretrofacial neurones in the cat. *J. Physiol. (Lond.),* 395: 41 – 56.

Dean, C. and Coote, J.H. (1986) A ventromedullary relay involved in the hypothalamic and chemoreceptor activation of sympathetic postganglionic neurones to skeletal muscle, kidney and splanchnic area. *Brain Res.,* 377: 279 – 285.

Dembowsky, K., Czachurski, J., Amendt, K. and Seller, H. (1980) Tonic descending inhibition of the spinal somato-sympathetic reflex from the lower brainstem. *J. Auton. Nerv. Syst.,* 2: 157 – 182.

Dembowsky, K., Lackner, K., Czachurski, J. and Seller, H. (1981) Tonic catecholaminergic inhibition of the spinal somato-sympathetic reflexes originating in the ventrolateral medulla oblongata. *J. Auton. Nerv. Syst.,* 3: 277 – 290.

Du, H.J. and Chao, Y.F. (1976) Localisation of central structures involved in descending inhibitory effect of acupuncture on viscero-somatic reflex. *Scientia Sinica,* 20: 137 – 148.

Duggan, A.W. and Morton, C.R. (1983) Periaqueductal grey stimulation: an association between selective inhibition of dorsal horn neurones and changes in peripheral circulation. *Pain,* 15: 237 – 248.

Fardin, V., Oliveras, J.L. and Besson, J.M. (1984) A reinvestigation of the analgesic effects induced by stimulation of the periaqueductal grey matter in the rat. I. The production of behavioural side effects together with analgesia. *Brain Res.,* 306: 105 – 123.

Foong, F. and Duggan, A.W. (1986) Brainstem areas tonically inhibiting dorsal horn neurones: studies with microinjection of the GABA analogue piperidine-4-sulphonic acid. *Pain,* 27: 361 – 371.

Futuro-Neto, H. and Coote, J.H. (1982) Desynchronised sleep-like pattern of sympathetic activity elicited by electrical stimulation of sites in the brainstem. *Brain Res.,* 252: 269 – 276.

Giradot, M.N., Brennan, J.J., Martindale, M.E. and Foreman, R.D. (1987) Effects of stimulating the subcoeruleus-parabrachial region on the non-noxious and noxious responses of T1-T5 spinothalamic tract neurones in the primate. *Brain Res.,* 409: 10 – 18.

Gray, B.G. and Dostrovsky, J.O. (1985) Descending inhibitory influences from periaqueductal gray, nucleus raphe magnus and adjacent reticular formation I. Effects on lumbar spinal cord nociceptive and non-nociceptive neurons. *J. Neuro-physiol.,* 49: 932 – 947.

Hall, J., Duggan, A.W., Morton, C. and Johnson, S. (1982) The location of brainstem neurones tonically inhibiting dorsal horn neurones in the cat. *Brain Res.,* 244: 215 – 224.

Hilton, S.M., Marshall, J.M. and Timms, R.J. (1983) Ventral medullary neurones in the pathway from the defence areas of the cat and their effect on blood pressure. *J. Physiol. (Lond.),* 345: 149 – 166.

Hoffmann, P. and Thoren, P. (1988) Electric muscle stimulation in the hind leg of the spontaneously hypertensive rat induces a long-lasting fall in blood pressure. *Acta Physiol. Scand.,* 133: 211 – 219.

Huangfu, D.H. and Li, P. (1985) The effect of deep peroneal nerve inputs on defence reaction elicited by brainstem stimulation. *Chin. J. Physiol. Sci.,* 1: 176 – 184.

Huangfu, D.H. and Li, P. (1986) Effect of deep peroneal nerve inputs on ventral medullary defence-related neurons. *Chin. J. Physiol. Sci.,* 2: 123 – 131.

Huangfu, D.H. and Li, P. (1988a) Role of nucleus raphe obscurus in the inhibition of defence reaction by deep peroneal nerve stimulation. *Chin. J. Physiol. Sci.,* 4: 77 – 83.

Huangfu, D.H. and Li, P. (1988b) The inhibitory effect of ARC-PAG-NRO system on the ventrolateral medullary neurones in the rabbit. *Chin. J. Physiol. Sci.,* 4: 115 – 125.

Huangfu, D.H., Huang, Q. and Li, P. (1987) Afferent connections of the ventrolateral medulla in the rabbit − studies with HRP technique. *Chin. J. Physiol. Sci.,* 3: 86 – 95.

Jennings, G.L., Nelson, L., Esler, M.D., Leonard, P. and Korner, P.L. (1984) Effects of changes in physical activity on blood pressure and sympathetic tone. *J. Hypertension,* 2: 139 – 141.

Katayama, Y., Watkins, L.R., Becker, D.P. and Hayes, R.L. (1984) Non-opiate analgesia induced by carbachol microinjection into the pontine parabrachial region of the cat. *Brain Res.,* 296: 263 – 283.

Lebedev, A.V., Krasiukov, A.V. and Nikitin, S.A. (1984) Neuronal organisation of the sympathoactivating structures of the bulbar ventrolateral surface. *Fiziol. Zh. USSR,* 70: 761 – 772.

Lewis, J.W., Baldrighi, G. and Akil, H. (1987) A possible interface between autonomic function and pain control: opioid analgesia and the nucleus tractus solitarius. *Brain Res.,* 424: 65 – 70.

Li, P. and Lovick, T.A. (1985) Excitatory projections from hypothalamic and midbrain defence areas to nucleus paragigantocellularis lateralis in the rat. *Exp. Neurol.,* 89: 543 – 553.

Liu, X., Zhu, B. and Zhang, S.X. (1986) Relationship between electroacupuncture analgesia and descending pain inhibitory mechanism of nucleus raphe magnus. *Pain,* 24: 383 – 396.

Loewy, A.D. and McKellar, S. (1981) Serotonergic projections from the ventral medulla to the intermediolateral cell column in the rat. *Brain Res.,* 21: 146 – 152.

Lovick, T.A. (1985a) Descending projections from the ventrolateral medulla and cardiovascular control. *Pflügers Arch.,* 404: 197–202.

Lovick, T.A. (1985b) Ventrolateral medullary lesions block the antinociceptive and cardiovascular responses elicited by stimulating the dorsal periaqueductal grey matter in rats. *Pain,* 21: 241–252.

Lovick, T.A. (1986a) Projections from brainstem nuclei to nucleus paragigantocellularis lateralis in the cat. *J. Auton. Nerv. Syst.,* 16: 1–11.

Lovick, T.A. (1986b) Analgesia and the cardiovascular changes evoked by stimulating neurones in nucleus paragigantocellularis lateralis in the rat. *Pain,* 25: 259–268.

Lovick, T.A. (1987a) Differential control of cardiac and vasomotor activity by neurones in nucleus paragigantocellularis lateralis in the cat. *J. Physiol. (Lond.),* 389: 23–35.

Lovick, T.A. (1987b) Tonic GABAergic and cholinergic influences on pain control and cardiovascular control neurones in nucleus paragigantocellularis lateralis in the rat. *Pain,* 31: 401–409.

Lovick, T.A. (1987c) Changes in motoneuronal excitability accompany analgesia evoked from the ventrolateral medulla in the rat. *J. Physiol. (Lond.),* 390: 51P.

Lovick, T.A. (1988) Convergent afferent inputs to neurones in nucleus paragigantocellularis lateralis in the cat. *Brain Res.,* 456: 483–487.

Lovick, T.A., Smith, P.R. and Hilton, S.M. (1984) Spinally-projecting neurones near the ventral surface of the medulla in the cat. *J. Auton. Nerv. Syst.,* 11: 27–33.

Lu, G.W. (1983) Characteristics of afferent fiber innervation on acupuncture points Zusanli. *Am. J. Physiol.,* 245: R606–612.

Lu, G.W., Xie, J.Q., Yang, J., Wang, Y.N. and Wan, Q.L. (1981) Afferent nerve fiber composition at point zusanli in relation of acupuncture analgesia: a functional morphological investigation. *Chin. Med. J.,* 94: 255–263.

Martin, G.F., Cabana, T., Humbertson, A.O., Laxson, L.C. and Panneton, W.M. (1981) Spinal projections from the medullary reticular formation of the North American opossum: evidence for connectional heterogeneity. *J. Comp. Neurol.,* 196: 663–682.

McAllen, R.M. (1986) Identification and properties of sub-retrofacial bulbospinal neurones: a descending cardiovascular pathway in the cat. *J. Auton. Nerv. Syst.,* 17: 151–164.

McAllen, R.M., Neil, J.J. and Loewy, A.D. (1982) Effects of kainic acid applied to the ventral surface of the medulla oblongata on vasomotor tone, the baroreceptor reflex and hypothalamic autonomic responses. *Brain Res.,* 238: 65–76.

Mraovitch, S., Kumada, M. and Reis, D.K. (1982) Role of the nucleus parabrachialis in cardiovascular regulation in the cat. *Brain Res.,* 232: 57–75.

Shyu, B.C. and Thoren, P. (1986) Circulatory events following spontaneous muscle exercise in normotensive and hypertensive rats. *Acta Physiol. Scand.,* 128: 515–524.

Steinbusch, H.W.M. (1981) Distribution of serotonin-immunoreactivity in the central nervous system of the rat-cell bodies and terminals. *Neuroscience,* 6: 557–618.

Terui, N., Saeki, Y. and Kumada, M. (1986) Barosensory neurons in the ventrolateral medulla and their responses to various afferent inputs from peripheral and central sources. *Jpn. J. Physiol.,* 36: 1141–1164.

Terui, N., Saeki, Y. and Kumada, M. (1987) Confluence of barosensory and non barosensory inputs at neurones in the ventrolateral medulla in rabbits. *Can. J. Physiol. Pharmacol.,* 65: 1584–1590.

Wall, P.D. (1967) The laminar organisation of dorsal horn and effects of descending impulses. *J. Physiol. (Lond.),* 188: 401–423.

Ward, D.G. (1988) Stimulation of the parabrachial nuclei with monosodium glutamate increases arterial pressure. *Brain Res.,* 462: 383–390.

Yao, T., Andersson, S. and Thoren, P. (1982) Long-lasting cardiovascular depression induced by acupuncture-like stimulation of the sciatic nerve in unanaesthetized hypertensive rats. *Brain Res.,* 240: 77–85.

J. Ciriello, M.M. Caverson and C. Polosa (Eds.)
Progress in Brain Research, Vol. 81
© 1989 Elsevier Science Publishers B.V. (Biomedical Division)

CHAPTER 18

The selectivity of descending vasomotor control by subretrofacial neurons

R.M. McAllen[1] and R.A.L. Dampney[2]

[1]Howard Florey Institute of Experimental Physiology and Medicine, University of Melbourne, Victoria 3052, Australia, and
[2]Department of Physiology, University of Sydney, N.S.W. 2006, Australia

Introduction

This chapter demonstrates that the notion is now widely accepted that neurons in the rostral ventrolateral medulla play an important part in cardiovascular control. What is not settled, however, is to what extent the various functions attributed to this interesting brain region might be subserved by a common pool of multipotent neurons. Our view is that the opposite is true, and that the ventrolateral medulla contains distinct neuron pools with highly specific connections and functions. We will focus on a compact group of spinally-projecting neurons termed the "subretrofacial nucleus" (SRF) and argue that this set of neurons is responsible for mediating the region's vasopressor actions. We will then discuss evidence that SRF neurons selectively drive "cardiovascular" sympathetic nerves (i.e. to heart, blood vessels and adrenal medulla). Finally, we will present data that support the view that within SRF there are neural subpopulations with even greater specificity of action, and that these may be functionally dedicated to control the vasomotor supply to single tissues.

The subretrofacial nucleus (SRF)

The SRF consists of a compact column of medium-small cells on either side of the medulla, ventral to, and separated from the retrofacial nucleus. In the cat, it extends for approximately 1.5 mm caudally from the caudal pole of the facial nucleus, and contains approximately 1000 cells. The densest formation is at its rostral pole, where it measures about 250 μm across; caudally it thins out and becomes less distinct. About 80% of its cells have been shown to stain immunohistochemically for tyrosine hydroxylase. They also stain for neuropeptide Y (but not substance P), and we may conclude that these form part – but only part – of the C1 group of adrenaline-synthesizing cells. Virtually all the neurons in this compact group appear to send axons to the spinal cord, where they terminate among preganglionic sympathetic neurons (Dampney et al., 1987a). Electrophysiological recordings (see below) also show that the spinally-projecting cells with cardiovascular function form a compact group at just this locus.

Functional localisation of vasomotor actions to SRF

In 1974, Guertzenstein and Silver showed that inhibition of superficial neurons at a restricted bilateral location in the ventrolateral medulla, caused the blood pressure of chloralose-anaesthetised cats to fall precipitously. This could be done with topically applied glycine (in which case it was reversible), electrolytic lesions or combinations of the two. The experiment illustrated in Fig. 1 essentially repeats their findings, but additionally shows

234

that these manoeuvres can reduce blood pressure and renal nerve activity to the level of the acute spinal animal. The lesions producing this effect destroyed the SRF, but not a great deal of the surrounding tissue.

Glycine inhibits cell bodies but is not believed to interrupt conduction in axons; therefore cell bodies in the region, rather than a passing fibre tract, were implicated in the maintenance of vasomotor tone. It would be elegant if this method could be adapted to a finer scale in order to map the responsible cells more precisely. Unfortunately, at least 50% of them (i.e. all the nucleus on one side) need to be inhibited before much change can be seen in blood pressure (Guertzenstein and Silver, 1974). By contrast, excitatory stimuli produce measurable effects when acting on relatively few cells. For this reason we have used the method of microinjecting excitant amino acids, which selec-

tively activate cell bodies (or dendrites) rather than passing axons (Goodchild et al., 1982), to map the vasomotor cells of this region more accurately (Dampney et al., 1985, 1987b; McAllen, 1986a).

Nanolitre quantities of 0.5 M sodium glutamate provide a strong stimulus to SRF cells, and 10 nl injections have been demonstrated to give a spatial resolution of 300 μm or better (Dampney and McAllen, 1988). Figure 2 shows representative records from such a mapping experiment, where three successive micropipette penetrations were made in the same coronal plane. Small quantities of horseradish peroxidase (HRP) were added to the glutamate so as to mark injection sites, and the spinally-projecting cells of SRF were also labelled by retrograde transport of wheat germ agglutinin-HRP, which had been injected 48 h previously into the thoracic spinal cord. (The two patterns of reaction product can be distinguished microscopically.) Focal injections of glutamate into SRF gave rise to brisk, large pressor responses: injections beyond effective diffusion range of SRF did not.

Electrophysiology

Electrophysiological recording experiments have also provided data to support the idea that SRF neurons form a descending vasomotor pathway. In the cat, studies from two laboratories have localized bulbospinal neurons with cardiovascular properties (principally barosensitivity) in a compact group ventral to the retrofacial nucleus (Barman and Gebber, 1985; McAllen, 1986c). Their distribution in the rabbit appears quite similar (Terui et al., 1987), though in the rat they may be relatively less compact with respect to neighbouring structures (Brown and Guyenet, 1984; Morrison et al., 1988). Detailed descriptions of the identification and properties of this class of neurons are presented in the articles quoted above, but the example shown in Fig. 3 illustrates the prime features: antidromic activation from dorsolateral funiculus or intermediolateral horn, axonal conduction velocity in the range of small myelinated

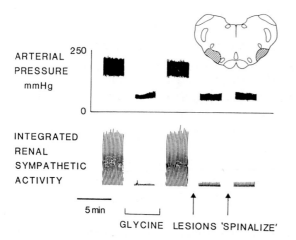

Fig. 1. The effect of bilateral inactivation of SRF neurons on arterial pressure and renal sympathetic activity (whole nerve recording) in the chloralose-anaesthetized, artificially ventilated cat. Panels show traces taken respectively before, during and after recovery from the application of 1 M glycine bilaterally to the ventral medullary surface over SRF, after making bilateral radio frequency lesions (see inset), and finally after ischaemically spinalizing the preparation by ligating the entire arterial supply to the brain. The inset shows the lesions (hatched) on a coronal section of medulla: they spread approximately 1 mm in from the surface, up to, but not involving the retrofacial nuclei (outlined). They extended 2 – 3 mm rostrocaudally. (Unpublished record from experiments reported by McAllen, 1985.)

fibres, spontaneous activity and inhibition by baroreceptors.

Cells of this type are most commonly encountered in groups, where, in recordings made with low impedance electrodes, it is possible to hear the entire background neural activity inhibited by baroreceptor stimuli. Multiple constant latency (presumably antidromic) potentials with the appropriate range of latencies on spinal stimulation, are encountered in the same place, and both features appear and disappear over about 200 μm of the microelectrode penetration.

The correspondence of the region where barosensitive bulbospinal neurons are found, with SRF, as localised by other means, is striking (Fig. 4). Evidence from lesions, neuroanatomical tracing, amino acid injections and electrophysiological recordings points to SRF as the cell group responsible for the vasomotor actions of the rostral ventrolateral medulla.

Range of SRF actions

Activation of neurons connected with the intermediolateral cell column might be expected to trigger other sympathetically-mediated responses besides increases in blood pressure. Therefore, a study was made to catalogue the extent of effects produced by moderate sized amino acid injections (30 – 50 nl of 0.2 M DL homocysteate or 0.5 M

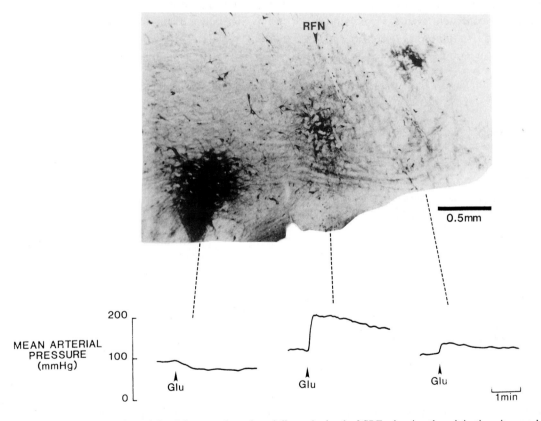

Fig. 2. Above: cross-section of the right ventrolateral medulla at the level of SRF, showing three injection sites marked by HRP. The spinally-projecting neurons are also labelled by a previous WGA-HRP injection (see text) centred on the ipsilateral intermediolateral horn at T2; the retrogradely labelled neurons are concentrated within the middle injection site. Dorsal to these is the retrofacial nucleus (RFN). Below: the corresponding records of arterial pressure in the chloralose-anaesthetized cat when 20 nl of 0.5 M sodium glutamate (Glu) were injected at each site.

glutamate) into SRF (McAllen, 1986b). In response to the injections the activity increased abruptly in all sympathetic nerves tested: cervical, inferior cardiac, splanchnic, renal and both cutaneous and muscle filaments in the hindlimb. All these nerves contain vasomotor (or cardiac) fibres, but some contain non-cardiovascular efferents as well. Effects on the latter were clarified by studying end-organ effects. Strong vasoconstriction was demonstrated directly in perfused mesenteric and femoral vascular beds, large increases were measured in circulating adrenaline and noradrenaline, and cardioacceleration was seen in vagotomized, adrenalectomized cats.

But the story was different for non-cardiovascular sympathetic actions. Pupils and nictitating membranes were not affected; piloerection was not seen; only small, inconsistent effects were seen on gut motility; and sudomotor (electrodermal) responses, while they could be obtained from an area rostromedial to SRF, were not evoked by focal injections into SRF (McAllen, 1986b). Respiratory effects could be evoked from neighbouring areas which were separated spatially from the vasomotor neurons of SRF. The absence of sympathetic eye signs matches the observation that this component of the "hypothalamic defence reaction" survives while the vasomotor component is blocked by kainic acid application to the ventral medulla (McAllen et al., 1982).

It therefore appears that SRF cells are selective in their actions on preganglionic neurons, in that they pick out those supplying the heart, blood vessels and adrenal medulla. This, of course, echoes the selectivity of the baroreceptor reflex, which is probably no accident. One would predict that the anatomy of preganglionic neuron innervation by SRF cells reflects the same functional selectivity.

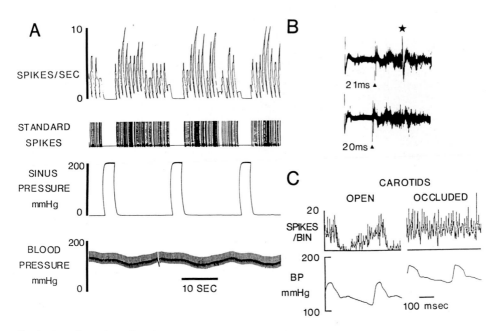

Fig. 3. Recordings of a bulbospinal SRF neuron in a chloralose-anaesthetized, paralyzed cat. (A) Chart record of spontaneous activity and its response to inflation of the ipsilateral carotid sinus (prepared as a blind sac). (B) Collision test. Electrical stimuli were delivered to the ipsilateral dorsolateral funiculus at C5 at delays after a spontaneous spike just longer (above, note antidromic spike marked by star) and shorter (below, note absence of antidromic spike) than "critical" delay. Each trace shows 10 superimposed sweeps. (C) Pulse-triggered histograms of spontaneous activity (each 510 cycles) before (left) and after (right) unloading the carotid baroreceptors. Aortic nerves and vagi were cut. (From McAllen, 1987.)

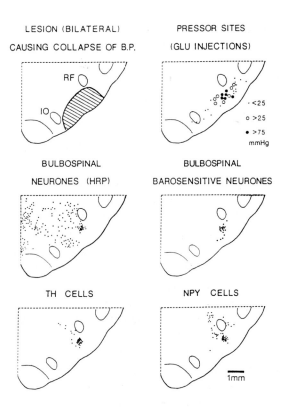

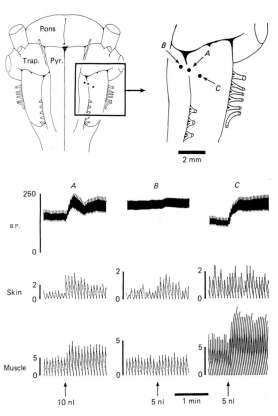

in chloralose-anaesthetized and artificially ventilated cats, and identified with the methods of Jänig (1985). The sinus and vago-aortic nerves were cut to remove the complication of reflex effects mediated by the arterial baroreceptors.

Figures 5 and 6 illustrate the principal, consistent finding: glutamate injections to the lateral side of SRF preferentially or exclusively activated the muscle vasoconstrictor fibre (MVC), and those to the medial side, the skin fibre. Intermediate injections activated both. These data avoid a number of problems of interpretation (secondary reflexes,

Fig. 4. Synthesis of different data on SRF. Diagrams of ventrolateral quadrant of medulla at the rostral pole of the inferior olive (I.O.); retrofacial nucleus (RF). Upper panels are from experiments illustrated in Figs. 1 and 2; middle panels show replotted data from Dampney et al. (1987a) and McAllen (1986c); lower panels show the locations of neurons that stained immunohistochemically for tyrosine hydroxylase (TH) and neuropeptide Y (NPY) (each taken from a separate representative experiment; avidin-biotin-peroxidase method). (Reproduced from McAllen and Dampney, 1988.)

Fig. 5. Above: ventral view of cat medulla showing pons, trapezoid body (Trap), pyramidal tract (Pyr) and three injection sites (not all from the same experiment). Below: chart records showing effects of glutamate microinjections at the three sites shown above on arterial pressure (B.P.), and the firing rate of single postganglionic vasoconstrictor fibres to skin and muscle, recorded simultaneously as described in text. Times and volumes of injections are indicated. (Reproduced from Dampney and McAllen, 1988.)

Functional subdivisions and topography of SRF

We have recently obtained clear evidence that subpopulations of SRF cells transmit their vasomotor drive to selected targets (Dampney and McAllen, 1988). In these experiments smaller injections of glutamate (2 – 10 nl) were used so as to improve spatial resolution. Simultaneous recordings were made of the electrical activity of postganglionic vasoconstrictor fibres supplying skin and muscle. These fibres were dissected from hindlimb nerves

238

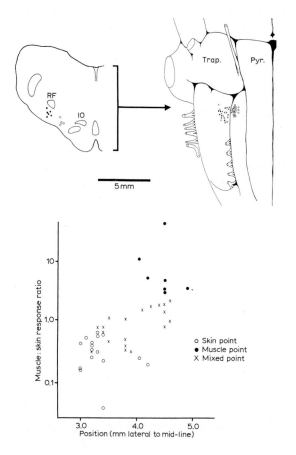

Fig. 6. Above: diagrammatic cross-section (left) and ventral view (right) of cat medulla showing pooled data of locations of injection sites. A ''skin point'' evoked a > 25% increase in activity of a skin vasoconstrictor unit but not of a muscle vasoconstrictor unit, a ''muscle point'' vice versa, and a ''mixed point'' caused the activity of both units to increase. Only dye-marked points are shown on the cross-section, but all effective sites on the ventral view. Below: the ratio of muscle vasoconstrictor unit to skin vasoconstrictor unit response (% increases in activity) to each effective injection has been plotted against its distance from the midline. The correlation is highly significant. (From Dampney and McAllen, 1988.)

different sensitivity or hormonally mediated responses of vascular smooth muscle, etc.) and show that the pathways from SRF to these tissues must be to some degree separate. They also strongly indicate that SRF is organized topographically.

Similar conclusions were drawn by Lovick

(1987), who showed that amino acid injections into the region of the rostral part of SRF preferentially reduced renal, compared to mesenteric or iliac vascular conductance. The latter responses were stronger with more caudal injections. We can confirm these findings.

We have previously inferred that the topography of SRF neurons corresponds to the type of tissue which is their functional target rather than the spinal segments to which they project. In an experiment to test this issue directly, brachial and femoral blood flows were recorded simultaneously from chloralose-anaesthetized, artificially ventilated cats whose adrenals had been removed, buffer nerves cut, and paws excluded from the circulation. Renal blood flow or renal nerve activity were also recorded, as an index of the vasomotor outflow from spinal segments intermediate between the other two. The results were clear: brachial vasoconstriction was evoked from the same parts of SRF as was femoral constriction (caudal and lateral). Renal effects followed glutamate injections into separate, rostral sites. We conclude that SRF neurons are arranged in terms of vascular beds rather than spinal segments.

Neurophysiological differentiation of SRF neurons

Most previous accounts of the properties of the bulbospinal neurons of this region have concentrated on their functional similarities. Nevertheless, differences have been noted. The cat lacks a significant subpopulation with unmyelinated spinal axons (Barman and Gebber, 1985; McAllen, 1986c) though these have been identified in rabbits (Terui et al., 1987) and rats (Brown and Guyenet, 1984; Morrison et al., 1988). A minority of SRF cells may be inhibited rather than excited by hypothalamic stimulation (Brown and Guyenet, 1985). Some SRF neurons show activity that is correlated better with external carotid than with renal nerve activity; others show the reverse, or no preference (Barman et al., 1984). The majority of SRF neurons show an activity peak coupled to the

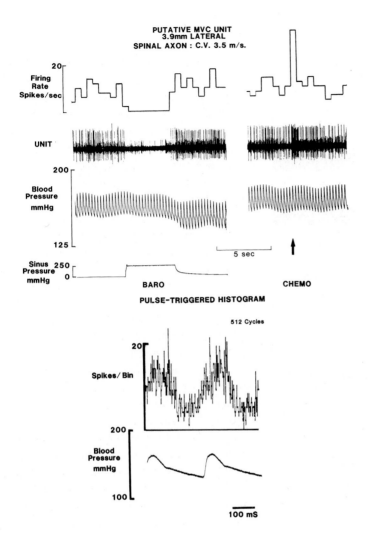

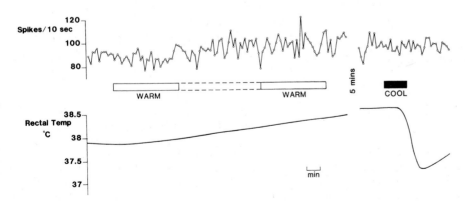

Fig. 7. (see p. 240 for legend).

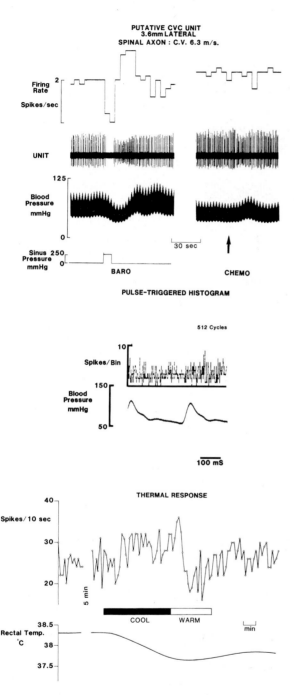

central inspiratory drive, a minority show the reverse pattern, while others still show no respiratory modulation (McAllen, 1987). Differences therefore exist between SRF neurons, but their functional significance has still to be evaluated.

Jänig and colleagues have developed a series of reflex tests which they apply to pre- and postganglionic sympathetic neurons. In most cases they have been able to classify each fibre into one of a small number of functional types, on the basis of its activity patterns (Jänig, 1985, 1988). In this way muscle (MVC), cutaneous (CVC) and visceral (VVC) vasoconstrictor neurons, as well as neurons with other functions, can be recognized in both post- and preganglionic fibre recordings (Jänig, 1988). If our hypothesis of functional dedication is true, the same may apply to SRF cells. (This would exclude characteristics known to be integrated within the spinal cord.)

Most CVC neurons are inhibited or not affected by carotid chemoreceptor stimulation, and this sets them apart from other vasoconstrictor neurons, which normally respond with excitation (Jänig, 1988). This stimulus was therefore used in a recent study to look for functional subclasses among SRF cells (McAllen, 1988). In chloralose-anaesthetized, paralyzed cats, SRF cells were identified by their antidromic response to spinal stimulation and their barosensitivity. Their responses were then tested to injections of CO_2-saturated saline, delivered close-arterially to the carotid body, while central respiratory drive was monitored from the phrenic nerve. Seven of 19 SRF cells were clearly inhibited by this stimulus, and four were excited. These were direct effects, and separable from any secondary reflex

Figs. 7 and 8. Records from two SRF bulbospinal neurons with properties suggesting respectively muscle vasoconstrictor (Fig. 7) and cutaneous vasoconstrictor (Fig. 8) function. The two units were recorded in separate experiments in chloralose-anaesthetized, paralyzed cats. Upper records show the effect of inflation of the ipsilateral carotid sinus (BARO), and of close arterial injection of approximately 0.1 ml CO_2-saturated saline to the contralateral carotid body (CHEMO). Middle records show pulse-triggered histograms of spontaneous activity. For these, only the contralateral sinus was providing a pulse-related baroreceptor signal; the ipsilateral sinus was deflated and the ipsilateral vago-aortic nerves cut. Lower records show the effect on firing rate and rectal temperature of warming and cooling the cat. This was done by peritoneal lavage with saline at approximately 43°C or 10 – 15°C.

changes. Three further cells showed enhanced inspiratory firing in parallel with the increased phrenic activity. The remainder were not affected.

The results suggest that a significant proportion of the neurons sampled in these experiments belonged to the CVC pathway. However, much firmer conclusions could be reached on the basis of a panel of tests, and experiments using this approach are in progress. Thermal stimuli have been added as a more definitive test for neurons in the CVC pathway (Jänig, 1988). Figures 7 and 8 show preliminary data from two SRF bulbospinal neurons with contrasting properties. One behaved like a peripheral CVC neuron and was clearly thermosensitive, the other showed the typical properties of a peripheral MVC (or renal vasoconstrictor) neuron, and little or no response to temperature.

Conclusion

Evidence has been presented which supports the following views:

(1) The vasomotor actions of the rostral ventrolateral medulla are in the main due to a compact column of neurons − the SRF. These cells have spinal axons which innervate the intermediolateral horn.

(2) The large majority of SRF cells contain catecholamine (adrenaline), and constitute part of the C1 cell group.

(3) SRF cells drive the sympathetic nerves that supply the heart, blood vessels and adrenal medulla, but not those which supply other organs.

(4) Subgroups of SRF cells are functionally dedicated to drive the vasomotor supply to one type of tissue, although the possibility that other SRF cells have a more generalized action cannot be excluded.

(5) SRF neurons are topographically organized with respect to function (target tissue).

(6) The differentiated response patterns of sympathetic vasoconstrictor neurons which supply different tissues are already discernible in SRF cells.

Acknowledgements

The authors' research was supported by the British Heart Foundation, Medical Research Council (U.K.), National Health and Medical Research Council (Australia) and the Australian Brain Foundation.

References

Barman, S.M. and Gebber, G.L. (1985) Axonal projection patterns of ventrolateral medullospinal sympathoexcitatory neurons. *J. Neurophysiol.*, 53: 1551 − 1566.

Barman, S.M., Gebber, G.L. and Calaresu, F.R. (1984) Differential control of sympathetic nerve discharge by the brain stem. *Am. J. Physiol.*, 247: R513 − R519.

Brown, D.L. and Guyenet, P.G. (1984) Cardiovascular neurons of brain stem with projections to spinal cord. *Am. J. Physiol.*, 247: R1009 − R1016.

Brown, D.L. and Guyenet, P.G. (1985) Electrophysiological study of cardiovascular neurons in the rostral ventrolateral medulla in rats. *Circ. Res.*, 56: 359 − 369.

Dampney, R.A.L. and McAllen, R.M. (1988) Differential control of sympathetic fibres supplying hindlimb skin and muscle by subretrofacial neurones in the cat. *J. Physiol.*, 395: 41 − 56.

Dampney, R.A.L., Goodchild, A.K. and Tan, E. (1985) Vasopressor neurons in the rostral ventrolateral medulla of the rabbit. *J. Auton. Nerv. Syst.*, 14: 239 − 254.

Dampney, R.A.L., Czachurski, J., Dembowsky, K., Goodchild, A.K. and Seller, H. (1987a) Afferent connections and spinal projections of the pressor region in the rostral ventrolateral medulla in the cat. *J. Auton. Nerv. Syst.*, 20: 73 − 86.

Dampney, R.A.L., Goodchild, A.K. and McAllen, R.M. (1987b) Vasomotor control by subretrofacial neurones in the rostral ventrolateral medulla. *Can. J. Physiol. Pharmacol.*, 65: 1572 − 1579.

Goodchild, A.K., Dampney, R.A.L. and Bandler, R. (1982) A method for evoking physiological responses by stimulation of cell bodies, but not axons of passage, within localized regions of the central nervous system. *J. Neurosci. Methods*, 6: 351 − 363.

Guertzenstein, P.G. and Silver, A. (1974) Fall in blood pressure produced from discrete regions of the ventral surface of the medulla by glycine and lesions. *J. Physiol.*, 242: 480 − 503.

Jänig, W. (1985) Organization of the lumbar sympathetic outflow to skeletal muscle and skin of the cat hindlimb and tail. *Rev. Physiol. Biochem. Pharmacol.*, 102: 119 − 213.

Jänig, W. (1988) Pre- and postganglionic vasoconstrictor neurons: differentiation, types and discharge properties. *Ann. Rev. Physiol.*, 50: 525 − 539.

242

Lovick, T.A. (1987) Differential control of cardiac and vasomotor activity by neurones in nucleus paragigantocellularis lateralis in the cat. *J. Physiol.,* 389: 23 – 35.

McAllen, R.M. (1985) Mediation of the fastigial pressor response and a somatosympathetic reflex by ventral medullary neurones in the cat. *J. Physiol.,* 368: 423 – 433.

McAllen, R.M. (1986a) Location of neurones with cardiovascular and respiratory function, at the ventral surface of the cat's medulla. *Neuroscience,* 18: 43 – 49.

McAllen, R.M. (1986b) Action and specificity of ventral medullary vasopressor neurones in the cat. *Neuroscience,* 18: 51 – 59.

McAllen, R.M. (1986c) Identification and properties of subretrofacial bulbospinal neurones: a descending cardiovascular pathway in the cat. *J. Auton. Nerv. Syst.,* 17: 151 – 164.

McAllen, R.M. (1987) Central respiratory modulation of subretrofacial bulbospinal neurones in the cat. *J. Physiol.,* 388: 533 – 545.

McAllen, R.M. (1988) The effects of arterial chemoreceptors on cat subretrofacial neurones. *J. Physiol.,* 399: 32P.

McAllen, R.M. and Dampney, R.A.L. (1988) Functional subdivisions among subretrofacial presympathetic neurons. In M. Sandler, A. Dahlstrom and R.H. Belmaker (Eds.), *Neurology and Neurobiology, Vol. 42, Progress in Catecholamine Research,* Alan R. Liss, New York, pp. 337 – 342.

McAllen, R.M., Neil, J.J. and Loewy, A.D. (1982) Effects of kainic acid applied to the ventral surface of the medulla oblongata on vasomotor tone, the baroreceptor reflex and hypothalamic autonomic responses. *Brain Res.,* 238: 65 – 76.

Morrison, S.F., Milner, T.A. and Reis, D.J. (1988) Reticulospinal vasomotor neurons of the rat rostral ventrolateral medulla: relationship to sympathetic nerve activity and the C1 adrenergic cell group. *J. Neurosci.,* 8: 1286 – 1301.

Sun, M.K., Young, B.S., Hackett, J.T. and Guyenet, P.G. (1988) Rostral ventrolateral medullary neurons with intrinsic pacemaker properties are not catecholaminergic. *Brain Res.,* 451: 345 – 349.

Terui, N., Saeki, Y. and Kumada, M. (1987) Confluence of barosensory and nonbarosensory inputs at neurons in the ventrolateral medulla in rabbits. *Can. J. Physiol. Pharmacol.,* 65: 1584 – 1590.

J. Ciriello, M.M. Caverson and C. Polosa (Eds.)
Progress in Brain Research, Vol. 81
© 1989 Elsevier Science Publishers B.V. (Biomedical Division)

CHAPTER 19

Role of the glycine sensitive area in the regulation of cardiac output

R.R. Campos Jr. and P.G. Guertzenstein

Departamento de Fisiologia, Escola Paulista de Medicina, Cx. Postal 20.393 (04034), São Paulo, SP, Brazil

Introduction

Dittmar had postulated a discrete location of the vasomotor center on the ventral part of the medulla at the end of the last century (Dittmar, 1873). For nearly half a century to follow the structures responsible for maintaining arterial blood pressure were thought to lie near the dorsal surface of the brainstem, on the floor of the fourth ventricle. In 1946, Alexander provided evidence suggesting that these structures were distributed throughout the entire medulla oblongata (Alexander, 1946). One should stress at this point that this localization of the vasomotor center was obtained through the use of electrical stimulation and as we know, electrical stimulation acts not only on nerve cell bodies but also on nerve fibers.

New evidence for a discrete localization of the vasomotor center appeared when Schlaefke and Loeschcke (1967), studying regions of the ventral surface of the medulla concerned with respiratory control, demonstrated that bilateral cooling of a small and superficial area of the ventral medulla produced not only respiratory changes but also a steep fall in blood pressure. Their experiment, however, did not exclude the possibility that this effect might be due to the inhibition of nerve fibers passing through this region, but having their cell bodies scattered throughout the medulla.

This problem was resolved when Feldberg and Guertzenstein found in a series of experiments that a number of substances, known to act on synapses were able to produce changes in blood pressure when applied through perspex rings to the same region in which localized cooling had produced hypotension. These substances were pentobarbitone sodium (Feldberg and Guertzenstein, 1972), cholinomimetics, leptazol, strychnine, tubocurarine and the amino acids glycine and GABA (Guertzenstein, 1973). Leptazol, strychnine and d-tubocurarine produced rises in arterial pressure, while pentobarbitone sodium, cholinomimetics, and the amino acids produced hypotension. A very interesting feature of these responses was the fact that high blood pressure could be obtained by unilateral application, whereas hypotension required bilateral application. Since both glycine and GABA are post-synaptic inhibitors, this combination of effects was strong evidence suggesting that the structures under the rings were responsible for the maintenance of arterial blood pressure, and that they must be cell bodies and not fibers of passage.

Using glycine as a tool it was possible to localize more precisely, within the areas covered by the perspex rings, the structures responsible for the maintenance of blood pressure (Guertzenstein and Silver, 1974). In these experiments, glycine was applied either unilaterally or bilaterally. Upper tracings of Fig. 1 illustrate unilateral applications of the drug, either on the right, or on the left side. Only slight falls in blood pressure were observed.

244

However, if the drug was applied subsequently to the contralateral side a severe hypotension was obtained, similar to that produced by bilateral applications.

In addition, as shown in Fig. 1, the unilateral electrolytic destruction of a small area within the left ring only produced a small blood pressure drop, but it potentiated the effect of glycine unilaterally applied to the opposite side, as shown in the lower panel of Fig. 1.

Bilateral electrolytic destruction of this glycine sensitive area (GSA), as shown in Fig. 2, produced a fall in arterial blood pressure to levels similar to those usually obtained in acute spinal animals, without signs of recovery for at least 6 h, which

was the longest period of time the animals were observed for.

These facts were used to localize more precisely within the area covered by the rings, the site of the cells responsible for the maintenance of the blood pressure. It was found that the GSA was restricted to a 1.5 mm wide strip extending from 1 to 2.5 mm caudal to the trapezoid bodies, and about 4 mm lateral to the midline. The maximum depth of this structure was found to be 0.8 mm below the ventral surface. The GSA appears to coincide with location of the C1 adrenergic cells studied by Reis and his colleagues (Ross et al., 1981).

Another ventral surface area concerned with maintenance of blood pressure has been recently described, at the medullary-spinal transition (Feldberg and Guertzenstein, 1986). As shown in the lower trace of Fig. 3, it responds to pentobarbitone

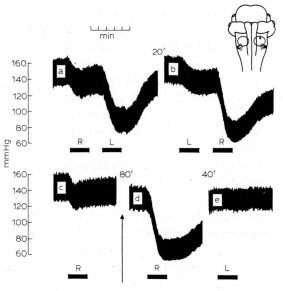

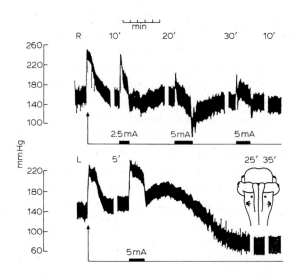

Fig. 1. Records of arterial blood pressure from an anesthetized cat artificially ventilated and atropinized. A 20% solution of glycine was applied to the ventral surface of the brainstem through perspex rings, the position of which is shown by the ovals in the diagram. Periods of application are indicated by the black bars. Glycine applied in a volume of 10 μl into either right (R) or left (L) ring. The arrow indicates electrolytic destruction on the glycine sensitive area on the left with a surface electrode placed 4 mm lateral to the midline and 2 mm caudal to the trapezoid bodies at the point indicated in the diagram by the black dot inside the left ring. Intervals between records indicated in minutes; interval between upper and lower tracing 20 min. (From Guertzenstein and Silver, 1974.)

Fig. 2. Records of arterial blood pressure from an anesthetized cat artificially ventilated and atropinized. The arrows mark the placing of an electrode (1 mm diameter) on the ventral surface of the brainstem, first on the right (R) and then on the left (L) side 4 mm lateral to the midline and 2 mm caudal to the trapezoid bodies, at the points indicated by the black dots in the diagram. Horizontal lines indicate that the electrode is kept in position until the end of the records. The black bars indicate periods of passage of 2.5 or 5 mA DC through the electrode. Intervals between records indicated in min, interval between upper and lower tracing 3 min. (From Guertzenstein and Silver, 1974.)

and leptazol in a manner similar to the GSA, but only in deeply anesthetized animals. The question of its role in blood pressure maintenance has been recently addressed. Apparently it exerts no important action in surgically anesthetized animals, where the GSA appears to maintain blood pressure by itself. However, in very deeply anesthetized cats, the GSA appears to require a drive coming from this more caudal area. Indications come from unpublished observations from our laboratory

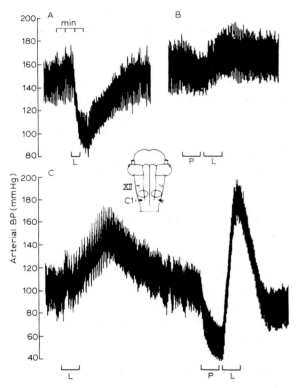

Fig. 3. Arterial blood pressure from a cat during surgical anesthesia following intravenous chloralose at a dosage of 60 mg/kg and atropine methylnitrate at 0.5 mg/kg; between (B) and (C) anesthesia was deepened by two additional intravenous injections of chloralose of 30 mg/kg. The interval between (A) and (B) was 40 min and between (B) and (C) was 200 min. Paired perspex rings placed across the exposed ventral surface of medulla oblongata for topical application of leptazol (200 mg/ml) (L) and sodium pentobarbitone (30 mg/ml) (P) as indicated by the bars marked L and P, respectively. The ovals in the diagram of the inset indicate the areas covered by the rings; the cat was breathing spontaneously during (A) and (B) but was artificially ventilated during (C) and (D). Time signal in minutes. (From Feldberg and Guertzenstein, 1986.)

(Andreatta and Campos), who found, in deeply anesthetized cats, that leptazol in the GSA still evokes its pressor effect after the hypotension induced by pentobarbitone in the caudal area; in contrast, leptazol loses its pressor ability in the caudal area, during hypotension produced by pentobarbitone in the GSA.

Although the GSA has been extensively studied during the last decade with respect to blood pressure and regional blood flow regulation, there are only a few studies about its role in the regulation of cardiac output (Hilton et al., 1983; Dampney et al., 1986; McAllen, 1986).

The present experiments describe the effects of excitation or inhibition of the GSA in connection to cardiac output (CO) control. The experiments were performed in α-chloralose anesthetized cats (80 mg/kg) artificially ventilated and given atropine methylnitrate (1 mg/kg, i.v.). Adrenergic blockage was obtained by means of an intravenous injection of propranolol (1 mg/kg) or phentolamine (repeated injections of 2.5 mg/kg to abolish the effect of noradrenaline in a dose that had increased blood pressure by 40 mmHg). Bilateral adrenalectomy was performed via a dorsal approach. Drugs were applied to the GSA through a perspex ring as previously described (Guertzenstein, 1973). Arterial blood pressure was recorded from the femoral artery, cardiac output was measured by thermodilution, and the blood temperature was monitored by means of a thermocouple placed at the root of the aorta. Room temperature saline (0.3 – 1.0 ml) was injected either in the left or in the right atrium. In eight experiments, left atrial pressure was also measured.

Pharmacological manipulation of the GSA and cardiac function

Excitation

As shown in Fig. 4, obtained from a group of 22 animals, leptazol (200 mg/ml) applied for 3 min to the GSA produced rises in mean arterial blood pressure (MABP), cardiac output (CO), heart rate (HR) and total peripheral resistance (TPR). The

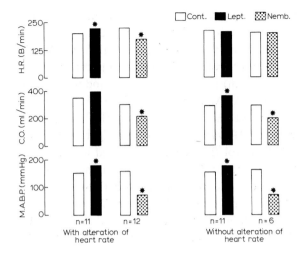

Fig. 7. Effects of a 3-min leptazol (200 mg/kg) and a 5 min pentobarbitone sodium (30 mg/kg) application to the glycine sensitive area on cardiac output and mean arterial blood pressure. On the left, animals with and on the right, animals without alterations of heart rate. An asterisk (*) indicates significant difference for pre-application values ($p < 0.05$). "$n = $" at the bottom of the figure indicates the number of animals in each group.

variations. This figure further shows that changes in MABP (bottom bars) produced by topical application of leptazol or pentobarbitone sodium to the GSA were the same in the two groups of animals independent of changes in HR.

Effects of intravenous adrenoceptor antagonists and adrenalectomy on the cardiovascular responses to leptazol and pentobarbitone sodium applications to the GSA

Figure 8 illustrates the influence of propranolol (i.v.), phentolamine (i.v.) and adrenalectomy on the cardiovascular effects of applications of leptazol (3 min), pentobarbitone sodium (5 min) and leptazol (3 min) just after a 5-min application of pentobarbitone sodium.

Beta-blockade by itself lowers MABP, CO and HR and raises TPR. During pharmacological manipulation of the GSA, β-blockade abolished the cardiac effects (CO and HR) but not MABP changes that were obtained in animals without propranolol. Thus, the changes in MABP in the animals after β-blockade were entirely due to changes in TPR.

Alpha-blockade by itself lowered the basal MABP due to a decrease in TPR. It also produced a rise in CO and HR. Leptazol stimulation of the GSA during α-blockade did not produce any changes in the above parameters; however, pentobarbitone sodium application lowered MABP, CO and HR but did not change TPR. Leptazol applied just after pentobarbitone sodium reversed its effects. The MABP fall due to pentobarbitone sodium application was due to a decrease in CO.

Adrenalectomy by itself did not change the cardiovascular parameters. However, it greatly reduced the effects of leptazol application either in relation to control values or in relation to values in animals where pentobarbitone sodium had been previously applied. Pentobarbitone sodium application produced the usual reductions in MABP, CO and HR as it did in untreated animals.

Discussion

The present experiments show that the glycine sensitive area plays a key role in CO regulation, apart from its well known function in the adjustment of blood pressure, peripheral resistance and HR (Ciriello et al., 1986; Millhorn et al., 1986).

These results support the findings of Hilton et al. (1983), who showed that during inhibition of the GSA, there was a decrease of $10-45\%$ in the values of CO. However, these authors did not analyze the cause of the decrease in the CO in terms of HR or filling pressure.

More recently, Dampney et al. (1985) in rabbits and McAllen (1986) in cats showed that microinjections of excitatory amino acids produced a rise in arterial blood pressure and a fall in CO. The difference between the effect of stimulation using microinjection and topical application can be explained by the fact that topical applications of drugs produce their effects in a much larger area than microinjection stimulation.

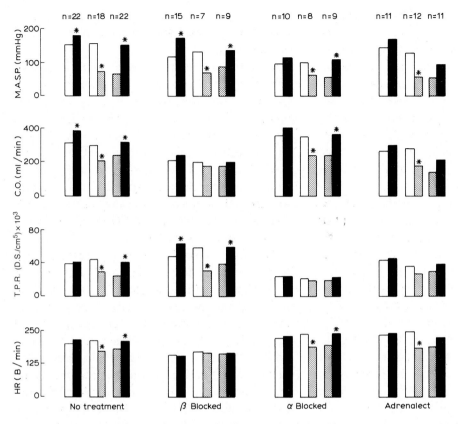

Fig. 8. Effects of system adrenoceptor antagonism and adrenalectomy on the mean changes in cardiovascular parameters due to topical application of leptazol for 3 min (■), pentobarbitone sodium for 5 min (▦) and leptazol just after pentobarbitone sodium to the glycine sensitive area. Open columns (□) denote pre-application values. "$n =$" at the top of the figure indicates number of animals in each experimental group. An asterisk (*) indicates significant difference from pre-application values or from values of leptazol in relation to the previous pentobarbitone sodium application ($p < 0.05$).

It is therefore conceivable that there are different neural structures, one responsible for the cardiac, and the other for peripheral resistance changes in the glycine sensitive area, although both are located in the areas covered by the rings. This hypothesis is supported by the findings of Lovick (1987) who showed that the nucleus paragigantocellularis lateralis, which lies within the areas covered by the rings in the present experiments, contains several populations of neurons which can preferentially control HR or blood flow to different vascular beds.

The experiments in animals after α- and β-adrenergic blockade favor the idea that the cardiac output changes produced by pharmacological manipulation of the glycine sensitive area are due to a change in the sympathetic activity to the heart and not to the vessels producing peripheral adjustments. This is because the main sympathetic adrenoceptors in the heart are the β-receptors and when these adrenoceptors were blocked the cardiac effects were completely abolished. Alpha-blockade on the other hand acts mainly on arteries and veins, and abolished the peripheral adjustments that might explain the observed CO changes. However, after α-blockade the CO was still dependent upon the activity of the glycine sensitive area, since the fall in arterial blood pressure produced by pentobarbitone sodium application was nearly primarily entirely due to a fall in CO. The absence

250

of a significant increase in arterial blood pressure, HR and CO during leptazol application may be due to the fact that phentolamine alone produces a fall in total peripheral resistance and blood pressure. This fall is a strong stimulus to cardiovascular reflexes which increases the sympathetic drive to the heart and consequently the cardiac output (Taylor et al., 1965). It is thus conceivable that in this situation a further sympathetic stimulus produced by leptazol application no longer produces clear effects.

Another interesting observation in animals treated with propranolol was the increase in peripheral resistance produced by leptazol application that was not observed in animals without pretreatment. The explanation for this finding may lie in the fact that microinjections of excitatory amino acids in some sites of the glycine sensitive area produce pressor responses accompanied by vasodilation in skeletal muscle (Lovick and Hilton, 1985).

Recently, it has also been shown that this vasodilation was nearly abolished by propranolol (Lovick, 1987). This muscle vasodilation could be the reason why leptazol application did not increase total peripheral resistance during a 3-min application in animals that had not received propranolol.

Although it is a well established fact that excitation of the glycine sensitive area elicits catecholamine release by the adrenal medulla, the role played by these hormones in the cardiovascular effects produced by this excitation is not well established (Ross et al., 1984; McAllen, 1986). In our experiments, adrenalectomy greatly diminished the increase of arterial blood pressure, HR and CO due to excitation of the glycine sensitive area with leptazol. This shows an important role of the adrenal hormones in this interaction. The sympathetic drive to the heart, however, was important to maintain the values of the CO and HR since inhibition of the glycine sensitive area by pentobarbitone sodium produced a fall of these parameters similar to that observed in animals with intact adrenals. The return of these values was only partial after a 3-min application of leptazol. This may

be explained by the synergism of the adrenal hormones with sympathetic function of the glycine sensitive area.

Although changes in CO were usually associated with changes in HR, in some animals the two parameters were dissociated. In fact, half of the animals in which leptazol was applied to the glycine sensitive area had an increase in CO without tachycardia and one third of the animals in which nembutal was applied had a decrease in cardiac output without bradycardia. This observation shows that, at least in the animals without HR alterations, the changes in CO were related to stroke volume and not to HR.

The other factor that could be responsible for the changes in cardiac output would be an increase or decrease in pre-load resulting in a rise or fall in the CO. This was not the cause of the CO variations since we showed that the changes in CO did not correlate with changes in mean atrial pressure.

The only other factor that could explain the changes in CO during pharmacological manipulation of the glycine sensitive area would be a variation in cardiac contractility. This could be due to direct sympathetic drive to the heart or through the release of catecholamines by the adrenals. The experiments in adrenalectomized animals show that both factors are acting.

Concluding remarks

The results obtained with pharmacological manipulation of the glycine sensitive area are a strong indication that this area controls CO, in addition to its well known role in the control of MABP, TPR and HR. This control is exerted most probably through the sympathetic innervation to the heart affecting its contractility.

Acknowledgements

This research was supported by CNPq, grant no. 405232/87.0/BF/FV. The authors wish to thank Prof. M. Rocha e Silva for critically reviewing the manuscript.

References

Alexander, R.S. (1946) Tonic and reflex functions of medullary sympathetic cardiovascular centers. *J. Neurophysiol.,* 9: 205 – 217.

Calaresu, F.R. and Yardley, C.P. (1988) Medullary basal sympathetic tone. *Ann. Rev. Physiol.,* 50: 511 – 524.

Ciriello, J., Caverson, Monica, M. and Polosa, C. (1986) Function of the ventrolateral medulla in the control of the circulation. *Brain Res. Rev.,* 11: 359 – 391.

Dampney, R.A.L., Goodchild, A.K. and Tan, E. (1985) Vasopressor neurons in the rostral ventrolateral medulla of the rabbit. *J. Auton. Nerv. Syst.,* 14: 239 – 254.

Dittmar, C. (1873) Uber die hage des sogenannten gefasscentrums in der medulla oblongata. *Ber. Sachs. Akad. Wiss.,* 25: 449 – 469.

Feldberg, W. and Guertzenstein, P.G. (1972) A vasodepressor effect of pentobarbitone sodium. *J. Physiol. (Lond.),* 224: 83 – 103.

Feldberg, W. and Guertzenstein, P.G. (1986) Blood pressure effects of leptazol applied to the ventral surface of the brainstem of cats. *J. Physiol.,* 372: 445 – 456.

Guertzenstein, P.G. (1973) Blood pressure effects obtained by drugs applied to the ventral surface of the brain stem. *J. Physiol. (Lond.),* 229: 395 – 408.

Guertzenstein, P.G. and Silver, A. (1974) Fall in blood pressure produced from discrete regions of the ventral surface of the medulla by glycine and lesions. *J. Physiol. (Lond.),* 242: 489 – 503.

Hilton, S.M., Marshall, J.M. and Timms, R.J. (1983) Ventral medullary relay neurones in the pathway from the defence areas of the cat and their effect on blood pressure. *J. Physiol. (Lond.),* 345: 149 – 166.

Lovick, T.A. (1987) Differential control of cardiac and vasomotor activity by neurones in nucleus paragigantocellularis lateralis in the cat. *J. Physiol.,* 389: 23 – 35.

Lovick, T.A. and Hilton, S.M. (1985) Vasodilator and vasoconstrictor neurones of the ventrolateral medulla in the cat. *Brain Res.,* 331: 352 – 357.

McAllen, R.M. (1986) Action and specificity of ventral medullary vasopressor neurones in the cat. *Neuroscience,* 18: 51 – 59.

Millhorn, D.E. and Eldridge, F.L. (1986) Role of ventrolateral medulla in regulation of respiratory and cardiovascular systems. *J. Appl. Physiol.,* 61: 1249 – 1263.

Ross, C.A., Armstrong, D.M., Ruggiero, D.A., Pickel, V.M., Joh, T.H. and Reis, D.J. (1981) Adrenaline neurons in the rostral ventrolateral medulla innervate thoracic spinal cord: a combined immunocytochemical and retrograde transport demonstration. *Neurosci. Lett.,* 25: 257 – 262.

Ross, C.A., Ruggiero, D.A., Park, D.H., Joh, T.H., Sved, A.F., Fernandez-Pardal, J., Saavedra, J.M. and Reis, D.J. (1984) Tonic vasomotor control by the rostral ventrolateral medulla: effect of electrical or chemical stimulation of the area containing C1 adrenaline neurons on arterial pressure, heart rate, and plasma catecholamines and vasopressin. *J. Neurosci.,* 4: 474 – 494.

Schlaefke, M. and Loeschcke, H.H. (1967) Lokalisation eines an der regulation von atmung und Kreislauf Beteiligten Gebietes an der ventralen oberflache der medulla oblongata durch Kalteblockade. *Pflügers Arch Gesamte Physiol.,* 297: 201 – 220.

Taylor, S.H., Sutherland, G.R., Mackenzie, G.J., Staunton, H.P. and Donald, K.W. (1965) The circulatory effects of intravenous phentolamine in man. *Circulation,* 31: 741 – 745.

J. Ciriello, M.M. Caverson and C. Polosa (Eds.)
Progress in Brain Research, Vol. 81
© 1989 Elsevier Science Publishers B.V. (Biomedical Division)

CHAPTER 20

Pressor responses to muscular contraction in the cat: contributions by caudal and rostral ventrolateral medulla

G.A. Iwamoto, T.G. Waldrop, R.M. Bauer and J.H. Mitchell

Departments of Veterinary Biosciences, Physiology and Biophysics, University of Illinois, Urbana-Champaign, Illinois, and Harry S. Moss Heart Center, University of Texas Southwestern Medical Center, Dallas, Texas, U.S.A.

Introduction

The portion of the ventrolateral medulla which is usually associated with regulation of blood pressure in the cat is known by a number of cytoarchitectonic names. Among the names utilized are the paragigantocellularis lateralis (in rats) and the subretrofacial region. Another way to refer to the region is by the designation "glycine sensitive area" which was introduced when agents were delivered to the ventrolateral medullary surface. However, the most general designation for this area is that it is contained in the rostral portion of the ventrolateral medulla. It is well known that cells of this region project to the intermediolateral cell column (IML) and comprise a key sympathoexcitatory pathway (see Ciriello et al., 1986b).

The research which will now be described has taken a more expansive view of the ventrolateral medulla, namely that more than the rostral portion may be involved in cardiovascular control, especially the case represented when muscular activity (exercise) stimulates the adjustments. The studies which will now be described are thus a cross between two fields, that of the neural control of the circulation and that of exercise physiology.

Cardiovascular responses induced by muscular contraction

Our main interests in studying central neural control of the cardiovascular system were the phenomena associated with cardiorespiratory adjustments during static exercise. These phenomena include changes in heart rate, blood pressure, regional blood flow and ventilation. Certainly, metabolic adjustments supporting the ability to contract muscles are basic to any form of animal life.

Neurally mediated cardiovascular adjustments during exercise are brought about by two general mechanisms: (1) a central neural drive in which the cardiovascular and motor systems are driven in parallel, often called "central command", and (2) a reflex initiated by activity in the contracting muscles which then activates the cardiovascular control system (Mitchell and Schmidt, 1983).

One convenient animal model which allows the study of the reflex mechanism utilizes the electrical stimulation of ventral roots (generally 3 times motor threshold, 0.1 msec pulses at 20 – 50 Hz) to elicit muscular contraction which, in turn, evokes increases in heart rate, blood pressure, appropriate changes in the pattern of blood flow and increases in ventilation. A schematic diagram of the experimental arrangement is shown on the left side of Fig. 1. Through the work of our laboratory group we have attempted to analyze what occurs during this reflex with emphasis on the neural circuitry underlying it. Many aspects have been considered, including the characteristics of afferents, the central pathway and the pattern of sympathetic outflow. For practical purposes, one might simply consider this a form of somatosympathetic reflex but originating from the actual contraction of muscle. For the sake of simplification, we have often referred to this response as the "exercise pressor reflex" with the full realization that this is only one component of the many control mechanisms underlying actual voluntary motor activity and accompanying cardiovascular responses.

The afferent input required for the reflex originates from small fibers in the A-delta and C fiber range, which in the case of muscle afferents are also known as the group III and IV afferents, respectively. There are two basic patterns of afferent discharge elicited by muscular contraction which have been elucidated (Kaufman et al., 1983). The group III afferents, as a rule, increase their firing at the onset of muscular contraction and show varying degrees of adaptation. This type of response appears to indicate that the afferents are mechanosensitive. The group IV afferents slowly increase their discharge during sustained contraction which is the pattern one would expect if the fibers were sensitive to the buildup of metabolites. These patterns should be kept in mind as they are echoed at higher levels of neural integration.

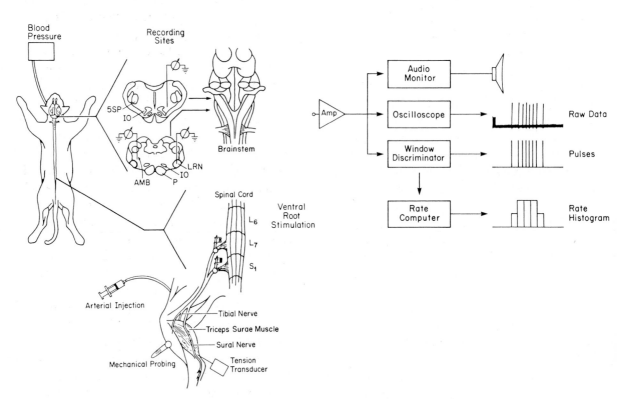

Fig. 1. Diagram showing the experimental preparation for studying the pressor response to muscular contraction and for investigation of single cells. The lower left side of the diagram shows the reflex paradigm. The L7 and S1 ventral roots are isolated in a cat following a laminectomy. Electrical stimulation is then applied, causing a static contraction of hindlimb muscles. The triceps surae is monitored for muscle tension. The upper left side of the diagram shows that the preparation can be used to monitor the discharge of medullary cells during static muscular contraction. On the right side of the diagram, the cell discharge can be displayed in various ways, as raw data, as window discriminator pulses or as a rate histogram.

Neural control of the cardiovascular response to muscular contraction

General localization of the supraspinal portions of the reflex

Our investigation of the reflex's central circuitry first included a series of serial transections which indicated that the reflex was essentially complete at medullary levels. There had been conflicting reports as to the nature of this reflex response versus that of other somatosympathetic responses already established in the literature (Iwamoto et al., 1985).

Using halothane anesthesia during surgical procedures, we were able to obtain experimental preparations for the study of the reflex following: (1) midcollicular decerebration, (2) medullary transection 5 mm rostral to the obex or (3) C1-spinal transection. Each of these preparations was free from anesthetic at the time of study.

Although we were able to obtain some blood pressure changes in the C1 spinal preparation we found that the medulla was required for a complete expression of the reflex including changes in blood pressure and heart rate. There was a supramedullary component present in the decerebrate preparations as the responses were somewhat diminished by the transection 5 mm rostral to the obex. Furthermore, although the non-anesthetized decerebrate preparations gave rise to somewhat larger pressor responses than intact anesthetized preparations, the difference in magnitude of the response was found to be due to the anesthetic. The decerebrate animals, once anesthetized, gave the same level of response as those initially anesthetized. These experiments indicated that despite evidence to the contrary, this reflex was much like any other somatosympathetic reflex in terms of its central circuitry.

Effects of lesioning and stimulation of central sites

Our search for the specific CNS sites involved in the reflex took us in two directions. We were, of course, interested in many of the sites which are of importance to all investigators who are examining sympathetic responses. This would include all of the areas designated as pressor sites. However, as we were interested in the fate of small fiber input from muscle, we were also obliged to consider the areas these signals were already known to affect in the medulla.

Caudal ventrolateral medulla. One such site of integration of high threshold muscle afferent activity is the caudal ventrolateral medulla (cVLM) in the region of the lateral reticular nucleus (LRN). This area had long been known from the work of investigators principally interested in motor control as a region receiving input from the higher threshold muscle afferents. The usual interpretation of cells in the area was that they were concerned mainly with relaying information from the "bilateral ventral flexor reflex tract" to the cerebellum (Oscarsson, 1973). However, a report from Ciriello and Calaresu (1977) indicated that cardiovascular reflexes, including responses to carotid sinus nerve stimulation and the somatosympathetic reflex in response to sciatic nerve stimulation were abolished by electrolytic lesions in this area.

We duplicated Ciriello and Calaresu's experiment in the case of the pressor response to muscular contraction (Iwamoto et al., 1982). Figure 2 shows that when bilateral electrolytic lesions were placed in or near the LRN in pentobarbital anesthetized cats, the pressor reflex was abolished. The precise lesion site in the cVLM was chosen using electrical stimulation. When a pressor area was reached in the cVLM at an appropriate depth, the site was lesioned. The existence of a pressor area in this region came as no surprise to us as Alexander's (1946) mapping of the pressor areas clearly included the cVLM.

However, this general result seemed at odds with studies (Reis et al., 1984) using chemical stimulation which appeared to indicate that the apparently equivalent area in the rat was a depressor zone. Our own work (Iwamoto et al., 1984) showed that areas in and near the LRN showed increased 2-

[^{14}C]deoxyglucose labelling (presumed to label cells and terminals) during muscular contraction. However, this did not demonstrate that the labelling was related to cardiovascular events.

Thus, this area of the cVLM was also investigated by the use of stimulation via glutamate microinjections (Iwamoto and Waldrop, 1986). In general, we found in decerebrate and chloralose anesthetized cats, using a variety of glutamate concentrations (1 M, 500 mM, 100 mM), that a pressor response could be evoked from stimulation in the cVLM adjacent to the dorsal border of the LRN and on the ventrolateral border of the medulla.

Figure 3 shows the effect of a 19 nl injection of 1 M glutamate into the cVLM just dorsal to the LRN on blood pressure and heart rate. Respiratory responses could be elicited from this area, consisting largely of increases in minute ventilation through increases in respiratory frequency.

Rostral ventrolateral medulla. Much evidence from a variety of experiments had indicated: (1) that cells from the rostral ventrolateral medulla (rVLM) project to the intermediolateral cell column (Amendt et al., 1979; Miura et al., 1983; Brown and Guyenet, 1984; Barman and Gebber,

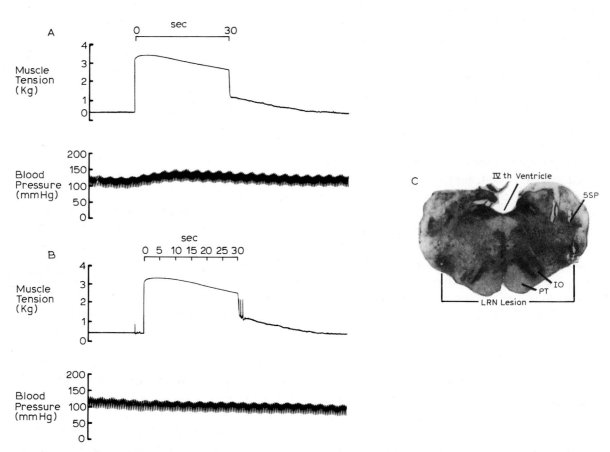

Fig. 2. Effects of bilateral lesions of the cVLM in the vicinity of the lateral reticular nucleus on the pressor response to static muscular contraction. Panel (A) shows the blood pressure response to muscular contraction evoked by electrical stimulation of the L7 and S1 ventral roots at 50 Hz, 3 times motor threshold. Panel (B) shows that as a result of the lesions shown in Panel (C), the pressor response to muscular contraction is abolished in Panel (B). PT = pyramidal tract; for all other abbreviations refer to Fig. 4. (From Iwamoto et al., 1982.)

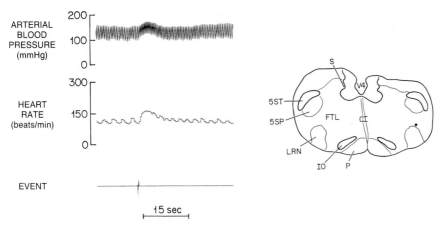

Fig. 3. Effect of L-glutamate microinjection on blood pressure and heart rate. A 19 nl injection of 1 M L-glutamate into the cVLM at the site shown at the right of the tracings, resulted in an increase of heart rate and blood pressure. For abbreviations refer to Fig. 4.

1985a; Ciriello et al., 1986b; Reis et al., 1984) and (2) that stimulation of this area elicits pressor responses (Alexander, 1946; Reis et al., 1984; Ciriello et al., 1986b; McAllen, 1986). We attempted to elucidate the possible role of this area in the reflex. Sun and Guyenet (1986) had established that a glutamate antagonist, kynurenic acid, was capable of blocking hypothalamic stimulus evoked responses mediated through this area. We used this glutamate antagonist to attempt to establish if the rVLM was active in the reflex responses evoked by muscular contraction (Bauer et al., 1988a).

In studies which included both the rVLM and cVLM it was found that kynurenic acid microinjected bilaterally (100 nl) could diminish the pressor response to muscular contraction. However, the response to stimulation in the posterior hypothalamus including the locomotor regions was unaffected by this antagonist (Iwamoto et al., 1988). These findings indicate that at least part of the pressor response to muscular contraction may be mediated by glutamatergic synapses in VLM.

Electrophysiological correlates of pressor responses to muscular contraction

One way in which it was established that the pressor activity in the cVLM could be related to the activity of cells rather than axons in the region was through single cell microelectrode recording (Iwamoto and Kaufman, 1987). These experiments also showed that the cells of the cVLM could be characterized according to their response to muscular contraction.

Using standard extracellular recording techniques, neuronal responses to muscular contraction were determined. Examination of waveforms demonstrated that the recordings were made from cell bodies rather than axons. We found that cells in the cVLM responded to: (1) ventral root stimulus-induced muscular contraction with a variety of discharge patterns, (2) intra-arterial injection of capsaicin (a selective small afferent fiber stimulant), and (3) probing of the somatic receptive fields.

The extent of the receptive fields was remarkable, often including all four limbs, with various inhibitory and facilitatory areas, much as had been described previously by motor neurophysiologists (Oscarsson, 1973). Nearly all of the cells tested were sensitive to capsaicin.

There were four patterns of responses observed on stimulation of the ventral roots with resulting muscular contraction: (1) inhibition of spontaneous discharge; (2) a brisk initial discharge followed by gradual adaptation; (3) a short-lived

258

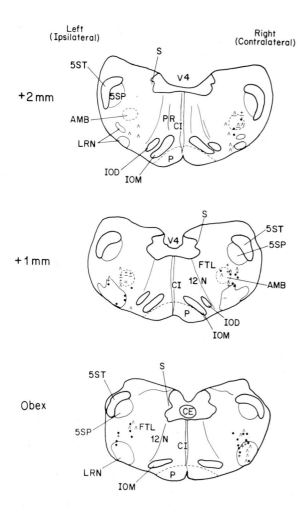

Fig. 4. Summary of cell responses to static muscular contraction according to recording site. Ipsilateral and contralateral sides are labelled with reference to hindlimb in which static muscular contraction was evoked. Each composite diagram is meant to encompass brain level indicated ± 0.5 mm. Dot = cell responding with initial brisk discharge and gradual return toward control levels (slow adaptation). Upward arrow = cell responding with an initial burst often accompanied by a burst at the cessation of contraction. Minus sign = cell inhibited during contraction. Plus sign = cell initially inhibited during contraction, later responding with slowly adapting discharge. Abbreviations: LRN = lateral reticular nucleus; P = pyramidal tract; CE = central canal; S = solitary tract; FTL = lateral tegmental field; IOM = medial accessory inferior olive; 5ST = spinal tract of trigeminal nerve; 5SP = parvocellular division, alaminar trigeminal nucleus; CI = nucleus centralis inferior; V4 = 4th ventricle; IOD = dorsal accessory inferior olive; AMB = nucleus ambiguus; PR = paramedian reticular nucleus; 12 N = hypoglossal nerve. (From Iwamoto et al., 1987.)

burst which accompanied the onset or cessation of contraction; and (4) a brief period of inhibition followed by excitation. A summary of cell locations and responses appears in Fig. 4.

Figure 5 shows a cell inhibited during muscular contraction. It seemed especially significant that some of the inhibited cells were located in the region of the nucleus ambiguous. This we have tentatively interpreted as the cellular correlate to observations which have suggested that vagal withdrawal (Mitchell and Schmidt, 1983) and perhaps inhibition of the baroreflex (Streatfeild et al., 1977) occurs during static muscular contraction. Other types of inhibition may be simply related to motor phenomena.

As mentioned, three general patterns of excitation were observed. Cells exhibiting each of these patterns may have some role to play in the reflex. Figure 6 shows an example of one cell on the ventrolateral border of the LRN, which exhibited a pattern of excitation followed by a gradual adaptation. This pattern of discharge appeared to us at the time to be perhaps the most significant of the three patterns of excitation. The same pattern had been observed in the group III afferents, primarily firing in response to the mechanical events of static muscular contraction. Thus, one could make a case for this type of cell participating in the reflex.

However, the pattern shown in Fig. 7 in which the cell demonstrates brief bursts at the onset and cessation of contraction may also be of importance. The most obvious interpretation is that these cells may give an added impetus to the onset of pressor responses accompanying muscular contraction. However, if one considers the case of actual static muscular contraction, it is possible that the asynchronous activation of motor units may provide what is interpreted by the brain as a series of onset and cessation responses.

At this time, we have no suitable explanation for the pattern of inhibition followed by sustained discharge. It is possible that the period of inhibition may reflect an interaction with the baroreflex which is later overwhelmed by the reflex elicited during muscular contraction.

Single cell recordings (Bauer et al., 1988b) were also carried out in chloralose-urethane anesthetized cats in the rVLM (2 mm rostral to the obex, 3.75 – 4.0 mm from the midline and 4.7 – 5.5 mm below the dorsal surface). The vast majority of cells monitored in the region (27/39) responded to muscular contraction by increasing their discharge (> 70%) over resting levels. The remainder of the cells (12/39) did not respond to muscular contraction or did not increase their discharge significantly.

We have continued to study the cells of the rVLM and cVLM. In an attempt to establish that the discharge of the contraction-sensitive cells is related to cardiovascular events, we have recently begun to apply spike-triggered averaging techniques in order to correlate the activity of the cells with the sympathetic outflow. The activity of these in both the rVLM and cVLM has been correlated with sympathetic nerve discharge using many of Barman and Gebber's (1985a,b) criteria for establishing this relationship. Our tentative conclusion is that these cells are likely to mediate resting sympathetic tone as well as acting to mediate pressor responses to muscular contraction.

Comparisons with other types of studies

Anatomical relationships. A great number of studies have shown that cells from the rVLM project to the spinal cord intermediolateral cell column (Amendt et al., 1979; Miura et al., 1983; Brown and Guyenet, 1984; Reis et al., 1984; Bar-

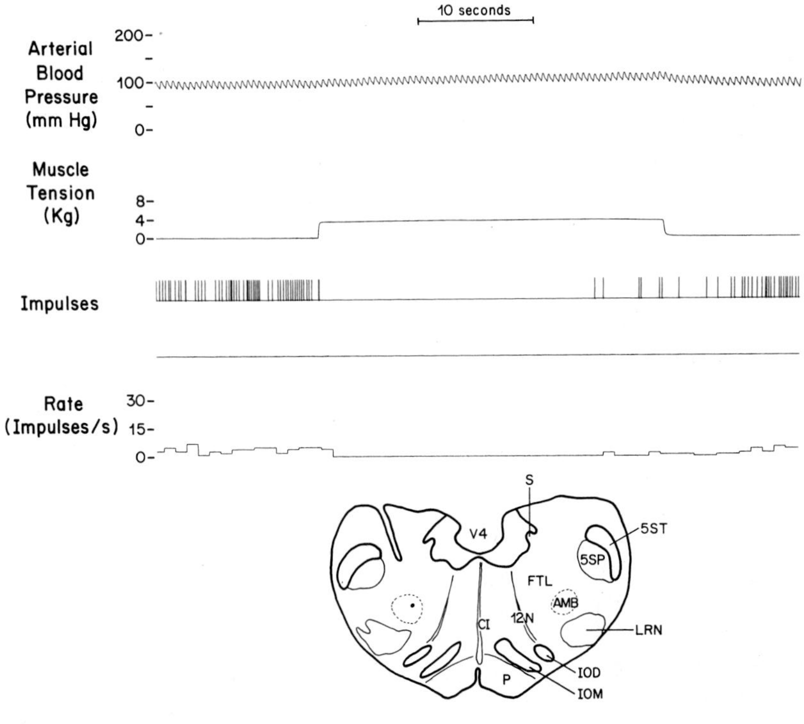

Fig. 5. Response to static contraction of cell within nucleus ambiguus region. Cell activity was recorded on side ipsilateral to the muscular contraction evoked by stimulation of L7 and S1 ventral roots at 3 times motor threshold with 0.1 msec monophasic pulses at 33.3 Hz for 30 sec. Upper traces show arterial blood pressure and muscle tension. Lower traces show output from window discriminator and a rate histogram computer. Note that a long period of inhibition results during muscular contraction. Similar pattern of inhibition occurs from the injection of capsaicin. Recording site is marked by a dot on the histology figure. For abbreviations refer to Fig. 4. (From Iwamoto and Kaufman, 1987.)

man and Gebber, 1985a; Ciriello et al., 1986b). Thus, it is easy to associate activity in these areas with pressor activity. A point which is often missed is that a small number of cells which are just dorsal to the LRN also project to the IML as demonstrated by retrograde labelling. This projection represents one way the information mediated in the cVLM could be relayed to the spinal cord. Another pathway by which the signals from the cVLM may affect sympathetic outflow is through possible connections with the rVLM which would, in turn, send the information to the spinal cord (Ciriello et al., 1986b).

Immunocytochemical studies. One controversial point in the literature deals with the question of phenylethanolamine *N*-methyltransferase (PNMT) and tyrosine hydroxylase (TH)-containing cells

and the processes they mediate in the medulla (Reis et al., 1984; Sun et al., 1988). The more rostral of the cell groups studied clearly may lie within the PNMT-containing areas. It was also of interest to us that based on the most recent studies of these areas in the cat (Marson and Loewy, 1985; Ciriello et al., 1986a; Ruggiero et al., 1986) the PNMT cells appear in the region just dorsal and ventral to the LRN. These cell groups, in part, are in the areas which we have identified as responsive to muscular contraction in the cVLM.

There are, of course, a host of additional transmitters which appear in these regions of the VLM which may play a role in this response. Glutamate (Bauer et al., 1988a), substance P (Marson and Loewy, 1985; Ciriello et al., 1986b, 1988), neurotensin, somatostatin and 5-HT (Ciriello et al., 1988) are all substances which may be involved

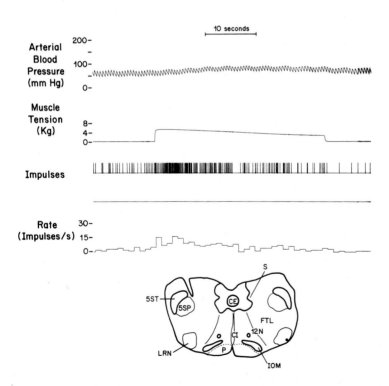

Fig. 6. Response of cVLM cell on the ventrolateral border of the LRN to static muscular contraction. Cell was recorded on side contralateral to stimulation of ventral roots at 3 times motor threshold with 0.1 msec monophasic pulses at 50 Hz for 30 sec. Format of figure is similar to that of Fig. 5. Note that there is a burst of activity at the onset of contraction followed by a gradual return toward resting levels. Receptive field of this cell included all four limbs. For abbreviations refer to Fig. 4. (From Iwamoto and Kaufman, 1987.)

in the modulation of neuronal activity mediating cardiovascular responses. The matter is further complicated by the possibility of co-localized substances (Lorenz et al., 1985).

Electrophysiological studies. Many studies support a possible role for rVLM and cVLM cells in the mediation of pressor responses to muscular contraction. Taken together with anatomical data, studies incorporating antidromic stimulation of cells projecting to the spinal cord have shown that cells of the rVLM may be involved in the mediation of resting blood pressure and the cardiovascular responses to somatic stimulation (Brown and Guyenet, 1984; Barman and Gebber, 1985a).

In examining this evidence, one must also consider other VLM areas which can be implicated in the reflex to muscular contraction. For example, the cells of the lateral tegmental field have been im-

plicated in the production of basal sympathetic nerve discharge (Barman and Gebber, 1985b). We have shown through 2-DG labelling that this area increases its activity level during the reflex (Iwamoto et al., 1984). This area will be a target of further investigation in our laboratory.

A final obvious question is what role higher centers may have in the modulation of these responses. It is clear that movement and accompanying cardiorespiratory responses may be evoked from stimulation of the posterior hypothalamus (Waldrop et al., 1988). While several studies have shown that posterior hypothalamic input impinges on these rVLM and cVLM cells, our most current evidence suggests that while the reflex evoked by muscular contraction might be diminished by the application of kynurenic acid, the response to posterior hypothalamic stimulation is not. This finding will also require further elucidation.

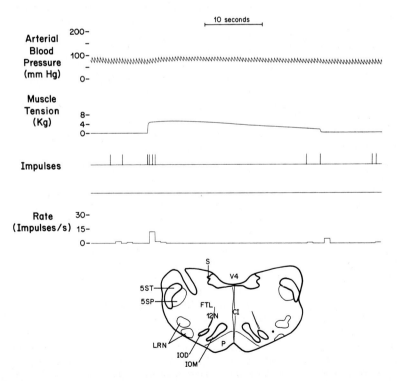

Fig. 7. Response of ventrolateral medullary cell recorded medial to LRN but 2 mm rostral to the obex on the side contralateral to the contracting limb. Format of figure is similar to that of Fig. 5. Response consists of a short burst at the onset and cessation of static contraction. For abbreviations refer to Fig. 4. (From Iwamoto and Kaufman, 1987.)

In summary, both the rVLM and cVLM exhibit characteristics which are consistent with a role for these areas in mediation of the pressor response evoked by muscular contraction. Further investigation will determine the precise role of these areas in somatosympathetic reflexes. The studies presteted have applied basic neuroscience to exercise physiology, and have further attempted to provide a complete understanding of the neural circuitry involved in circulatory adjustments to muscular activity.

Acknowledgements

This work was supported by NIH grants HL 06296, HL 37400 and HL 38726 and the American Heart Association.

References

Alexander, R.S. (1946) Tonic and reflex functions of medullary sympathetic cardiovascular centers. *J. Neurophysiol.,* 9: 205 – 217.

Amendt, K., Czachurski, J., Dembowsky, K. and Seller, H. (1979) Bulbospinal projections to the intermediolateral cell column: a neuroanatomical study. *J. Auton. Nerv. Syst.,* 1: 103 – 117.

Barman, S.M. and Gebber, G.L. (1985a) Axonal projection patterns of ventrolateral medullospinal sympathoexcitatory neurons. *J. Neurophysiol.,* 53: 1551 – 1566.

Barman, S.M. and Gebber, G.L. (1985b) Lateral tegmental field neurons of cat medulla: a potential source of basal sympathetic nerve discharge. *J. Neurophysiol.,* 54: 1498 – 1512.

Bauer, R.M., Iwamoto, G.A. and Waldrop, T.G. (1988a) Microinjections of a glutamate antagonist into the rostral ventrolateral medulla alters a somatosympathetic reflex. *FASEB J.,* 2: A1728.

Bauer, R.M., Iwamoto, G.A. and Waldrop, T.G. (1988b) Static muscular contraction alters the discharge frequency of neurons in the rostral ventrolateral medulla in cats. *Soc. Neurosci. Abstr.,* 14: 1318.

Brown, D.L. and Guyenet, P.G. (1984) Cardiovascular neurons of brain stem with projections to spinal cord. *Am. J. Physiol. (Reg. Int. Comp. Physiol.),* 247: R1009 – 1016.

Ciriello, J. and Calaresu, F.R. (1977) Lateral reticular nucleus: a site of somatic and cardiovascular regulation in the cat. *Am. J. Physiol. (Reg. Int. Comp. Physiol.)* 233: R100 – 109.

Ciriello, J., Caverson, M.M. and Park, D.H. (1986a) Immunohistochemical identification of noradrenaline and adrenaline synthesizing neurons in the cat ventrolateral medulla. *J. Comp. Neurol.,* 253: 216 – 230.

Ciriello, J., Caverson, M.M. and Polosa, C. (1986b) Function of the ventrolateral medulla in the control of the circulation. *Brain Res. Rev.,* 11: 359 – 391.

Ciriello, J., Caverson, M.M., Calaresu, F.R. and Krukoff, T.L. (1988) Neuropeptide and serotonin immunoreactive neurons in the cat ventrolateral medulla. *Brain Res.,* 440: 53 – 66.

Iwamoto, G.A. and Kaufman, M.P. (1987) Characteristics of caudal ventrolateral medullary cells responsive to muscular contraction. *J. Appl. Physiol.,* 62: 149 – 157.

Iwamoto, G.A. and Waldrop, T.G. (1986) Stimulation of caudal ventrolateral medulla by L-glutamate in the cat. *Soc. Neurosci. Abstr.,* 12: 685.

Iwamoto, G.A., Kaufman, M.P., Botterman, B.R. and Mitchell, J.H. (1982) Effects of lateral reticular nucleus lesions on the exercise pressor reflex in cats. *Circ. Res.,* 51: 400 – 403.

Iwamoto, G.A., Parnavelas, J.G., Kaufman, M.P., Botterman, B.R. and Mitchell, J.H. (1984) Activation of caudal brainstem cell groups during the exercise pressor reflex in the cat as elucidated by 2-[^{14}C] deoxyglucose. *Brain Res.,* 304: 178 – 182.

Iwamoto, G.A., Waldrop, T.G., Kaufman, M.P., Botterman, B.R., Rybicki, K.J. and Mitchell, J.H. (1985) Pressor reflex evoked by muscular contraction: contributions by neuraxis levels. *J. Appl. Physiol.,* 59: 459 – 467.

Iwamoto, G.A., Bauer, R.M. and Waldrop, T.G. (1988) Effects of medullary microinjections of a glutamate antagonist upon cardiorespiratory responses to posterior hypothalamic stimulation. *FASEB J.,* 2: A1727.

Kaufman, M.P., Longhurst, J.C., Rybicki, K.J., Wallach, J.H. and Mitchell, J.H. (1983) Effects of static muscular contraction on impulse activity of groups III and IV afferents in cats. *J. Appl. Physiol.,* 55: 105 – 112.

Lorenz, R.G., Saper, C.B., Wong, D.I., Ciaranello, R.D. and Loewy, A.D. (1985) Co-localization of substance P and phenylethanolamine-*N*-methyl-transferase-like immunoreactivity in neurons of ventrolateral medulla that project to the spinal cord: potential role in control of vasomotor tone. *Neurosci. Lett.,* 55: 255 – 260.

Marson, L. and Loewy, A.D. (1985) Topographical organization of substance P and monoamine cells in the ventral medulla of the cat. *J. Auton. Nerv. Syst.,* 14: 271 – 285.

McAllen, R.M. (1986) Location of neurones with cardiovascular and respiratory function, at the ventral surface of the cat's medulla. *Neuroscience,* 18: 43 – 49.

Mitchell, J.H. and Schmidt, R.F. (1983) Cardiovascular reflex control by afferent fibers from skeletal muscle receptors. In *Handbook of Physiology, The Cardiovascular System, Peripheral Circulation and Organ Blood Flow, Sect. 2, Vol. III,* Am. Physiol. Soc., Bethesda, MD, pp. 623 – 650.

Miura, M., Onai, T. and Takayama, K. (1983) Projections of upper structure to the spinal cardioacceleratory center in cats: an HRP study using a new microinjection method. *J. Auton. Nerv. Syst.,* 7: 119–139.

Oscarsson, O. (1973) Functional organization of spinocerebellar paths. In: A. Iggo (Ed.), *Handbook of Sensory Physiology, Somatosensory System, Vol. II,* Springer-Verlag, Berlin, pp. 381–488.

Reis, D.J., Granata, A.R., Joh, T.H., Ross, C.A., Ruggiero, D.A. and Park, D.H. (1984) Brainstem catecholamine mechanisms in tonic and reflex control of blood pressure. *Hypertension,* 6, Suppl. II: II7–15.

Ruggiero, D.A., Gatti, P., Gillis, R.A., Norman, W.P., Anwar, M. and Reis, D.J. (1986) Adrenaline synthesizing neurons in the medulla of the cat. *J. Comp. Neurol.,* 252: 532–542.

Streatfeild, K.A., Davison, N.S. and McCloskey, D.I. (1977) Muscular reflex and baroreflex influences on heart rate during isometric contractions. *Cardiovasc. Res.,* 11: 87–93.

Sun, M-K. and Guyenet, P.G. (1986) Hypothalamic glutamatergic input to medullary sympathoexcitatory neurons in rats. *Am. J. Physiol. (Reg. Int. Comp. Physiol.),* 251: R798–810.

Sun, M-K., Young, B.S., Hackett, J.T. and Guyenet, P.G. (1988) Rostral ventrolateral medullary neurons with intrinsic pacemaker properties are not catecholaminergic. *Brain Res.,* 451: 345–349.

Waldrop, T.G., Bauer, R.M. and Iwamoto, G.A. (1988) Microinjection of GABA antagonists into the posterior hypothalamus elicits locomotor activity and a cardiorespiratory activation. *Brain Res.,* 444: 84–94.

J. Ciriello, M.M. Caverson and E. Polosa (Eds.)
Progress in Brain Research, Vol. 81
© 1989 Elsevier Science Publishers B.V. (Biomedical Division)

CHAPTER 21

Cardiovascular control by the rostral ventrolateral medulla in the conscious dog

Kenneth J. Dormer and Toby G. Bedford

Department of Physiology and Biophysics, University of Oklahoma Health Sciences Center, P.O. Box 26901, Oklahoma City, OK 73190, U.S.A.

Introduction

Concentrated efforts have been made in the last few years to understand the anatomical and physiological constructs of a group of adrenaline-containing cells in the rostral ventrolateral medulla. This area, since its earliest discovery over 100 years ago, has recently again been suggested to be a major component of the "vasomotor center" of the brainstem (Loewy et al., 1981; Dampney et al., 1985; Ciriello et al., 1986; Ruggiero et al., 1986; Calaresu, 1988; Reis et al., 1988). Indeed, bilateral ablation of this area is reportedly equivalent to spinal cord transection and autonomic collapse. Both the generation of tonic vasomotor tone through the control of sympathetic preganglionic activity and its modulation by cardiovascular reflexes emanating from the arterial baroreceptors have shown the area to be an integrative site with direct projections to sympathetic preganglionic neurons. It has also been shown that this area affects plasma levels of catecholamines and vasopressin which also influence the maintenance of arterial pressure and heart rate (Ross et al., 1984).

Evolving anatomical terminology and commingling of cardiovascular cells in this region with respiratory control neurons has made some of the functional identification of this area difficult. First, it had been established that only a subpopulation of the noradrenergic A1 group described by Hökfelt had demonstrated this vasomotor function and these adrenaline-containing cells correspond to his adrenergic C1 group. The C1 cell group is also a portion of the nucleus paragigantocellularis lateralis which others have described as having vasomotor function (Sun and Guyenet, 1986). Earlier application of drugs to the ventral surface of the brainstem caused cardiorespiratory changes, suggesting that commingling of cardiovascular and respiratory cells existed with different function (Feldberg, 1976). Such commingling has been recently confirmed and associations made between the ventral medullary surface and the deeper vasomotor neurons (Gatti et al., 1986). This "glycine-sensitive area" of Feldberg (1976) was primarily located over the intermediate or "S" chemosensitive zone of the ventral medulla that affected respiration (Schlaefke and See, 1980; Feldman and Ellenberger, 1988). In addition, this same group of tonic vasomotor neurons in the rostral ventrolateral medulla has been referred to as the "VLM", "RVLM" and "RVMM" and was recently given a specific identity by two investigative groups: the nucleus reticularis rostroventrolateralis or "nRVL" (Ross et al., 1984) and the nucleus subretrofacialis (McAllen, 1986). For the purposes of uniformity in this chapter, RVLM will be used to designate the adrenergic cell group affecting cardiovascular control and in particular, the lateral portion of this group.

Because of the integrative activities in the RVLM, any confirmation of the physiological role of this area will necessarily be carried out in the unanesthetized animal models. We still do not know if decreased tonic vasomotor activity seen in anesthetized animal models will reflect in lowered arterial pressure in the conscious state. The present experiments, therefore, were conducted on the chronically instrumented dog to provide information on the role of RVLM in generating vasomotor tone in the absence of anesthetics and in the presence of normal hormonal, blood volume and reflex regulatory mechanisms which also influence the maintenance of arterial pressure. Additional information on the functional specificity of neurons within RVLM can also be obtained by measuring cardiac output and regional blood flows. Finally, respiratory changes can be observed in the spontaneously breathing, relaxed animal.

It was first necessary to document the presence of homologous cells in the canine containing the enzyme for adrenaline synthesis, phenyl-ethanolamine *N*-methyltransferase (PNMT) (Dormer et al., 1988b). Next, the location of the pressor area was functionally mapped using ventral surface application (Dormer et al., 1988a) and then microinjection of L-glutamate or its analog kainic acid. Finally, unilateral lesions were placed in RVLM of instrumented dogs that had been previously observed during everyday cardiovascular stressors such as exercise and postural change. Following recovery from lesions the tests were repeated and the results indicate that partial lesion of RVLM can lower resting arterial pressure without affecting motor or apparent cognitive performance. Bilateral lesions, on the other hand, were incompatible with life due to hypotension and apnea.

Methods

Microinjection of L-glutamic acid in RVLM of anesthetized dogs

Adult mongrel dogs of either sex (16.5 – 29.0 kg) were anesthetized with aqueous α-chloralose (110 mg/kg, i.v.) and intubated with an endotracheal tube. The omocervical or femoral artery was cannulated for measurement of arterial pressure and the heart rate was determined by a biotachometer (Gould Biotach) sensing the arterial pressure waveform. Respiration was spontaneous and monitored by induction plethysmography (Respitrace, Inc.). An induction coil was placed around the chest at the 4th rib for qualitative measurements of chest excursions (relative tidal volume). Respiratory rate was obtained from the volume signal and all variables were continuously recorded on a chart recorder (Gould 2800).

A craniotomy was performed and the dorsal surface of the medulla exposed by removal of a portion of the supraoccipital bone above the foramen magnum. Using a high speed drill with irrigation the bone was removed 5 – 6 mm lateral to midline, the dura reflected and the dorsal medulla visualized. The obex, partially covered by the vermis of the cerebellum, was used as the reference midline and the dog was placed in a stereotaxic apparatus (Kopf Instruments) to establish horizontal zero. Standard stereotaxic coordinates were not used but rather an angular approach to the RVLM was made with an obex reference. When a 26-gauge microsyringe was inserted at 55 degrees from horizontal zero at 4 mm lateral and 1 – 3 mm rostral to obex, the RVLM is reached at 9 – 10 mm depth in most mongrel dogs (excluding those with excessively long or short snouts). A 1 μl syringe (Hamilton) was placed on a stereotaxic microinjection unit (Kopf Model 5000) for microinjection of drugs. L-glutamic acid (monosodium, pH = 7.3, 100 or 200 mM) was injected in volumes of 50 or 100 nl as the cannula approached the RVLM. A response, if present, usually occurred within 20 sec of injection and waiting 5 – 10 min allowed sufficient recovery for repeat injections. The rostral caudal area 4 mm lateral to obex was explored and the maximal pressor site marked for subsequent histological verification by injecting 50 nl of 2% Pontamine Blue dye through the same microsyringe. Kainic acid (pH = 7.4, 100 mM) was occasionally injected in 50 nl volumes for comparison.

The brainstem was removed after each dog was

euthanized in the anesthetized state by 10 ml injection of euthanizing solution (T61, National Labs). Following 10 days in 10 buffered formalin the brainstem was sectioned in 55 μm frozen slices on a sliding microtome. Sections were stained with thionin to distinguish cell bodies and the injection site identified, then drawn by camera lucida or photographed.

Kainic acid lesions in the RVLM of the chronically instrumented dog

Conditioned, heart worm-free dogs (n = 6) of either sex and weighing 14 – 19 kg were first conditioned to the laboratory by multiple visits over 5 – 10 days. During this time, adaptation began to occur to a motorized treadmill, tilting laboratory table and face mask. Vitamin supplementation and daily oral antibiotics (trimethoprim, 80 mg, p.o.) were begun prior to surgery. Dogs were then preanesthetized with Na-thiamylal (30 mg/kg, i.v.) and using sterile technique under halothane anesthesia (1 – 1.5% in O_2) a left thoracotomy was performed. A pulse-transit time, ultrasonic blood flowmeter (Transonic Systems, Inc.) was implanted on the ascending aorta at the base of the heart for volumetric measurement of aortic flow and cardiac output. A 4 mm diameter semiconductor strain gauge, pressure transducer (Konigsberg Instruments) was implanted into the wall of the descending aorta for measurement of aortic pressure. All wires were tunneled subcutaneously to percutaneous skin connectors and the chest closed.

The dogs were attended to daily for a 14-day recovery period during which laboratory adaptation continued and they became accustomed to resting quietly in the identical environment with the same handler at approximately the same time of day. They also learned to breathe through a face mask connected to a regulator capable of switching between room air or 10% O_2 and 90% N_2. They were conditioned to voluntarily complete a submaximal exercise tolerance test (ETT) on a motorized treadmill. In addition, they became accustomed to being passively tilted on a laboratory table with supports to sustain a 75 degree head-up tilt for 1 – 3 min without struggling or displaying observable restlessness. Every effort was made to eliminate anxiety or restlessness in the dog so that recording cardiorespiratory variables in the conscious state was not confounded by psychological status.

Dogs were recorded from for 10 – 14 days following recovery. A minimum of three ETTs were performed between days off. Multiple daily tilt-training sessions (4 – 18) were performed before recording 3 – 6 responses to 75 degree tilt over 2 – 3 days. Resting data were recorded on 8 – 15 occasions, almost on a daily basis and prior to each exercise recording session. Resting response to 6 min of breathing the above hypoxic gas mixture was recorded on 2 – 4 separate days of this 2-week recording period, both preceded and followed by breathing of room air through the same demand regulator. The dogs were comfortable, relaxed and often fell asleep during this testing. All recordings of aortic pressure (AP), heart rate (HR), cardiac output (CO), respiratory rate (RR) and relative tidal volume were made on the same chart recorder.

Next the dogs were anesthetized with α-chloralose (110 mg/kg, i.m.), intubated and a sterile craniotomy was performed using the techniques described for acute microinjection of L-glutamate. Aortic pressure, HR and respirations were monitored during this lesion surgery. The RVLM was identified by the injection of sterile 100 mM L-glutamate using the obex as a reference coordinate as described above. Then kainic acid was injected over 3 – 5 min in volumes of 50 nl per site over 1 – 2 mm distance in the horizontal plane. Medication for pain was again administered postoperatively (Talwin 1 – 5 mg/lb, i.m.) and the dogs allowed to recover for 5 – 10 days.

Following recovery the above experiments were repeated at approximately the same time of day and at the same intervals and numbers of repetitions. Data for prelesion tests were averaged together for each dog and likewise for postlesion data. Each dog served as its own control but in addition one sham lesion control was performed with the same conditions except for the microsyringe cannula being inserted only through 2 – 3 mm of brainstem during the sterile lesion procedure. Prelesioned and postlesion data were compared with Student's paired t-test and the criterion of significance set at $P < 0.05$.

Results

Effects of L-glutamate in RVLM of anesthetized dogs

Earlier studies on anesthetized beagles had established that the region on the ventral surface of the brainstem corresponding to the intermediate or "S" chemosensitive zone and portions of the rostral "M" region reflected the rostral medullary position of the vasomotor neurons. When cotton pledgets containing 40 mM kainic acid were placed on the ventral surface or radiofrequency lesions were placed bilaterally, then mean arterial pressure decreased and the pressor response to electrical stimulation of the rostral fastigial nucleus was reduced or ablated (Dormer et al., 1988a). Thus, when glutamate was injected from the dorsal surface to this same rostral location it was found that 4.0 ± 0.3 mm lateral to midline produced the optimal pressor response. Further anatomical identification was a necessary second step in the development of the canine model for RVLM studies and this was supported by immunocytochemistry in the region for adrenaline-containing neurons (Dormer et al., 1988). Now physiological responses can be compared with the PNMT-containing cell locations. The dorsal approach to RVLM was necessary in the dog to avoid extensive neck surgery and the angular approach allows for the avoidance of penetrating vital nuclei that may confound the interpretation of the results.

The distribution of PNMT-containing cells in the canine RVLM is more diffuse than in other species, nevertheless, the mechanical effect alone of the cannula entering the RVLM was often sufficient indication of the vasomotor region. The pressor effect from entering the RVLM is shown in Fig. 1 where driving of the microsyringe barrel had no effect until the depth of 9 mm which was at the rostral extent of the inferior olive, near retrofacial nucleus. It is probable that the glutamate solution was continually diffusing from the end of the 26-gauge barrel, perhaps activating cell bodies without injection taking place. Nevertheless, with the injection of glutamate there followed increased mean arterial pressure (MAP) and coronary blood flow velocity with decrease in HR. Larger pressor responses were accompanied by greater bradycardia. Changes in respiration were also coincident with the glutamate response lasting about 1 min, namely; increased respiratory rate and decreased depth. It was not determined if the minute ventilation actually increased because only relative changes were measured by plethysmography. When kainic acid was injected through the same cannula system the excitatory phase of the response was considerably greater than that of glutamate and lasted for 30 – 40 min, whereupon the arterial pressure and respiratory rate and depth began to decrease. Heart rate also decreased and this exacerbated the hypotensive state. Positive pressure ventilation was usually necessary to support the dog through the kainate depressor phase (lesion process) but often a spontaneous, cluster breathing pattern developed that could provide sufficient ventilation for the unilateral kainic acid lesion to survive. This pattern demonstrated a shortened inspiratory time compared to the prelesion state.

The combined results from glutamate injection in 10 dogs is shown in Fig. 3 revealing significant cardiorespiratory changes in response to 114 nl of 100 mM L-glutamate. The HR decreased an average of 15 beats/min (14% of the control values). Mean arterial pressure increased 20 mmHg or an average of 20% from the control. The range of pressor responses to 100 ± 50 nl injections was between 5 and 40 mmHg. Respiratory rate increased an average of 3 breaths/min representing 25% above the average preinjection rate and this was accompanied by a decrease of 21% in the relative tidal volume. The RVLM sites that produced these changes ranged from 5 to 7 mm rostral to obex in this series of mongrel dogs. A representative 55 μm section and drawing of an RVLM pressor site is shown in Fig. 4. The greatest responses were obtained 5 – 7 mm rostral to obex and 4 – 4.5 mm

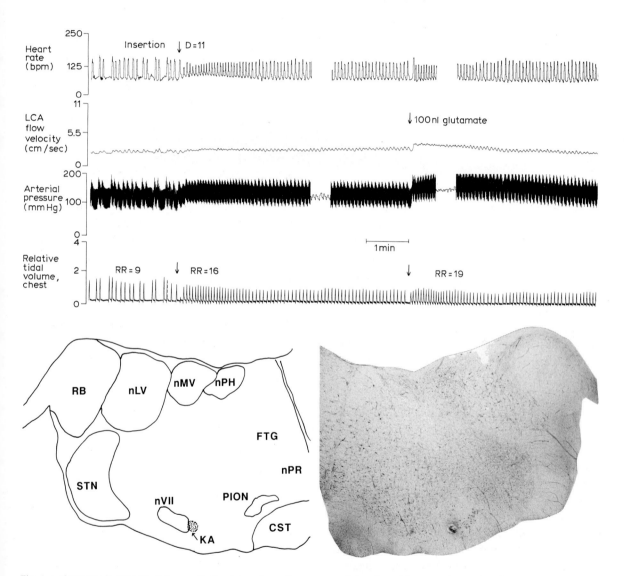

Fig. 1. L-glutamate in RVLM of the anesthetized dog. A continuous record showing a 26-gauge microsyringe first entering the RVLM at a target depth of 11 mm (first arrow) and then injecting 100 nl of 20 mM L-glutamate (second arrow). Location was 6.1 mm rostral to obex and 4 mm right of midline as shown in the histological section. This section represents the most rostral area from which the pressor response could be obtained by glutamate or kainate. Abbreviations: CST = corticospinal tract; FTG = gigantocellular tegmental field; LCA = left circumflex coronary artery; nLV = lateral vestibular nucleus; nMV = medial vestibular nucleus; nPH = nucleus praepositus hypoglossi; nRP = nucleus raphe pontis; nVII = facial nucleus; PION = principal lamellae of inferior olive; RB = restiform body; RR = respiratory rate; STN = spinal trigeminal nucleus; X = vagus nerve.

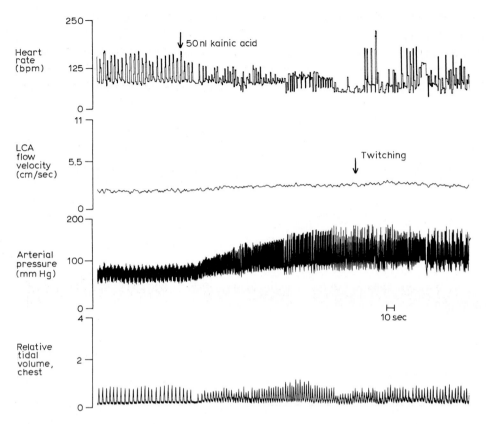

Fig. 2. Kainic acid in RVLM of the anesthetized dog. When 50 nl of 100 mM kainate in phosphate buffered saline was injected (first arrow) into the same region of the dog in Fig. 1 a stronger response was elicited. Bradycardia always accompanied the pressor response. Twitching of facial vibrissae began (second arrow) several minutes following injection indicating activation of facial nerve.

from midline at the rostral pole of the inferior olive, ventromedial to the retrofacial nucleus. Injections caudal to this area, approximately 2 – 4 mm rostral to obex, were depressor in nature with decreased MAP and HR. In 9 of 10 dogs the resting HR was lower following several cannula penetrations in this unilateral series, suggesting that the nucleus ambiguus was not affected to reduce vagal motor tone and increase resting HR. Sufficient information was gained from these acute series of dogs to enable location of the RVLM usually in 1 or 2 passes of the barrel of a microcannula into the medulla of a mongrel dog.

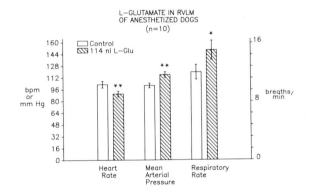

Fig. 3. Averaged results from glutamate in anesthetized dogs. An average injection of 114 nl in RVLM at typical levels of 5 – 7 mm rostral to obex produced these changes. Mean ± S.E.M. where ** $p < 0.01$ and * $p < 0.05$.

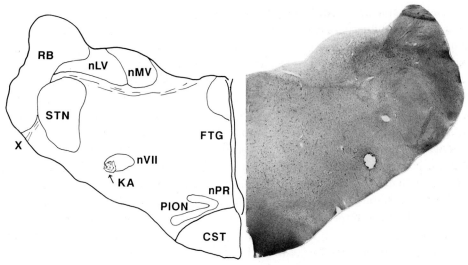

Fig. 4. Representative brainstem section from kainic acid lesion in instrumented dog. This section represents the more rostral (6.5 mm rostral to obex) of two kainic acid injection sites, 1 mm apart. Fifty nanoliters was injected at each site and all dogs received 100 nl total. Abbreviations: (see Fig. 1).

Unilateral kainic acid lesions of the RVLM in the instrumented dog

During the actual lesion production and the first few days of recovery there was a noticeable difference in respiratory pattern. Unfortunately, we have only begun to monitor this pattern recently. The cluster breathing that was obvious at first, where triplets or doublets of inspirations occurred between periods of apnea, progressively disappeared and respirations became more regular with more normal inspiratory times. A substantial decrease in arterial pressure was not always evident during the lesion procedure. There, in fact, appeared to be a partial recovery during the 1–3 h of monitoring after the lesion placement. No motor deficits appeared in any of the dogs and they were able to perform treadmill exercise following 3–4 days of recovery. After 6 or 9 days the testing resumed and postlesion data were obtained. Behaviorally, the dogs seemed more calm and less excitable, according to untrained observers. Yet, they were alert and responsive to commands. Dogs were tested for up to 3 weeks following recovery and as Table I indicates, there

was a significant decrease in the resting MAP accompanied by a significant increase in resting HR. These are the averaged results for each dog's individual averages, serving as its own control, recorded during the prelesion and postlesion

TABLE I

Combined results from kainic acid lesions in six dogs are shown in comparison with one sham lesion dog. The sham lesion only penetrated the medulla but all other testing was comparable to the lesion group

	RVLM kainic acid lesion resting conscious dogs ($n = 6$; $\bar{x} \pm$ S.E.)		
	Heart rate (bpm)	Mean arterial pressure (mmHg)	Cardiac output (l/min)
Prelesion	81 ± 5	105 ± 5	2.0 ± 0.4
Postlesion	94 ± 7	88 ± 5	2.2 ± 0.5
	($p < 0.05$)	($p < 0.05$)	($p < 0.05$)
	Sham lesion control ($n = 1$)		
Prelesion	81 ± 4	98 ± 4	1.3 ± 0.05
Postlesion	73 ± 5	104 ± 7	1.4 ± 0.2

periods. A sham lesion dog did not show comparable results, having been subjected to thoracotomy, craniotomy and similar laboratory exposure and adaptation. A trend was present for cardiac output (CO) to be increased as well, probably as a result of the increased HR.

Three dogs had received bilateral injections, 50 – 100 nl, of 100 mM kainic acid into the RVLM region using the same sterile techniques described above. Either they could not be weaned from the ensuing apnea that began about 40 min after injection or after weaning from the respirator and stimulating respiration by administration of respiratory stimulants (e.g. doxapram, 2.5 – 5.0 mg/lb) they could not maintain adequate ventila-

tion to sustain life. Hypotensive crisis was not the apparent cause of death in these animals.

All lesions were drawn and photographed from 55 μm sections of the brainstems and stained with thionin for cell differentiation. The Pontamine Blue dye was differentiated and along with the scarred cannula track was used to identify the site of lesion. As in the acute series, the lesion sites were confined to the rostral extent of the inferior olive either located between the lateral and medial portions of the lateral reticular nucleus or ventromedial to the caudal pole of the retrofacial nucleus. These sites were 5 – 7 mm rostral to obex allowing for some variability in the sizes of the dogs' heads.

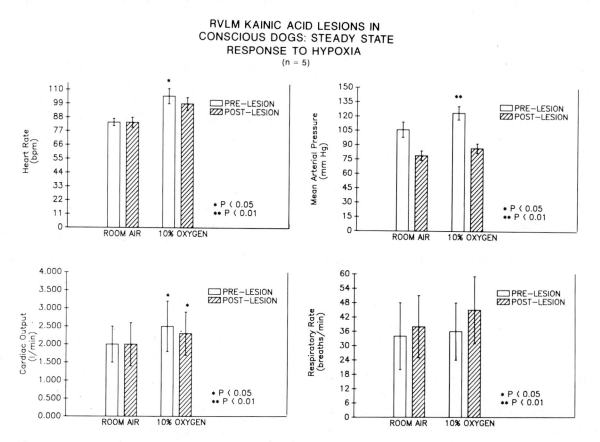

Fig. 5. Conscious dog response to hypoxia before and after RVLM lesion. The mean ± S.E.M. steady state responses to breathing room air followed by 6 min of 10% O_2 is shown for five dogs. Minute volume (not shown) was substantially increased though respiratory rate was not.

The dogs were again randomly subjected to the stressors of cerebral hypoxia, tilt table postural changes and treadmill exercise again and the results averaged among dogs are shown in the subsequent figures. The response to breathing a hypoxic gas mixture in the relaxed state while lying down is shown in Fig. 5. Prior to receiving unilateral RVLM lesions breathing the 10% O_2, 90% N_2 gas mixture caused significant increases in HR, MAP and CO but not respiratory rate. Six minutes was selected for this protocol because beyond this limit respiratory rate began to fall and pressure rise precipitously. Imperceptively, the dogs would simply cease to breathe, so at 6 min the mixture was switched to room air without the dog's knowledge and then the test repeated after a recovery time. Unfortunately, relative tidal volume was not recorded in all dogs but it increased around 100%. Hence the slight increase in rate of respiration does not reflect the tremendous change in minute ventilation that undoubtedly occurred in response to the hypoxic challenge. Following recovery from the lesion placement there remained a noticeable but non-significant increase in HR, MAP and CO in response to the 6 min hypoxia.

A different type of stressor presented to the awake dogs before and following the kainic acid lesions involved the passive change in posture where the investigator tilted the awake, relaxed and conditioned dog to a 75 degree head-up tilt on a tilting table. This maneuver elicits cerebello-vestibular reflexes as well as peripheral baroreflexes to re-establish and maintain arterial pressure at normal set points. We have previously shown the conscious dog to be a reasonable model for this type of stressor even though head-up tilt in the dog is less frequently elicited than in the human. This is a difficult stressor to demonstrate onset and effectiveness of sympathetic cardiovascular responses because alerting and anxiety associated with the tilt must be minimized. Repetition training of the tilt over several weeks was used to habituate the dogs to the procedure such that the rapid onset changes observed were not associated with fear or anxiety responses or adrenomedullary activation but

rather with the reflex adjustments that normally occur during everyday postural adjustments. The usual response during a 1 to 5-min tilt is a significant increase in arterial pressure (and peripheral resistance), a decrease in CO and no change in HR (Bedford and Dormer, 1988). Comparing the prelesion to postlesion responses at 1 and 3 min into sustained head-up tilt we see in Fig. 6 that the HR response is not changed in the dogs but MAP cannot be sustained during the tilt and drops slightly below the resting levels. Change in cardiac output was unaffected by unilateral lesion in these dogs.

Submaximal treadmill exercise was the most rigorous of the stressors presented to the dogs on at least three occasions before and following recovery from lesion surgery. The averaged responses to MAP and CO are shown in Fig. 7. No motor deficits were observed in the dogs and they exercised willingly while lightly tethered (to protect instrumentation wires) on the treadmill. Arterial pressure but not HR was significantly different before and during exercise as a result of unilateral lesions. Decrease in the magnitude of arterial pressure was evident but also the early rise in

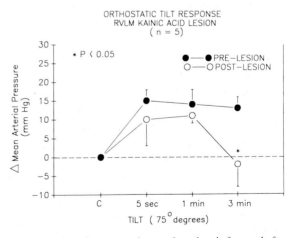

Fig. 6. Head-up tilt response in conscious dogs before and after RVLM lesion. No significant changes were observed in heart rate or cardiac output during this 1–3 min 75-degree tilt, however, elevated arterial pressure was not maintained after recovery to lesion. The averaged change from MAP immediately prior to tilting is shown ± S.E.M.

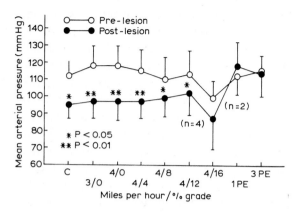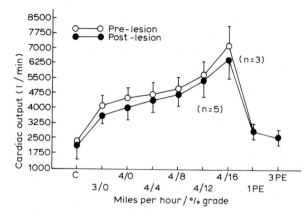

Fig. 7. Response to submaximal exercise before and after RVLM lesion. Dogs voluntarily exercised up to 4 miles/h at 16% grade in 3-min intervals (for each stage of exercise). Averaged results for five dogs ± S.E.M. are shown for MAP and CO. No changes were observed in HR or CO, though both were elevated. MAP was lower than in the prelesion state except during the 1 and 3 min recovery periods (resting).

pressure during the first 6 min of exercise was attenuated. No significant change occurred in CO but it was consistently higher at rest and all levels of exercise, supporting the evidence of decreased afterload with no change in HR. Subjective observations by the technicians indicated that the dogs looked less energetic at the higher workloads and had to increase their effort to complete the submaximal ETT. Some were unable to complete the test and is a reason for fewer data points at the highest workload.

Conclusions

These results represent the first study showing the effects of discrete partial RVLM lesions in a conscious animal. The catecholaminergic anatomical substrate for RVLM in this region is comparable to what has been described in other species (Barnes et al., 1988; Dormer et al., 1988). The concept of a group of tonically active neurons, the "tonic vasomotor center" of Kumada et al. (1979), dedicated to the production of vasomotor tone is supported by the decreased MAP observed during rest and active states. This confirms the predictions regarding RVLM from many studies using anesthetized models (Reis et al., 1984). One unique observation in the dog, however, is that HR is not decreased along with MAP but rather is increased.

Since the dog displays vagomotor tone closer to that of the human than the rat or cat, this probably represents normal baroreceptor reflex compensation for the lower arterial pressure and demonstrates the intact parasympathetic cardiomotor pathway. Not supported is the concept that the reticular formation of the lower brainstem is a common system as a whole and that the cardiovascular and respiratory systems exert an influence on nearly all neurons (Langhorst et al., 1983). On the other hand, our results cannot defend the RVLM as the sole vasomotor center since bilateral RVLM lesions extending 2 mm in the rostrocaudal plane only reduced arterial pressure to 60 – 70 mmHg and the ultimate cause of death was apnea. There was also a certain amount of recovery to the unilateral kainate lesion hypotension in the conscious dogs suggesting plasticity in the remaining RVLM or support from other systems such as increased blood volume. Others have suggested that anesthetic complications may have contributed to the lethal hypotension observed in the rat (Cochrane et al., 1988) and that the RVLM is not the only area of the central nervous system capable of maintaining vasomotor tone.

The fact that every glutamate RVLM activation in the acute dogs and every kainate lesion in the chronic dogs affected respiratory as well as cardiovascular status is not surprising but emphasizes the commingling of cells in this vital area (Loeschcke et al., 1970; Trouth et al., 1973; Feldman, 1986). It also supports the physiological observations in humans and animals that during exercise, for example, there is a functional coordination between cardiovascular and respiratory changes (Feldman, 1988). Heart beat and respiration coordination (Weckenmann et al., 1988) and entrainment of ventilation frequency to exercise rhythm in humans (Paterson et al., 1986), as well as basic studies on animals (Eldridge et al., 1985; Millhorn and Eldridge, 1986) support the concept of cardiorespiratory control in a coordinated manner. Cox and Brody (1988) suggested that the mechanics of respiration actually affected the results of RVLM lesions in the rat. This observation is consonant with the data of McAllen (1987) which indicate that central respiratory neurons may modulate the activity of subretrofacial (RVLM) neurons. The RVLM may be the site where this coordination takes place. Kainic acid lesions in this area cannot affect vasomotor tone alone because of the commingling of cells from nucleus ambiguus, Botzinger complex of the ventral respiratory group and the RVLM (Feldman and Ellenberger, 1988).

The impaired hypoxic response in conscious dogs, analogous to cerebral ischemia which was shown by Guyton (1948) to produce a pressor response, indicates that the lesion impaired the resulting sympathoexcitation. Although the mechanism of the response to hypoxia may not be the same as the chemoreceptor reflex attributable to this region and the ventral surface of the brainstem, the association of respiratory and cardiovascular control is made. When Kumada et al. (1979) found that the vasomotor component of the cerebral ischemic response was abolished by lesions in the dorsal outflow track from RVLM, this confirmed the early work of Amendt et al. (1978) that neurons within this chemosensitive area projected to the intermediolateral cell column. Central chemosensitivity apparently is relegated to the ventral surface of the rostral medulla and in particular the intermediate zone (Schlaefke, 1981) with some

overlap into the rostral zone (Nattie et al., 1988). Such areas directly underlie the RVLM (portions of nucleus paragigantocellularis lateralis). Therefore, if removal of this chemosensitive zone also ablates the vasomotor component to decreases in pH, then our observations of less superficial kainic acid lesions affecting the response to hypoxia are consistent with the cardiorespiratory role of this vital area.

Finally, higher brainstem influences on the RVLM would also be expected if it were to function as a true vasomotor center. The reduced MAP during exercise along with the consistent trend of increased CO and HR suggests that if there is a central command for the neural control of arterial pressure during exercise as some have suggested (Eldridge et al., 1985), it was prevented from increasing pressure to prelesion levels in the exercising dogs. Others have described topographical arrangement of RVLM cells affecting skin and muscle vasoconstriction, projections or relays from hypothalamic, cardiopulmonary and baroreceptor regions to the RVLM and impaired pressor responses from activation of fastigial nucleus (Ciriello et al., 1985; Porter and Brody, 1985; Dampney and McAllen, 1988; Dormer et al., 1988). Since all of these mechanisms presumably would be called into play during the highly integrative activity of exercise, it would be predicted that some impairment in exercise performance should be evident in dogs with RVLM lesions even to the extent of not being as "energetic" in finishing the submaximal workload.

In summary, the combined observations of rest and activity in conscious dogs that have received partial lesions of neurons in RVLM show that the lower arterial pressure and impaired responses to specific stressors is consistent with what has been shown in anesthetized animal models.

Acknowledgements

We gratefully recognize the expert technical help of Mr. Brian A. Barkan and Ms. Susan R. Ashlock, without whose help these studies would have been extremely difficult. This work was supported in part by the Presbyterian Health Foundation of Oklahoma City.

References

Amendt, K., Czachurski, J., Dembowsky, K. and Seller, H. (1978) Neurones within the "chemosensitive area" on the ventral surface of the brainstem which project to the intermediolateral column. *Pflügers Arch.*, 375: 289 – 292.

Barnes, K.L., Chernicky, C.L., Block, C.H. and Ferrario, C.M. (1988) Distribution of catecholaminergic neuronal systems in the dog. *J. Comp. Neurol.*, 274: 127 – 141.

Bedford, T.G. and Dormer, K.J. (1988) Arterial hemodynamics during head up tilt in conscious dogs. *J. Appl. Physiol.*, 65: 1556 – 1562.

Calaresu, F.R. (1988) Medullary basal sympathetic tone. *Ann. Rev. Physiol.*, 50: 511 – 524.

Ciriello, J., Caverson, M.M. and Calaresu, F.R. (1985) Lateral hypothalamic and peripheral cardiovascular afferent inputs to ventrolateral medullary neurons. *Brain Res.*, 347: 173 – 176.

Ciriello, J., Caverson, M.M. and Polosa, C. (1986) Function of the ventrolateral medulla in the control of the circulation. *Brain Res. Rev.*, 11: 359 – 391.

Cochrane, K.L., Buchholz, R.A., Hubbard, J.W., Keeton, T.K. and Nathan, M.A. (1988) Hypotensive effects of lesions of the rostral ventrolateral medulla in rats are anesthetic-dependent. *J. Auton. Nerv. Syst.*, 22: 181 – 187.

Cox, B.F. and Brody, M.J. (1988) Tidal volume affects the response to inactivation of the rostral ventrolateral medulla. *Hypertension*, 11 Suppl. I: I-186 – I-189.

Dampney, R.A.L. and McAllen, R.M. (1988) Differential control of sympathetic fibres supplying hindlimb skin and muscle by subretrofacial neurones in the cat. *J. Physiol.*, 395: 41 – 56.

Dampney, R.A.L., Kumada, M. and Reis, D.J. (1979) Central neural mechanisms of the cerebral ischemic response: characterization, effect of brainstem and cranial nerve transections, and simulation by electrical stimulation of restricted regions of medulla oblongata in rabbit. *Circ. Res.*, 44: 48 – 62.

Dampney, R.A.L., Goodchild, A.K. and Tan, E. (1985) Vasopressor neurons in the rostral ventrolateral medulla of the rabbit. *J. Auton. Nerv. Syst.*, 14: 239 – 254.

Dormer, K.J., Ruggiero, D.A., Anwar, M. and Ashlock, S.R. (1986) Functional mapping of the canine rostral ventrolateral medulla (RVL) with L-glutamate and phenylethanolamine *N*-methyltransferase (PNMT) immunohistochemistry. *Soc. Neurosci. Abst.*, 14: 191.

Dormer, K.J., Person, R.J., Andrezik, J.A., Foreman, R.D. and Braggio, J.A. (1988) Rostral ventrolateral medullary lesions abolish the fastigial cardiovascular response in beagles.

Am. J. Physiol., 256: H1200 – H1208, 1989.

Eldridge, F.L., Millhorn, D.E., Kiley, J.P. and Waldrop, T.G. (1985) Stimulation by central command of locomotion, respiration and circulation during exercise. *Respir. Physiol.*, 59: 313 – 339.

Feldberg, W. (1976) The ventral surface of the brain stem: a scarcely explored region of pharmacological sensitivity. *Neuroscience*, 1: 427 – 441.

Feldman, J.L. (1986) Neurophysiology of breathing in mammals. In *Handbook of Physiology, The Nervous System, Intrinsic Regulatory System of the Brain, Vol. IV, Sect. 1*, Am. Physiol. Soc., Bethesda, MD, pp. 463 – 524.

Feldman, J.L. and Ellenberger, H.H. (1988) Central coordination of respiratory and cardiovascular control in mammals. *Ann. Rev. Physiol.*, 50: 593 – 606.

Gatti, P.J., Norman, W.P., DaSilva, A.M.T. and Gillis, R.A. (1986) Cardiorespiratory effects produced by microinjecting L-glutamic acid into medullary nuclei associated with the ventral surface of the feline medulla. *Brain Res.*, 381: 281 – 228.

Granata, A.R., Ruggiero, D.A., Park, D.H., Joh, T.H. and Reis, D.J. (1983) Lesions of epinephrine neurons in the rostral ventrolateral medulla abolish vasopressor components of baroreflex and cardiopulmonary reflex. *Hypertension*, 5 (Suppl. V): V80 – V84.

Guyton, A.C. (1948) Acute hypertension in dogs with cerebral ischemia. *Am. J. Physiol.*, 154: 45 – 54.

Kumada, M., Dampney, R.A.L. and Reis, D.J. (1979) Profound hypotension and abolition of the vasomotor component of the cerebral ischemic response produced by restricted lesions of medulla oblongata in rabbit. *Circ. Res.*, 45: 63 – 70.

Langhorst, P., Shulz, B., Shulz, G. and Lambertz, M. (1983) Reticular formation of the lower brainstem. A common system for cardiorespiratory and somatomotor functions: discharge patterns of neighboring neurons influenced by cardiovascular and respiratory afferents. *J. Auton. Nerv. Syst.*, 9: 411 – 432.

Loeschcke, H.H., De Lattre, J., Schlaefke, M.E. and Trouth, C.O. (1970) Effects on respiration and circulation of electrically stimulating the ventral surface of the medulla oblongata. *Respir. Physiol.*, 10: 184 – 197.

Loewy, A.D., Wallach, J.H. and McKellar, S. (1981) Efferent connections of the ventral medulla oblongata in the rat. *Brain Res. Rev.*, 3: 63 – 80.

McAllen, R.M. (1986) Location of neurones with cardiovascular and respiratory function, at the ventral surface of the cat's medulla. *Neuroscience*, 18: 43 – 49.

McAllen, R.M. (1987) Central respiratory modulation of bulbospinal neurones in the cat. *J. Physiol.*, 388: 533 – 545.

Millhorn, D.E. and Eldridge, F.L. (1986) Role of ventrolateral medulla in regulation of respiratory and cardiovascular systems. *J. Appl. Physiol.*, 61: 1249 – 1263.

Nattie, E.E., Mills, J.W., Ou, L.C. and St. John, W.M. (1988) Kainic acid on the rostral ventrolateral medulla inhibits phrenic output and CO$_2$ sensitivity. *J. Appl. Physiol.*, 65: 1525 – 1534.

Paterson, D.J., Wood, G.A., Morton, A.R. and Henstridge, J.D. (1986) The entrainment of ventilation frequency to exercise rhythm. *Eur. J. Appl. Physiol.*, 55: 530 – 537.

Porter, J.P. and Brody, M.J. (1985) Neural projections from paraventricular nucleus that subserve vasomotor functions. *Am. J. Physiol.*, 248 (*Reg. Integrative Comp. Physiol.* 17): R271 – R281.

Reis, D.J., Ross, C.A., Ruggiero, C.A., Granata, A.R. and Joh, T.H. (1984) Role of adrenaline neurons of ventrolateral medulla (the C1 group) in the tonic and phasic control of arterial pressure. *Clin. Exp. Hypertension*, A6: 221 – 241.

Reis, D.J., Morrison, S. and Ruggiero, D.A. (1988) The C1 of the brainstem in tonic and reflex control of blood pressure. State of the Art Lecture. *Hypertension, Suppl. 1*, 11: I8 – I13.

Ross, C.A., Ruggiero, D.A., Park, D.H., Joh, T.H., Sved, A.F., Fernandez-Pardal, J., Saavedra, J.M. and Reis, D.J. (1984) Tonic vasomotor control by the rostral ventrolateral medulla: effect of electrical or chemical stimulation of the area containing C1 adrenaline neurons on arterial pressure, heart rate, and plasma catecholamines and vasopressin. *J. Neurosci.*, 4: 274 – 494.

Ruggiero, D.A., Gatti, P.J., Gillis, R.A., Norman, W.P., Anwar, M. and Reis, D.J. (1986) Adrenaline-synthesizing neurons in the medulla of the cat. *J. Comp. Neurol.*, 252: 532 – 542.

Schlaefke, M. (1981) Central chemosensitivity: a respiratory drive. *Rev. Physiol. Biochem. Pharmacol.*, 90: 172 – 244.

Schlaefke, M.E. and See, W.R. (1980) Ventral medullary surface stimulus response in relation to ventilatory and cardiovascular effects. In H.P. Koepchen, S.M. Hilton and A. Trzebski (Eds.), *Central Interaction Between Respiratory and Cardiovascular Control Systems*, Springer-Verlag, Berlin, pp. 56 – 63.

Sun, M.K. and Guyenet, P.G. (1986) Hypothalamic glutamatergic input to medullary sympatho-excitatory neurons in rats. *Am. J. Physiol.*, 251: R798 – R810.

Trouth, C.O., Loeschcke, H.H. and Berndt, J. (1973) Topography of the circulatory responses to electrical stimulation in the medulla oblongata. Relationship to respiratory responses. *Pflügers Arch.*, 339: 185 – 201.

Weckenmann, M., Adam, G., Rauch, E. and Schulenberg, A. (1988) The coordination of heart beat and respiration during ergometric stress in patients with functional cardiovascular diseases. *Basic Res. Cardiol.*, 83: 452 – 458.

Control of Neurohypophysial Hormone Release by Ventrolateral Medullary Neurons

J. Ciriello, M.M. Caverson and C. Polosa (Eds.)
Progress in Brain Research, Vol. 81
© 1989 Elsevier Science Publishers B.V. (Biomedical Division)

CHAPTER 22

Organization of ventrolateral medullary afferents to the hypothalamus

Monica M. Caverson and John Ciriello

Department of Physiology, Health Sciences Centre, The University of Western Ontario, London, Ontario, Canada N6A 5C1

Introduction

There has been a considerable amount of experimental evidence suggesting that pathways from the ventrolateral medulla (VLM) ascending to the hypothalamus function as important components of neuronal circuits controlling autonomic and neuroendocrine function (for reviews see Ciriello et al., 1986b, and Sawchenko and Swanson, 1982). In particular, it has been suggested that VLM neurons exert a direct influence on the release of arginine vasopressin (AVP) by magnocellular neurosecretory neurons in the paraventricular (PVH) and supraoptic (SON) nuclei of the hypothalamus. This suggestion was based on the observation that electrical stimulation of neurons in the lateral medullary reticular formation caused an increase in the release of AVP (Mills and Wang, 1964a,b). The subsequent observations that topical application of the cholinergic agonist nicotine (Feldberg et al., 1975), and of the GABA and glycine antagonists bicuculline and strychnine (Feldberg and Rocha e Silva, 1978), to the VLM surface, resulted in an increase in AVP secretion, and that application of GABA or glycine to the caudal region of the VLM inhibited AVP release caused by carotid artery occlusion (Feldberg and Rocha e Silva, 1981), further supported the suggestion that neurons in the VLM were involved in the control of AVP release. Recently, it has been

shown that selective excitation of VLM neurons following microinjection of L-glutamate into the caudal VLM resulted in an increase in plasma levels of AVP (Blessing and Willoughby, 1985).

We have used neuroanatomical tract tracing and electrophysiological extracellular single unit recording techniques in the cat to delineate the organization of ascending projections from the VLM to regions of the PVH and SON where magnocellular neurosecretory neurons containing vasopressin have been demonstrated in this species (Caverson et al., 1987). This chapter summarizes this morphological and functional evidence, some of which has previously been published (Caverson and Ciriello, 1984; Ciriello and Caverson, 1984a,b,c).

Anatomical organization of VLM afferent projections to the PVH and SON

The precise organization of afferent projections from the VLM to the PVH and SON was investigated using two neuroanatomical tract tracing techniques. The technique of fluorochrome histochemistry was used in the first series of experiments to demonstrate the location of retrogradely labelled neuronal perikarya in the VLM after placement of two different fluorescent tracers in the regions of the PVH and SON. To eliminate the possibility that the retrogradely

282

labelled neurons in the VLM were the result of up-take of the fluorochromes by fibers coursing through the injection sites in the PVH and SON and not terminating in these hypothalamic nuclei, a second series of experiments was done in which tritiated amino acids (which are selectively incorporated into cell bodies and transported anterogradely to the terminals) were injected into the VLM and the autoradiographic technique was used to demonstrate projection fields resulting from the anterograde transport of the amino acids.

As a result of localized injections of the retrogradely transported fluorochromes Granular Blue (GB) and Nuclear Yellow (NY) into the regions of the PVH and/or SON, retrogradely labelled neuronal perikarya were observed primari-

ly throughout the caudal VLM (Fig. 1) bilaterally, but with an ipsilateral predominance.

Retrogradely labelled cells resulting from the injection of different fluorochromes into the PVH and SON had a similar distribution in the VLM. The majority of these neurons were found at the level of the obex, primarily in the region dorsal and lateral to the lateral reticular nucleus (LRN) and ventral to the nucleus ambiguus. Fewer labelled neurons were found ventral to the LRN, some of which were located adjacent to the ventral surface, near the intramedullary rootlets of the hypoglossal nerve. Immediately rostral to the LRN, fluorescent labelled neurons were observed in the nucleus paragigantocellularis lateralis.

In addition to neurons in the VLM labelled

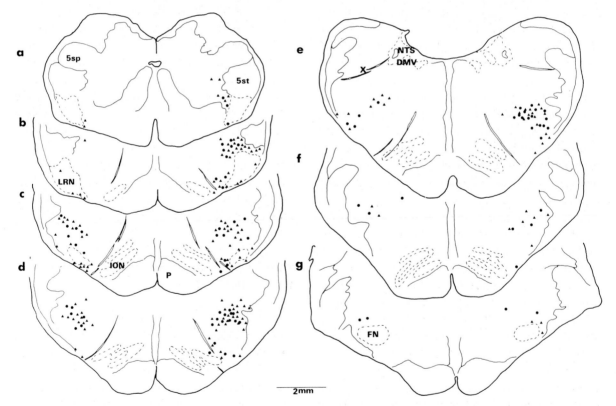

Fig. 1. Series of transverse sections of the ventral brainstem at approximately 0.5 mm intervals showing the location of labelled neurons in the VLM after injection of Granular Blue in the PVH (▲) and Nuclear Yellow in the SON (●) region. Each symbol represents one labelled neuron found on the section drawn. 5sp = spinal trigeminal nucleus; 5st = spinal trigeminal tract; DMV = dorsal motor nucleus of the vagus; FN = facial nucleus; ION = inferior olivary nucleus; LRN = lateral reticular nucleus; NTS = nucleus of the solitary tract; X = vagus nerve.

283

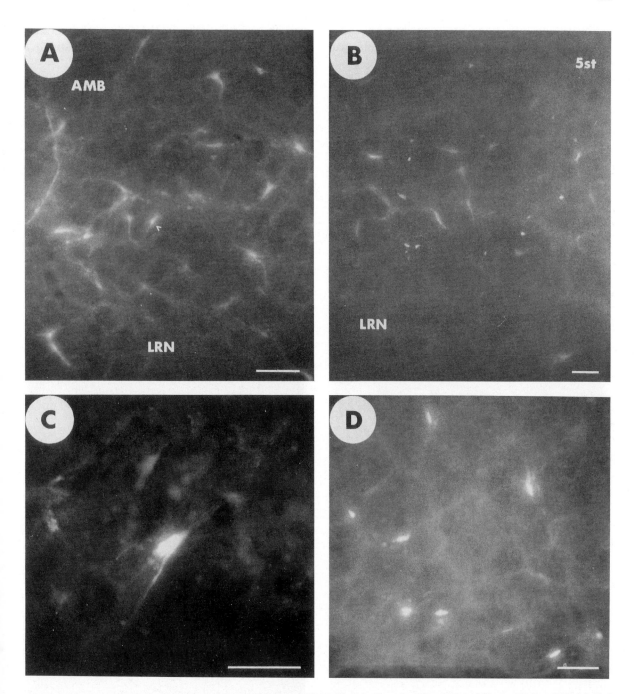

Fig. 2. Photomicrographs through the region of the ipsilateral VLM showing Granular Blue (GB) and Nuclear Yellow (NY) labelled cells after injections of these fluorochromes into the PVH and SON, respectively. (A) Single- and double-labelled neurons after GB injection in the PVH region and NY injection in the SON region. Arrow points to double-labelled neuron shown in (C). (B) Single GB and NY labelled neurons in VLM at a more rostral level. (D) NY labelled neurons in VLM after an injection in the SON region. AMB = nucleus ambiguus. Scale in (A, B, D), 100 μm and in (C), 50 μm.

284

following an injection into one hypothalamic nucleus, a small population of cells was found that was labelled after injection of different fluorescent markers into the PVH and SON. These double-labelled cells were interspersed among single-labelled neurons in the caudal VLM and provided evidence for the existence of a small population of VLM neurons that sent collateral axons to the PVH and SON (Fig. 2).

In the second study, injections of a mixture of [³H]proline and leucine were made in regions of the VLM shown in the previous study to contain retrogradely labelled cells and the precise distribution of anterogradely labelled fibers and presumptive nerve terminals in the regions of the PVH and SON was determined. Anterograde labelling was found throughout the PVH and SON (Fig. 3) bilaterally, but with an ipsilateral predominance. The greatest concentration of terminal labelling

was observed over the medial aspect of the caudal PVH (Fig. 3B) and over the ipsilateral caudal extent of the SON (Fig. 3D).

The distribution of retrogradely labelled neurons in this study is in agreement with previously published reports indicating a similar distribution of VLM neurons projecting to the PVH and SON in the rat (Loewy et al., 1981; Sawchenko and Swanson, 1982) and rabbit (Blessing et al., 1982). In addition, the location of retrogradely labelled neurons in the VLM described in this study corresponds to the location of neurons that have previously been shown to contain the catecholamine synthesizing enzyme dopamine β-hydroxylase (DBH) in the cat (Ciriello et al., 1986a). This finding is supported by reports in the rat and rabbit of retrogradely labelled cells in the VLM that also contain DBH (Blessing et al., 1982; Sawchenko and Swanson, 1982). Taken together,

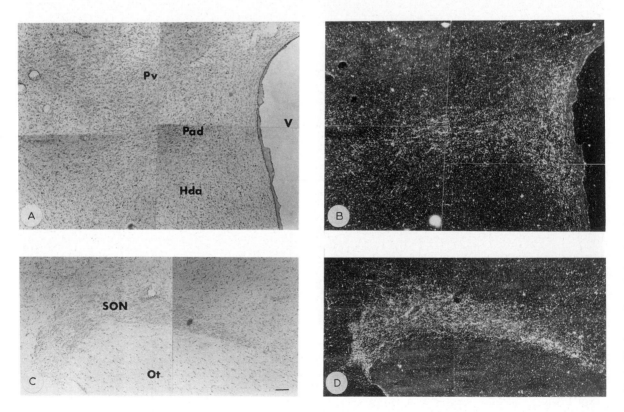

Fig. 3. Photomicrographs of thionin counterstained autoradiographs through the region of the PVH (A,B) and SON (C,D) ipsilateral to the site of injection in the VLM. (B) and (D) are darkfield photomicrographs of (A) and (C), respectively. Scale, 0.1 mm.

these data suggest that most VLM neurons sending afferent projections to the PVH and SON are likely to be noradrenergic and correspond to the A_1 cell group described originally by Dahlstrom and Fuxe (1964). Catecholaminergic fibers from the VLM have been described to join the ascending longitudinal catecholamine bundle from the locus coeruleus in the rostral brainstem (Jones and Friedman, 1983). This tract contributes fibers to thalamic and subthalamic regions. In addition, VLM ascending catecholaminergic fibers have been shown to contribute to the dense innervation of hypothalamic and telencephalic regions via the medial forebrain bundle (Jones and Friedman, 1983).

The projection from the VLM to the PVH and SON was confirmed in the second study using the autoradiographic anterograde transport technique. In addition, the distribution of terminal labelling observed in the PVH and SON is in agreement with previous results obtained using this technique in the rat (Loewy et al., 1981; McKellar and Loewy, 1981; Sawchenko and Swanson, 1982). The fact that most of the anterograde labelling in the PVH and SON also coincides closely with the distribution of noradrenergic fibers and terminals in the PVH and SON (McNeill and Sladek, 1980; Swanson et al., 1981) supports the suggestion that A_1 neurons in the VLM are the likely source of this innervation. However, recent evidence that neurons in the VLM of the cat contain other neuropeptides (see chapter by Ciriello and Caverson, this volume) and that fibers and presumptive nerve terminals containing these neuropeptides are also found in the magnocellular and parvocellular regions of the PVH and in the SON in the cat (Caverson et al., 1985) suggests that the ascending projection from the VLM may not exclusively contain catecholamines.

Electrophysiological studies on VLM neurons projecting to the PVH and SON

Previous studies have shown that activation of sensory afferent fibers, originating in peripheral baroreceptors and chemoreceptors, and stimulation of the nucleus of the solitary tract, the primary site of termination of cardiovascular afferent fibers (Crill and Reis, 1968; Ciriello and Calaresu, 1981), evokes short-latency single-unit responses in the PVH and SON (Calaresu and Ciriello, 1980) and influences the release of AVP (Share and Levy, 1962, 1966). This evidence, combined with the finding that application of glycine or GABA to the caudal VLM inhibits the release of AVP as a result of "unloading" baroreceptors (Feldberg and Rocha e Silva, 1981), suggested that the VLM may be a site of origin of an ascending cardiovascular pathway through which peripheral baroreceptor afferent information is relayed to the PVH and SON. This suggestion was further supported by the finding that neurons in the VLM altered their firing frequency during activation of cardiovascular afferent fibers (Ciriello and Calaresu, 1977; Calaresu and Ciriello, 1980; Caverson et al., 1983a,b, 1984), and during selective activation of baroreceptors and chemoreceptors (Caverson et al., 1984; Ciriello and Calaresu, 1977). However, it remained equivocal whether VLM neurons relayed cardiovascular afferent information directly to the PVH and SON. Therefore, two series of experiments were done to obtain electrophysiological evidence regarding this issue.

In the first series, the region of the VLM that had been shown in the neuroanatomical tract tracing studies to contain retrogradely labelled neurons was systematically explored for single units antidromically activated by electrical stimulation of the PVH and/or SON. In addition, these units were tested for their orthodromic response to stimulation of sensory afferent fibers in the carotid sinus and aortic depressor nerves carrying information from baroreceptors and chemoreceptors. The second series of experiments examined the orthodromic response of PVH neurons, identified as magnocellular neurosecretory neurons by antidromic activation from the neurohypophysis, to stimulation of VLM neurons.

All single units in the VLM that responded to

stimulation of hypothalamic sites were assessed for antidromic activation using previously established criteria (Lipski, 1981). Antidromic action potentials evoked by electrical stimulation of either the PVH and/or SON were recorded from 195 histologically verified single units in the VLM of chloralose-anesthetized cats. These units were subdivided into three groups on the basis of their antidromic responses; one group was activated by stimulation of the PVH ($n = 100$); the second group responded antidromically to stimulation of the SON ($n = 69$; Fig. 4); and the third group was antidromically activated by stimulating both the PVH and SON ($n = 26$; Table I; Fig. 5). All units that were classified as antidromic were tested for their orthodromic response to electrical stimula-

tion of sensory afferent fibers in the carotid sinus and aortic depressor nerves.

Single units responding antidromically to stimulation of the PVH had onset latencies corresponding to a mean conduction velocity of 4.3 ± 0.3 m/sec (range 0.5 to 12.5 m/sec; Table I). There appeared to be two distinct groups of units in the VLM projecting to the PVH identified on the basis of their conduction velocities. One group contained units whose axons conducted in the range of 0.5 to 3.3 m/sec (mean 1.9 ± 0.1 m/sec; $n = 44/100$), and the second group contained units that responded with latencies cor-

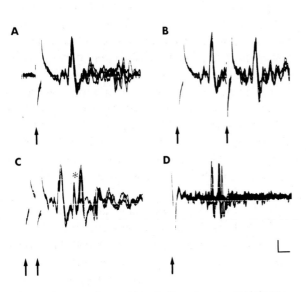

Fig. 4. Response of an antidromically activated unit in VLM to different frequencies of stimulation of SON (A – C) and to stimulation of the CSN (D). Each record is five superimposed sweeps, and the stimuli were delivered at the arrows. (A) Note the constant latency and 2 component (initial segment and somatodendritic) spike in record at 0.5 Hz. (B) Action potentials evoked with two stimuli applied at 116 Hz. (C) Note the separation of the initial segment-somatodendritic components (*) and the occasional failure of the somatodendritic component of the spike after the second stimulus at 500 Hz. (D) Orthodromic response of same unit to stimulation of the CSN. Calibrations, 2 msec and 100 μV (A – C), and 5 msec and 100 μV (D).

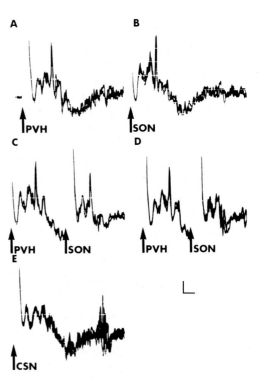

Fig. 5. VLM neuron antidromically activated by electrical stimulation of both the PVH and SON. Each record is five superimposed sweeps. Stimuli delivered at arrows. (A) Response of VLM neuron to stimulation of PVH at 0.5 Hz (0.1 msec and 0.6 mA). (B) Response of VLM neuron to stimulation of SON at 0.5 Hz (0.1 msec and 0.8 mA). (C) When two stimuli are applied 10 msec apart, both antidromic potentials are present. (D) When the interval between stimuli is reduced to 8.8 msec, the SON potential is cancelled. (E) Orthodromic response of unit to electrical stimulation of the CSN. Calibration, 2 msec and 200 μV.

TABLE I

Electrophysiological characteristics of single units in VLM antidromically activated by stimulation of PVH and SON

Site of stimulation	No. of units	Conduction velocity of antidromic units (m/sec)	Spike duration (msec)	Following frequency (Hz)	% Units responding to CSN and/or ADN
PVH	100	4.3 ± 0.3	2.1 ± 0.1	289 ± 15	65
SON	69	7.8 ± 0.6	2.0 ± 0.2	276 ± 15	38
PVH		5.0 ± 0.5	1.6 ± 0.1	269 ± 22	
+	26				38
SON		5.3 ± 0.6	1.6 ± 0.1	272 ± 18	

Values are mean ± S.E. ADN = aortic depressor nerve; CSN = carotid sinus nerve; VLM = ventrolateral medulla; PVH = paraventricular nucleus of the hypothalamus; SON = supraoptic nucleus of the hypothalamus.

responding to conduction velocities of greater than 3.6 m/sec (mean 6.2 ± 0.3 m/sec; $n = 56/100$). In addition, 10 of the 100 antidromically activated single units to stimulation of the ipsilateral PVH were also activated by stimulation of the contralateral PVH with similar conduction velocities (3.5 ± 0.6 m/sec to ipsilateral PVH stimulation; 3.7 ± 0.8 m/sec to contralateral PVH stimulation). Of the 100 VLM units antidromically activated from the PVH, 65% were also orthodromically excited by stimulation of carotid sinus and/or aortic depressor nerves. The axons of antidromically activated units responding to sensory afferent inputs conducted at slower velocities (mean 3.4 ± 0.5 m/sec; $n = 65$) than those of nonresponsive units (mean 6.0 ± 0.6 m/sec; $n = 35$).

The second group of single units in the VLM responded antidromically following electrical stimulation of the SON (Fig. 4) with onset latencies corresponding to a mean conduction velocity of 7.8 ± 0.6 m/sec ($n = 69$; Table I). Similar to the observation reported above for VLM units projecting to the PVH, single units antidromically activated by SON stimulation could also be subdivided into two groups on the basis of their conduction velocities. The first group conducted in the range of 1 to 7 m/sec (mean 4.4 ± 0.3 m/sec; $n = 36/69$), and the second contained neurons

whose axons conducted at velocities greater than 7 m/sec (mean, 11.5 ± 0.6 m/sec; range 7.2 to 27 m/sec; $n = 33/69$). Thirty-eight percent (26/69) of these units responded with excitation to activation of cardiovascular afferent fibers. Single units orthodromically excited by stimulation of cardiovascular afferent fibers responded antidromically to stimulation of the SON with latencies corresponding to a mean conduction velocity of 5.7 ± 0.4 m/sec (range 1.7 to 9.5 m/sec), whereas the mean conduction velocity of units that were non-responsive to the tested inputs was significantly faster (mean 9.1 ± 0.8 m/sec; range 1.4 to 27 m/sec).

The third group of VLM single units responded antidromically to stimulation of both the PVH and SON (Figs. 5 and 6). In each case the antidromic potential evoked by stimulation of one site was cancelled by stimulation of the other site. The conduction velocities of the collateral axons were not significantly different (combined mean 5.1 ± 0.4 m/sec; Table I). As shown in Fig. 5D, cancellation of an antidromic potential occurred when the stimuli were applied to the SON and PVH at an interval (8.8 m/sec) that was less than the sum of the latencies of the two antidromic potentials (9.6 m/sec). This observation suggested that this neuron likely possessed two long axons with the branching point for the two axons occurring close

288

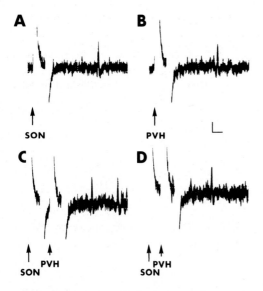

Fig. 6. Response of VLM unit antidromically activated by electrical stimulation of both the SON (A: 0.1 msec and 0.4 mA) and PVH (B: 0.1 msec and 0.4 mA) at 0.5 Hz. When two stimuli are delivered at 4.5 msec apart, both antidromic potentials are present, but when the stimulus interval is reduced to 2.7 msec the PVH potential is cancelled. Each record is five superimposed sweeps. Stimuli delivered at arrows. Calibration, 2 msec and 50 μV.

to the soma. However, in most cases a short time interval was required between the two stimuli for cancellation of the evoked antidromic spikes (Fig. 6), suggesting that the majority of neurons likely possessed two short axon collaterals with the branch point for the axons located close to their terminal sites. Of the 26 neurons with collateral axons, 38% (10/26) were excited orthodromically by stimulation of cardiovascular afferent fibers and the remaining 16 units were unresponsive to the tested inputs.

The anatomical distribution of the antidromically activated units in the VLM corresponded closely to that reported in the retrograde transport study suggesting that the activity recorded from single units likely originated in cell bodies and not in fibers of passage. The majority of the single units were located at medullary levels extending from approximately 0.5 mm caudal to obex to 4 mm rostral to obex, primarily in a region dorsal and

lateral to the LRN at caudal levels and near the ventral surface at rostral levels.

These electrophysiological data provide evidence that neurons in the VLM relay sensory afferent information from peripheral cardiovascular receptors to the PVH and SON. Although the question of whether VLM single units responded to selective activation of peripheral baroreceptors or chemoreceptors was not addressed in this study, the fact that L-glutamate stimulation of neurons in the VLM has been shown to increase the release of AVP (Blessing and Willoughby, 1985), that peripheral chemoreceptor activation has also been shown to increase AVP release (Share and Levy, 1966), and that all antidromically activated units recorded in VLM that responded to the carotid sinus and antidepressor nerves were excited suggests that the neurons recorded from in this study most likely responded to peripheral chemoreceptor activation. Whether VLM single units also relay baroreceptor afferent information to the PVH and SON remains equivocal for the following reasons. First, the location of VLM single units in this study corresponded closely with the distribution of neurons previously shown to contain DBH (Ciriello et al., 1986a), suggesting that some of the units recorded from were likely noradrenergic neurons belonging to the A_1 cell group in the VLM. Second, a dense plexus of noradrenergic fibers and nerve terminals have been demonstrated in regions of the PVH and SON containing AVP magnocellular neurosecretory neurons (McNeill and Sladek, 1980; Sawchenko and Swanson, 1981), and application of noradrenaline to AVP magnocellular neurosecretory neurons has been shown to excite these neurons and to stimulate AVP release (see chapter by Day, this volume). Third, most of the retrogradely labelled cells after an injection of a tracer into the PVH and SON have been shown to contain DBH immunoreactivity (Sawchenko and Swanson, 1982). However, destruction of noradrenergic terminals in the PVH and SON does not alter the effects of baroreceptor activation of AVP cells (Day and Renaud, 1984; Day et al., 1984). Therefore, there is increasing evidence to suggest that A_1 noradrenergic cells in the VLM that project to the PVH and SON most likely do not relay baroreceptor inhibitory information to AVP cells. The possibility remains, however, that some of the VLM single units activated from the PVH and SON in this study were non-noradrenergic, on the basis of their coincident anatomical distribution to that of peptidergic neurons in the VLM (see chapter by Ciriello and Caverson, this volume). Whether non-noradrenergic VLM neurons are involved in relaying baroreceptor inhibitory information to PVH and SON AVP neurons has not been determined.

An unexpected finding was that axons of neurons in the VLM relaying cardiovascular afferent information conducted at significantly slower velocities than axons of neurons which were non-responsive to buffer nerve stimulation. These data suggested that there are at least two functionally different populations of VLM neurons that project directly to the PVH and SON. It is not surprising to find that some of the neurons in the VLM antidromically activated by stimulation of the PVH and SON were not responsive to cardiovascular afferent inputs, as this area has been shown also to relay visceral sensory information unrelated to the cardiovascular system (for reviews see Ciriello et al., 1986b, and Sawchenko and Swanson, 1982). Some of these units were found close to the ventral surface of the brainstem in an area known to be sensitive to [H^+] and pCO_2 (for reviews see Ciriello et al., 1986b, and Schlaefke, 1981). In addition, activation of central CO_2 chemoreceptors has been shown to alter the metabolic activity of the VLM and of the PVH and SON (Ciriello et al., 1985) and influence the release of vasopressin (Tenney, 1960), suggesting that some of these neurons are involved in mediating central chemoreceptor information to the PVH and SON.

Although the previous evidence suggested that VLM single units projected directly to PVH and SON magnocellular neurosecretory neurons, electrophysiological evidence in support of this suggestion was unavailable in the cat. Therefore, a series

of extracellular single unit recording experiments was done in which single unit activity was recorded from magnocellular neurosecretory neurons in the PVH antidromically activated from the neurohypophysis and the orthodromic response of these units to VLM stimulation was determined. Experiments were done in chloralose anesthetized cats using the transpharyngeal approach to access the PVH and the neurohypophysis. The orthodromic response to stimulation of the VLM of 20 single units in the PVH that were classified as magnocellular neurosecretory neurons was exclusively excitatory (Fig. 7). The onset latency of

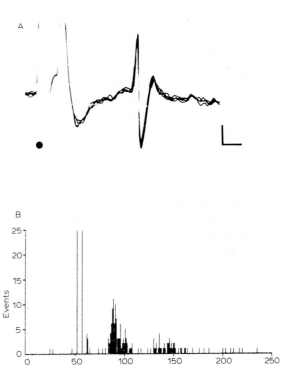

Fig. 7. Orthodromic response of PVH single unit antidromically activated by electrical stimulation of the neurohypophysis to stimulation of the VLM. (A) Response of PVH neuron to stimulation of neurohypophysis. Stimulus delivered at dot. Calibration 5 msec and 50 μV. (B) Peristimulus time histogram of orthodromic response of this unit in PVH to electrical stimulation (2 pulses at 50 msec) of VLM. Bin width 1 msec. Stimuli delivered at arrows.

the orthodromic input to these PVH neurons from the VLM was 19.8 ± 4 msec (range 10 to 80 msec). The anatomical location of the neurons in the PVH responding to VLM stimulation corresponded closely to that of previously described AVP-containing neurons in the dorsal component of the PVH of the cat (Caverson et al., 1987).

Summary

In summary, these anatomical and electrophysiological data have provided evidence to support the suggestion that VLM neurons project directly to regions of the hypothalamus that contain magnocellular neurosecretory neurons. In addition, these results support the suggestion that pathways ascending from the VLM to the hypothalamus function, in part, in the control of the release of the neurohypophyseal hormones by PVH and SON magnocellular neurosecretory neurons during activation of peripheral cardiovascular receptors.

Acknowledgements

This work was supported by the Medical Research Council of Canada and Heart and Stroke Foundation of Ontario. M.M. Caverson is a Heart and Stroke Foundation of Canada Scholar and J. Ciriello is a Career Investigator of the Heart and Stroke Foundation of Ontario.

References

Blessing, W.W. and Willoughby, J.O. (1985) Excitation of neuronal function in rabbit caudal ventrolateral medulla elevates plasma vasopressin. *Neurosci. Lett.*, 58: 189–194.

Blessing, W.W., Jaeger, C.B., Ruggiero, D.A. and Reis, D.J. (1982) Hypothalamic projections of medullary catecholamine neurons in the rabbit: a combined catecholamine fluorescence and HRP transport study. *Brain Res. Bull.*, 9: 279–286.

Calaresu, F.R. and Ciriello, J. (1980) Projections to the hypothalamus from buffer nerves and nucleus tractus solitarius in the cat. *Am. J. Physiol.*, 239: R130–R136.

Caverson, M.M. and Ciriello, J. (1984) Electrophysiological identification of neurons in ventrolateral medulla sending collateral axons to paraventricular and supraoptic nuclei in the cat. *Brain Res.*, 305: 375–379.

Caverson, M.M., Ciriello, J. and Calaresu, F.R. (1983a) Direct pathway from cardiovascular neurons in the ventrolateral medulla to the region of the intermediolateral nucleus of the upper thoracic cord: an anatomical and electrophysiological investigation in the cat. *J. Auton. Nerv. Syst.*, 9: 451–475.

Caverson, M.M., Ciriello, J. and Calaresu, F.R. (1983b) Cardiovascular afferent inputs to neurons in the ventrolateral medulla projecting directly to the central autonomic area of the thoracic cord in the cat. *Brain Res.*, 274: 354–358.

Caverson, M.M., Ciriello, J. and Calaresu, F.R. (1984) Chemoreceptor and baroreceptor inputs to ventrolateral medullary neurons. *Am. J. Physiol.*, 247: R872–879.

Caverson, M.M., Ciriello, J., Calaresu, F.R. and Krukoff, T.L. (1985) Distribution of peptide and serotonin immunoreactive fibers and terminals in paraventricular nucleus of the cat. *Soc. Neurosci. Abstr.*, 11: 826.

Caverson, M.M., Ciriello, J., Calaresu, F.R. and Krukoff, T.L. (1987) Distribution and morphology of vasopressin, neurophysin II and oxytocin immunoreactive cell bodies in the forebrain of the cat. *J. Comp. Neurol.*, 259: 211–236.

Ciriello, J. and Calaresu, F.R. (1977) Lateral reticular nucleus: a site of somatic and cardiovascular integration in the cat. *Am. J. Physiol.*, 233: R100–R109.

Ciriello, J. and Calaresu, F.R. (1981) Projections from buffer nerves to the nucleus of the solitary tract: an anatomical and electrophysiological study in the cat. *J. Auton. Nerv. Syst.*, 3: 299–310.

Ciriello, J. and Caverson, M.M. (1984a) Organization of ventrolateral medullary (VLM) afferents to the paraventricular (PVH) and supraoptic (SON) nuclei in the cat. *Fed. Proc.*, 43: 401.

Ciriello, J. and Caverson, M.M. (1984b) Direct pathway from neurons in the ventrolateral medulla relaying cardiovascular afferent information to the supraoptic nucleus in the cat. *Brain Res.*, 292: 221–228.

Ciriello, J. and Caverson, M.M. (1984c) Ventrolateral medullary neurons relay cardiovascular inputs to the paraventricular nucleus. *Am. J. Physiol.*, 247: R968–R978.

Ciriello, J. and Caverson, M.M. (1989) Relation of enkephalin-like immunoreactive neurons to other neuropeptide and monoamine containing neurons in the ventrolateral medulla. In *Progress in Brain Research*, this volume.

Ciriello, J., Rohlicek, C.V. and Polosa, C. (1985) 2-Deoxyglucose uptake in the central nervous system during systemic hypercapnia in the peripherally chemodenervated rat. *Exp. Neurol.*, 88: 673–687.

Ciriello, J., Caverson, M.M. and Park, D.H. (1986a) Immunohistochemical identification of noradrenaline- and adrenaline-synthesizing neurons in the cat ventrolateral medulla. *J. Comp. Neurol.*, 253: 216–230.

Ciriello, J., Caverson, M.M. and Polosa, C. (1986b) Function of ventrolateral medulla in the control of the circulation.

Brain Res. Rev., 11: 359 – 391.

Crill, N.E. and Reis, D.J. (1968) Distribution of carotid sinus and depressor nerves in cat brain stem. *Am. J. Physiol.*, 214: 269 – 276.

Dahlstrom, A. and Fuxe, K. (1964) Evidence for the existence of monoamine containing neurons in the central nervous system. I. Demonstration of monoamines in the cell bodies of brain stem neurons. *Acta Physiol. Scand.*, 62, Suppl. 232: 1 – 55.

Day, T.A. and Renaud, L.P. (1984) Electrophysiological evidence that noradrenergic afferents selectively facilitate the activity of supraoptic vasopressin neurons. *Brain Res.*, 303: 233 – 240.

Day, T.A., Ferguson, A.V. and Renaud, L.P. (1984) Facilitatory influence of noradrenergic afferents on the excitability of rat paraventricular nucleus neurosecretory cells. *J. Physiol. (Lond.)*, 355: 237 – 249.

Feldberg, W. and Rocha e Silva, M. (1978) Vasopressin release produced in anaesthetized cats by antagonists of GABA and glycine. *Br. J. Pharmacol.*, 62: 99 – 106.

Feldberg, W. and Rocha e Silva, M. (1981) Inhibition of vasopressin release to carotid occlusion by gamma amino butyric acid and glycine. *Br. J. Pharmacol.*, 72: 17 – 24.

Feldberg, W., Guertzenstein, P.G. and Rocha e Silva, M. (1975) Vasopressin release by nicotine: the site of action. *Br. J. Pharmacol.*, 54: 463 – 474.

Jones, B.E. and Friedman, L. (1983) Atlas of catecholamine perikarya, varicosities and pathways in the brainstem of the cat. *J. Comp. Neurol.*, 215: 382 – 396.

Lipski, J. (1981) Antidromic activation of neurones as an analytical tool in the study of the central nervous system. *J. Neurosci. Methods*, 4: 1 – 32.

Loewy, A.D., Wallach, J.H. and McKellar, S. (1981) Efferent connections of the ventral medulla oblongata in the rat. *Brain Res. Rev.*, 3: 63 – 80.

McKellar, S. and Loewy, A.D. (1981) Organization of some brain stem afferents to the paraventricular nucleus of the hypothalamus in the rat. *Brain Res.*, 217: 351 – 357.

McNeill, T.H. and Sladek, J.R., Jr. (1980) Simultaneous monoamine histofluorescence and neuropeptide immunocytochemistry: correlative distribution of catecholamine varicosities and magnocellular neurosecretory neurons in the rat supraoptic and paraventricular nuclei. *J. Comp. Neurol.*, 193: 1023 – 1033.

Mills, E. and Wang, S.C. (1964a) Liberation of antidiuretic hormone: location of ascending pathways. *Am. J. Physiol.*, 207: 1399 – 1404.

Mills, E. and Wang, S.C. (1964b) Liberation of antidiuretic hormone: pharmacologic blockade of ascending pathways. *Am. J. Physiol.*, 207: 1404 – 1410.

Sawchenko, P.E. and Swanson, L.W. (1982) The organization of noradrenergic pathways from the brainstem to the paraventricular and supraoptic nuclei in the rat. *Brain Res. Rev.*, 4: 275 – 325.

Schlaefke, M.E. (1981) Central chemosensitivity: a respiratory drive. *Rev. Physiol. Biochem. Pharmacol.*, 90: 171 – 244.

Share, L. and Levy, M.N. (1962) Cardiovascular receptors and blood titer of antidiuretic hormone. *Am. J. Physiol.*, 203: 425 – 428.

Share, L. and Levy, M.N. (1966) Effect of carotid chemoreceptor stimulation on plasma antidiuretic hormone titer. *Am. J. Physiol.*, 210: 157 – 161.

Swanson, L.W., Sawchenko, P.E., Berod, A., Hartman, B.K., Helle, K.B. and Vanorden, D.E. (1981) An immunohistochemical study of the organization of catecholaminergic cells and terminal fields in the paraventricular and supraoptic nuclei of the hypothalamus. *J. Comp. Neurol.*, 196: 271 – 285.

Tenney, S.M. (1960) The effect of CO_2 on neurohumoral and endocrine mechanisms. *Anesthesiology*, 21: 674 – 685.

J. Ciriello, M.M. Caverson and C. Polosa (Eds.)
Progress in Brain Research, Vol. 81
© 1989 Elsevier Science Publishers B.V. (Biomedical Division)

CHAPTER 23

Involvement of caudal ventrolateral medulla neurons in mediating visceroreceptive information to the hypothalamic paraventricular nucleus

H. Yamashita, H. Kannan and Y. Ueta

Department of Physiology, University of Occupational and Environmental Health, School of Medicine, Yahatanishi-ku, Kitakyushu 807, Japan

Introduction

The paraventricular nucleus (PVN) of the hypothalamus is well known to be involved in the release of the neurohypophyseal hormones, vasopressin and oxytocin from the posterior pituitary gland. In addition, the PVN has been demonstrated morphologically to have "direct" connections not only to the neurohypophysis but also to various sites in the central nervous system, such as the median eminence, the brainstem and spinal cord, which are involved in the control of adenohypophyseal hormone release and of autonomic nervous function, respectively (Swanson and Sawchenko, 1983).

The PVN neurons, including neurosecretory cells projecting to the neurohypophysis have been shown to receive information from receptors in the cardiovascular system and viscera (Barker et al., 1971; Koizumi and Yamashita, 1978; Calaresu and Ciriello, 1980; Kannan and Yamashita, 1983). The pathways through which afferent impulses from these visceroreceptors reach the PVN have been studied morphologically (Swanson and Sawchenko, 1983) but have not been well documented functionally. The primary sensory afferents from these peripheral visceroreceptors run through the carotid sinus nerves and vagi and reach the nucleus of the tractus solitarius (NTS) in the dorsomedial medulla (Spyer, 1982). It has been suggested that a "direct" pathway mediates the visceroreceptive information from the NTS to the PVN (Ciriello and Calaresu, 1980; Kannan and Yamashita, 1985). However, other "indirect" pathways should be considered as well. Neuroanatomical studies have shown that NTS and adjacent neurons project to the caudal ventrolateral medulla (CVLM) (Cottle and Calaresu, 1975; Loewy and Burton, 1978). Furthermore, neurons in the CVLM including the A1 catecholaminergic cell group have been shown to project to the PVN (Sawchenko and Swanson, 1981; Tribollet and Dreifuss, 1981; Blessing et al., 1982; McKellar and Loewy, 1982), and in turn neurons in the CVLM receive afferent inputs from the cardiovascular system and the splanchnic region (Ciriello and Calaresu, 1977; Perrin and Crousillat, 1983). These studies suggest that the CVLM may be an important relay station for afferent neural signals from cardiovascular and visceral receptors on their way to the PVN.

In this chapter, we present results of studies in which the characteristics of neurons in the CVLM which project to the PVN have been assessed by electrophysiological and pharmacological means. Most data have been previously published (Kannan et al., 1984, 1986, 1987).

Synaptic inputs from the CVLM to neurohypophyseal and tuberoinfundibular neurosecretory neurons

The effects of electrical stimulation of the CVLM on discharge activity of neurohypophyseal neurosecretory neurons, i.e. cells which were antidromically fired by stimulation of the pituitary stalk, were studied in male Wistar rats anesthetized with urethane (600 mg/kg, i.p.) and α-chloralose (60 mg/kg, i.p.). Criteria for identifying an antidromically conducted action potential were: constant latency; ability to follow stimuli at 200 Hz in one-to-one fashion; and collision with a spon-

taneously occurring spike (Fig. 1Aa). Stimulation of the CVLM (single pulses, 0.2 msec, 0.2 mA) produced synaptically mediated excitation in 10 (Fig. 1Ac,d), among 35 phasically firing neurosecretory neurons (Fig. 1Ab). The latency, on the basis of peristimulus time histograms, ranged from 30 to 60 msec, with a median at 40 – 45 msec. To compare the responsiveness of the phasic neurons with that of the non-phasic neurons, we also tested 81 continuously firing neurons. Stimulation of the CVLM excited 32 neurons and inhibited one neuron. Of the continuous firing neurons showing the excitatory responses, we tested 12 for their response to baroreceptor activa-

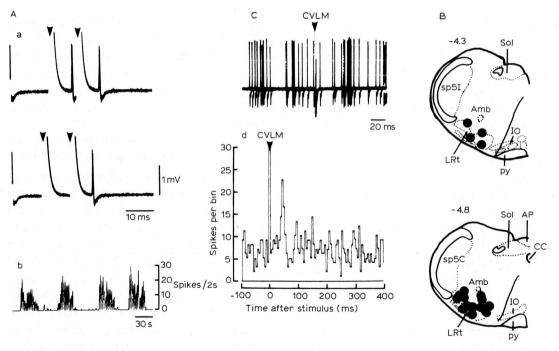

Fig. 1. (A) A Phasically firing neurosecretory neuron of the paraventricular nucleus (PVN) that was excited in response to caudal ventrolateral medulla (CVLM) stimulation. (Aa) Antidromic invasion test. Each panel shows five superimposed oscilloscope traces. Upper panel: constant latency of the antidromic action potentials evoked by double shocks (arrowheads). Lower panel: action potential evoked by the first stimuli was cancelled by collision with spontaneous action potentials occurring at the beginning of the trace. (Ab) Ratemeter record shows phasic pattern of spontaneous activity of the neuron. (Ac) Superimposed oscilloscope records of the response to 50 single pulse stimuli (0.2 msec and 0.2 mA) applied to the CVLM (arrow). (Ad) Peristimulus time histogram of the response to CVLM stimulation derived from 300 sweeps with bin width of 5 msec. Stimulus parameters, 0.2 msec and 0.2 mA. (B) Location of stimulating electrodes tips in the CVLM plotted on drawings of frontal sections. Filled circles indicate stimulation sites that yielded excitatory responses from PVN neurons. Amb = nucleus ambiguus; AP = area postrema; CC = central canal; LRt = lateral reticular nucleus; py = pyramidal tract; sp5C = nucleus of the spinal tract of the trigeminal nerve, caudal part; sp5I = nucleus of the spinal tract of the trigeminal nerve, intermediate part; Sol = nucleus solitary tract.

tion induced by intravenous injections of phenylephrine (8 μg). Of the 12 continuous firing neurons 6 were inhibited and 6 were unresponsive (Fig. 2).

Vasopressin-secreting neurons in the PVN have been tentatively identified as those which display a phasic firing pattern and show inhibitory responses to baroreceptor activation (Harris, 1979; Poulain and Wakerley, 1982). The present study demonstrates that PVN neurosecretory neurons which fulfill these criteria, such as vasopressin-secreting neurons, receive an excitatory synaptic input from the CVLM. The data obtained from continuously firing cells that were unresponsive to baroreceptor activation and excited by CVLM stimulation suggests the possibility that PVN oxytocin-secreting neurons also receive excitatory synaptic inputs from the CVLM.

We also examined the effects of electrical and chemical stimulation of the CVLM on the discharge activity of PVN tuberoinfundibular (TI) neurons. Cells which could be antidromically ac-

tivated by stimulation of the median eminence but not by the neurohypophysis were classified as TI neurons. Electrical stimulation of the CVLM excited 14 TI neurons out of 28 tested (Fig. 3A,B). The remaining 14 neurons were not affected by the stimulus. Threshold current and onset latency for the excitatory responses of these neurons were similar to those of neurohypophyseal neurosecretory neurons. In order to confirm that the excitatory response of the TI neurons was produced by activation of CVLM neurons and not by nerve fibers travelling through the area, we tested the same TI neurons which had been excited by electrical stimulation with chemical stimulation of the CVLM. For chemical and electrical stimulation of the same site of the CVLM, 3-barrelled glass micropipettes (tip size, 60 – 80 μm) were used. Microinjection of glutamate into the CVLM increased the firing rate of 7 out of 8 cells (Fig. 3C) and produced no effect in one cell. The chemical stimulus was consistently associated with a rapid decrease of arterial blood pressure and heart rate,

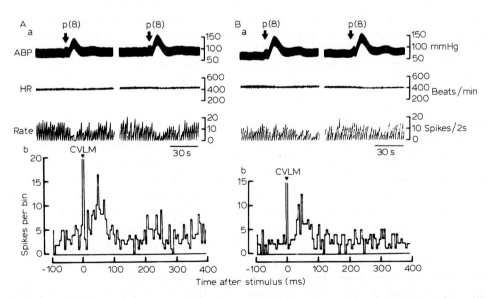

Fig. 2. Effects of baroreceptor stimulation on two (A,B) PVN continuously firing neurosecretory neurons that were excited by CVLM stimulation. In (Aa) and (Ba), traces from top to bottom: arterial blood pressure (ABP), heart rate (HR) and ratemeter record of neural activity (Rate). Arrows indicate i.v. injection of phenylephrine (8 μg). (Ab) and (Bb) are peristimulus time histograms (bin width, 5 msec; number of sweeps, 100). Single pulse stimuli (0.2 msec and 0.2 mA) were applied to the CVLM. Note that cell A was inhibited by baroreceptor stimulation, but not cell B.

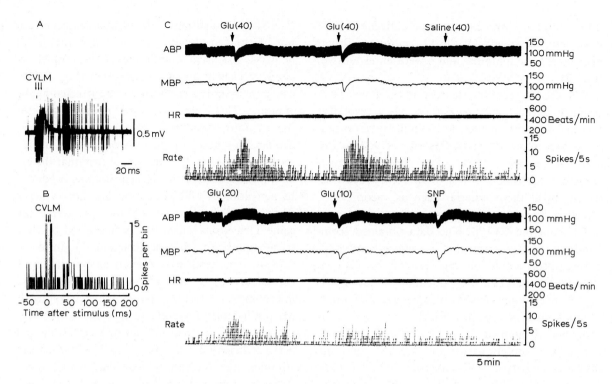

Fig. 3. An example of a TI neuron in the PVN that was excited in response to electrical and chemical stimulation of the CVLM. (A) Oscilloscope record of 400 superimposed sweeps. Three pulses of 200 Hz, 0.5 msec duration and 50 μA intensity were applied to the CVLM (marked by arrows). (B) Peristimulus time histogram of data shown in (A). (C) Records of arterial blood pressure (ABP), mean blood pressure (MBP), heart rate (HR) and ratemeter record of neural activity (Rate). Microinjection of L-glutamate (0.5 M, marked by Glu, with the volume, in nl, indicated in parentheses) evoked transient hypotension, bradycardia and an increase in firing rate, while saline did not produce significant changes. Upper and lower panels are continuous. Intravenous administration of the vasodilator, sodium nitroprusside (SNP, 8 μg) produced hypotension similar to that of glutamate, but no significant change in unit firing rate. (From Kannan et al., 1987.)

as previously reported by other investigators (Blessing and Reis, 1982). Injections of the same volume of saline had no effect on the firing rates of these cells. To exclude the possibility that the excitatory response observed was secondary to hypotension and/or bradycardia, a vasodilator, sodium nitroprusside (8 – 16 μg per animal), was injected intravenously. The drug produced hypotension similar to that caused by glutamate microinjection into the CVLM, but no change in the units' firing rates were observed. The TI neurons which were affected by electrical or chemical stimulation of the CVLM were also inhibited by i.v. administration of phenylephrine. These results suggest that the TI neurons receive

inhibitory inputs from arterial baroreceptors.

The functional and chemical identity of the TI cells responsive to baroreceptor and CVLM afferents remains uncertain so far. However, the parvocellular population of the PVN contains large numbers of CRF- and TRH-immunoreactive perikarya and the majority of these cells project to the median eminence (Lechan and Jackson, 1982; Antoni et al., 1983; Swanson et al., 1983; Nishiyama et al., 1985). In view of the evidence that hypovolemia and/or hypotension evoke an increase in plasma ACTH and thyroid-stimulating hormone (TSH) levels (Cameron et al., 1984; Plotsky and Vale, 1984; Hamamura et al., 1985), it is reasonable to assume that some of TI neurons responding to stimulation of baroreceptors and the CVLM are CRF- or TRH-secreting neurons.

Characteristics of neurons in the CVLM projecting to the PVN

In this series of experiments, we have attempted: (1) to describe some of the electrophysiological and pharmacological properties of neurons in the CVLM which project to the PVN; and (2) to determine whether these CVLM neurons receive synaptic inputs from visceral receptors.

Extracellular recordings were obtained from neurons located in the CVLM. Stimulation of the PVN evoked antidromically conducted action potentials in 71 neurons. From their antidromic spike

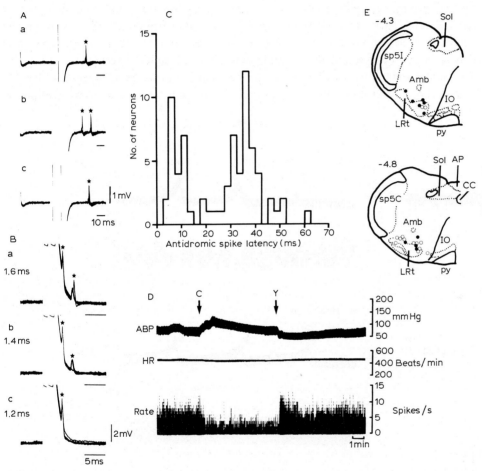

Fig. 4. Characteristics of CVLM neurons that project directly to the PVN. (A,B) Antidromic responses of cells in the CVLM to PVN stimulation. Records are 5 superimposed oscilloscope tracings. Asterisks indicate antidromically evoked action potentials. (A) Antidromic responses of a slow-conducting cell. (Aa) Constant latency: (Ab) and (Ac) paired-pulse stimulation at 100 Hz and collision test. Note the absence of the first evoked spike by collision with spontaneous action potentials (Ac). Spontaneous action potentials were used to trigger stimulation of the PVN. (B) Antidromic responses of a fast-conducting cell. Paired-pulse stimulation at various interpulse intervals (indicated by number in each figure). (C) Frequency distribution of antidromic spike latencies in CVLM neurons following PVN stimulation. (D) Effects of clonidine (C) and yohimbine (Y) on neural activity of a slow-conducting cell. The record was obtained from a baroreceptor-denervated rat. Clonidine injection (18 µg/kg, i.v.) inhibited the neuron, an effect which could be antagonized by yohimbine (0.48 mg/kg). (E) Approximate locations of CVLM neurons which were antidromically activated by PVN stimulation. Open and closed circles indicate location of slow- and fast-conducting cells, respectively. Abbreviations as in Fig. 1.

latencies, these neurons could be divided into two groups; one had longer antidromic spike latencies (35.8 ± 8.5 msec, mean ± S.D., n = 47), than the other group (7.8 ± 3.0 msec, n = 24) (Fig. 4C). Assuming the distance between the recording and the stimulating electrodes to be 15 mm, the mean axon conduction velocities in the two groups were estimated to be 0.45 and 2.2 m/sec, respectively. Neurons of the first group, referred to as slow-conducting cells, had long duration action potentials (Fig. 4B). By contrast, neurons of the second group, referred to as fast-conducting cells, were characterized by action potentials with a sharp rising phase and a shorter duration (Fig.

4A). Slow-conducting cells fired irregularly at a slow rate, while the majority of the fast-conducting cells showed no spontaneous discharges. The spontaneous activity of 8 of 9 slow-conducting cells tested was reduced by i.v. clonidine administration (9–18 μg/kg). Clonidine injection produced a transient hypertension followed by delayed, long-lasting hypotension. The effects of clonidine could be consistently reversed by administration of the α_2-adrenergic antagonist, yohimbine (0.48 mg/kg). Clonidine and yohimbine had similar effects in baroreceptor-denervated and in normal rats, suggesting that the responses are not attributable to peripheral

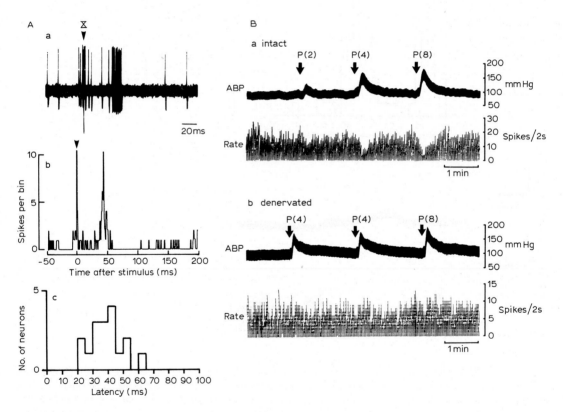

Fig. 5. Synaptic responses evoked by the cervical vagus nerves and the arterial baroreceptors in CVLM neurons which were antidromically activated by PVN stimulation. (A) Effect of stimulation of the vagus nerve on the firing rate of a slow-conducting cell. Arrowheads indicate time of stimulation. (Aa) An oscilloscope record of 20 superimposed sweeps; stimulus parameters were 100 μA and 0.5 msec. (Ab) Peristimulus time histogram of 75 sweeps obtained from the same cell. (Ac) Frequency distribution of onset latencies of excitatory responses of CVLM neurons to stimulation of the vagus nerves. (B) Effects of baroreceptor activation. Upper trace shows arterial blood pressure (ABP) and lower trace, ratemeter record of neural activity (Rate). (Ba) Example of a slow-conducting neuron which was inhibited by i.v. injection of phenylephrine (marked by P; numbers in parentheses indicate the amount of μg injected). (Bb) Example of a neuron in a baroreceptor-denervated rat which was unaffected by phenylephrine injection.

baroreceptor activation (Fig. 4D). Figure 4E shows the approximate location of neurons in the CVLM which were activated by PVN stimulation. These neurons were found particularly in the dorsolateral region of the lateral reticular nucleus; there was no difference in the locations of slow-conducting and fast-conducting neurons.

Cervical vagus nerve stimulation produced excitation in 16 of 20 slow-conducting cells tested (Fig. 5A). This response consisted of either a single spike or a burst of 2 – 3 spikes. Baroreceptor activation induced by i.v. administration of phenylephrine inhibited 10 of 21 slow-conducting cells tested (Fig. 5Ba). A similar elevation of blood pressure in baroreceptor-denervated rats was without effect on these cells, indicating that the responses were due to peripheral baroreceptor activation and not to direct effects of the drug on the recorded cells (Fig. 5Bb). The findings demonstrate that neurons in the rat CVLM project directly to the PVN and that some of these receive synaptic input from the vagus nerve and the baroreceptors.

Discussion

The present study demonstrates that putative vasopressin-secreting neurons in the PVN receive excitatory synaptic input from the CVLM. Histological examination showed that in order to be effective stimulation electrodes had to be located within or adjacent to the lateral reticular nucleus. The cell bodies of A1 catecholamine neurons have been shown to be situated in this area (Dahlstrom and Fuxe, 1964). Numerous catecholamine-containing axons terminate within the PVN (McNeill and Sladek, 1980; Swanson et al., 1981). By combined catecholamine fluorescence and retrograde transport studies, the catecholamine innervation of the PVN has been shown to be derived mainly from the A1 catecholamine cell group in the CVLM (Blessing et al., 1982; Sawchenko and Swanson, 1984). Studies of the role of catecholamines, especially noradrenaline, in the regulation of vasopressin

release have produced conflicting results (Sklar and Schrier, 1983). It has, however, been established in in vitro experiments that noradrenaline excites, via α_1-receptors, vasopressin-secreting neurons in the PVN and the supraoptic nucleus (SON) (Randle et al., 1984; Inenaga et al., 1986). Thus, it is possible that the excitatory responses observed in neurosecretory neurons of the PVN are, at least in part, mediated through catecholaminergic afferents of A1 origin. Our data agrees with the results of other investigators (Day et al., 1984). Presumed oxytocin-secreting cells were also excited by stimulation of the CVLM. In this regard, our results contrast with those of Day et al. (1984), who reported that electrical stimulation of the A1 area in the CVLM did not affect the neural activity of oxytocin-secreting neurons. The reason for the discrepancy between that report and the present results is not clear at present.

Tuberoinfundibular neurons, some of which might be CRF- or TRH-secreting cells (Lechan and Jackson, 1982; Antoni et al., 1983; Swanson et al., 1983; Nishiyama et al., 1985), were excited by electrical and chemical stimulation of the CVLM. This result agrees with a previous report (Day et al., 1985). While the functional role of catecholamines in the regulation of ACTH and TSH secretion remains controversial (Weiner and Ganong, 1978), our observations support the proposed facilitatory role of catecholamines acting at central sites on the secretion of these hormones (Smyth et al., 1983; Tapia-Arancibia et al., 1985).

CVLM neurons which project directly to the PVN could be subdivided into two different populations on the basis of their electrophysiological and pharmacological properties. The properties of slow-conducting cells were similar to those previously reported for catecholaminergic cells in other parts of the brain (Guyenet, 1980; Segal et al., 1983; Byrum et al., 1984). Thus, there is a possibility that some of the slow-conducting cells are catecholaminergic cells. Fast-conducting cells, on the other hand, may be non-catecholaminergic. In fact, anatomical studies have suggested that CVLM contains both catecholaminergic and non-catecholaminergic neurons which project directly to the PVN region (Loewy and Burton, 1978; Sawchenko and Swanson, 1981; Blessing et al., 1982).

The slow-conducting cells received inhibitory and excitatory inputs from the baroreceptors and from the vagus nerves, respectively. Neurons in the ventrolateral medulla projecting to the PVN have been reported, in cats, to receive synaptic inputs from buffer nerves (Ciriello and Caverson, 1984). Activation of baroreceptors and electrical stimulation of the vagus nerves have been shown to inhibit and excite PVN neurosecretory cells, respectively (Barker et al., 1971; Koizumi and Yamashita, 1978; Kannan and Yamashita, 1983). Latencies of antidromically evoked action potentials recorded from slow-conducting cells in the CVLM by PVN stimulation were similar to those of orthodromic excitatory responses evoked by CVLM stimulation. From these observations, it may be concluded that the slow-conducting cells in the CVLM, presumed to represent A1 catecholaminergic cells, which receive excitatory inputs from the vagus nerves and inhibitory inputs from baroreceptors, influence, in turn, PVN neurons via a monosynaptic excitatory pathway. The hypothesis is supported by evidence which shows that local application of the inhibitory neurotransmitters, γ-aminobutyric acid (GABA) and glycine, to the ventral surface of the medulla blocks the increase in plasma vasopressin concentration elicited by bilateral carotid occlusion (Feldberg and Rocha e Silva, 1981). Furthermore, direct injection of muscimol, a GABA agonist, into the CVLM completely abolished the secretion of vasopressin in response to hemorrhage and to constriction of the inferior vena cava (Blessing and Willoughby, 1985). On the other hand, depletion of catecholaminergic terminals, induced by 6-hydroxydopamine injection into the PVN, did not suppress the inhibitory responses of PVN neurosecretory cells to baroreceptor activation (Day et al., 1984). This finding indicates that catecholamines are not directly involved in most baroreceptor-induced inhibition of PVN neurosecretory cells. Recently, the local application of bicuculline, a GABA antagonist, has been reported to block the baroreceptor-induced inhibition of neurosecretory neurons in the PVN and SON (Jhamandas and Renaud, 1986; Kasai et al., 1987), suggesting a possible involvement of local GABAergic neurons. However, the possibility must be kept in mind that non-catecholaminergic, slow-conducting cells in the CVLM may also mediate baroreceptor-related information to the PVN neurons.

Summary

Both neurohypophyseal and tuberoinfundibular neurosecretory neurons in the PVN received excitatory synaptic inputs from the CVLM. We electrophysiologically identified neurons in the CVLM which project to the PVN. On the basis of antidromic spike latencies, two different populations of neurons could be differentiated: slow- and fast-conducting cells. Slow-conducting cells which were presumed to be A1 catecholaminergic cells, received inhibitory and excitatory synaptic inputs from arterial baroreceptors and the cervical vagus nerve, respectively. Our results suggest that slow conducting cells in the CVLM which cause excitation of PVN neurons via a monosynaptic pathway, mediate visceroreceptive information to the PVN.

Acknowledgements

The works presented in this chapter were supported in part by Grants-in-Aids for Scientific Research, nos. 57570056, 58440022, 62570078 and 63480118 from the Ministry of Education, Japan.

References

Antoni, F.A., Palkovits, M., Makara, G.B., Linton, E.A., Lowry, P.J. and Kiss, J.Z. (1983) Immunoreactive corticotrophin-releasing hormone in the hypothalamoinfundibular tract. *Neuroendocrinology*, 36: 415 – 423.

Barker, J.L., Crayton, J.W. and Nicoll, R.A. (1971) Antidromic and orthodromic responses of paraventricular and supraoptic neurosecretory cells. *Brain Res.*, 33: 353 – 366.

Blessing, W.W. and Reis, D.A. (1982) Inhibitory cardiovascular function of neurons in the caudal ventrolateral medulla of the rabbit: relationship to the area containing A1 noradrenergic cell. *Brain Res.*, 253: 161–171.

Blessing, W.W. and Willoughby, J.O. (1985) Inhibiting the rabbit caudal ventrolateral medulla prevents baroreceptor-initiated secretion of vasopressin. *J. Physiol. (Lond.)*, 367: 253–265.

Blessing, W.W., Jaeger, C.B., Ruggiero, D.A. and Reis, D.J. (1982) Hypothalamic projections of medullary catecholamine neurons in the rabbit: a combined catecholamine fluorescence and HRP transport study. *Brain Res. Bull.*, 9: 279–286.

Byrum, C.E., Stornetta, R. and Guyenet, P.G. (1984) Electrophysiological properties of spinally-projecting A5 noradrenergic neurons. *Brain Res.*, 303: 15–29.

Calaresu, F.R. and Ciriello, J. (1980) Projections to the hypothalamus from buffer nerves and nucleus tractus solitarius in the cat. *Am. J. Physiol.*, 239: R130–136.

Cameron, V., Espiner, E.A., Nicholls, M.G., Donald, R.A. and MacFarlane, M.R. (1984) Stress hormones in blood and cerebrospinal fluid of conscious sheep: effect of hemorrhage. *Endocrinology,* 115: 1460–1465.

Ciriello, J. and Calaresu, F.R. (1977) Lateral reticular nucleus: a site of somatic and cardiovascular integration in the cat. *Am. J. Physiol.*, 233: R100–R109.

Ciriello, J. and Calaresu, F.R. (1980) Monosynaptic pathway from cardiovascular neurons in the nucleus tractus solitarii to the paraventricular nucleus in the cat. *Brain Res.*, 193: 529–533.

Ciriello, J. and Caverson, M.M. (1984) Ventrolateral medullary neurons relay cardiovascular inputs to the paraventricular nucleus. *Am. J. Physiol.*, 246: R968–R978.

Cottle, M.K.W. and Calaresu, F.R. (1975) Projections from the nucleus and tractus solitarius in the cat. *J. Comp. Neurol.*, 161: 143–158.

Dahlstrom, A. and Fuxe, K. (1964) Evidence for the existence of monoamine-containing neurons in the central nervous system. I. Demonstration of monoamines in the cell bodies of brain stem neurons. *Acta Physiol. Scand.*, 62 Suppl. 232: 1–55.

Day, T.A., Ferguson, A.V. and Renaud, L.P. (1984) Facilitatory influence of noradrenergic afferents on the excitability of rat paraventricular nucleus neurosecretory cells. *J. Physiol. (Lond.)*, 355: 237–249.

Day, T.A., Ferguson, A.V. and Renaud, L.P. (1985) Noradrenergic afferents facilitate the activity of tuberoinfundibular neurons of the hypothalamic paraventricular nucleus. *Neuroendocrinology*, 41: 17–22.

Feldberg, W. and Rocha e Silva, M., Jr. (1981) Inhibition of vasopressin release to carotid occlusion by γ-aminobutyric acid and glycine. *Br. J. Pharmacol.*, 72: 17–24.

Guyenet, P.G. (1980) The coerulospinal noradrenergic neurons: anatomical and electrophysiological studies in the rat. *Brain Res.*, 189: 121–133.

Hamamura, M., Onaka, T. and Yagi, K. (1986) Parvocellular neurosecretory neurons: converging inputs after saphenous nerve and hypovolemic stimulations in the rat. *Jpn. J. Physiol.*, 36: 921–933.

Harris, M.C. (1979) Effects of chemoreceptor and baroreceptor stimulation on the discharge of hypothalamic supraoptic neurones in rats. *J. Endocrinol.*, 82: 115–125.

Inenaga, K., Dyball, R.E.J., Okuya, S. and Yamashita, H. (1986) Characterization of hypothalamic noradrenaline receptors in the supraoptic nucleus and periventricular region of the paraventricular nucleus of mice in vitro. *Brain Res.*, 369: 37–47.

Jhamandas, J.H. and Renaud, L.P. (1986) A γ-aminobutyric-acid-mediated baroreceptor input to supraoptic vasopressin neurones in the rat. *J. Physiol. (Lond.)*, 381: 595–606.

Kannan, H. and Yamashita, H. (1983) Electrophysiological study of paraventricular nucleus neurons projecting to the dorsomedial medulla and their responses to baroreceptor stimulation in rats. *Brain Res.*, 279: 31–40.

Kannan, H. and Yamashita, H. (1985) Connections of neurons in the region of the nucleus tractus solitarius with hypothalamic paraventricular nucleus: their possible involvement in neural control of the cardiovascular system in rats. *Brain Res.*, 329: 205–212.

Kannan, H., Yamashita, H. and Osaka, T. (1984) Paraventricular neurosecretory neurons: synaptic inputs from the ventrolateral medulla in rats. *Neurosci. Lett.*, 51: 183–188.

Kannan, H., Osaka, T., Kasai, M., Okuya, S. and Yamashita, H. (1986) Electrophysiological properties of neurons in the caudal ventrolateral medulla projecting to the paraventricular nucleus of the hypothalamus in rats. *Brain Res.*, 376: 342–350.

Kannan, H., Kasai, M., Osaka, T. and Yamashita, H. (1987) Neurons in the paraventricular nucleus projecting to the median eminence: a study of their afferent connections from peripheral baroreceptors, and from the A1-catecholaminergic area in the ventrolateral medulla. *Brain Res.*, 409: 358–363.

Kasai, M., Osaka, T., Inenaga, K., Kannan, H. and Yamashita, H. (1987) γ-Aminobutyric acid antagonist blocks baroreceptor-activated inhibition of neurosecretory cells in the hypothalamic paraventricular nucleus of rats. *Neurosci. Lett.*, 81: 319–324.

Koizumi, K. and Yamashita, H. (1978) Influence of atrial stretch receptors on hypothalamic neurosecretory neurons. *J. Physiol. (Lond.)*, 285: 341–358.

Lechan, R.M. and Jackson, I.M.D. (1982) Immunohistochemical localization of thyrotropin-releasing hormone in the rat hypothalamus and pituitary. *Endocrinology*, 111: 55–65.

Loewy, A.D. and Burton, H. (1978) Nuclei of the solitary tract: efferent projections to the lower brain stem and spinal cord of the cat. *J. Comp. Neurol.*, 181: 421–450.

302

McKellar, S. and Loewy, A.D. (1982) Efferent projections of the A1 catecholamine cell group in the rat: an autoradiographic study. *Brain Res.*, 241: 11 – 29.

McNeill, T.H. and Sladek, Jr., J.R. (1980) Simultaneous monoamine histofluorescence and neuropeptide immunocytochemistry. II. Correlative distribution of catecholamine varicosities and magnocellular neurosecretory neurons in the rat supraoptic and paraventricular nuclei. *J. Comp. Neurol.*, 193: 1023 – 1033.

Nishiyama, T., Kawano, H., Tsuruo, Y., Maegawa, M., Hisano, S., Adachi, T., Daikoku, S. and Suzuki, M. (1985) Hypothalamic thyrotropin-releasing hormone (TRH)-containing neurons involved in the hypothalamic-hypophysial thyroid axes. Light microscopic immunohistochemistry. *Brain Res.*, 345: 205 – 218.

Perrin, J. and Crousillat, J. (1983) Splanchnic afferent input to the lateral reticular nucleus of the cat. *J. Auton. Nerv. Syst.*, 8: 383 – 393.

Plotsky, P.M. and Vale, W. (1984) Hemorrhage-induced secretion of corticotropin-releasing factor-like immunoreactivity into the rat hypophysial portal circulation and its inhibition by glucocorticoids. *Endocrinology*, 114: 164 – 169.

Poulain, D.A. and Wakerley, J.B. (1982) Electrophysiology of hypothalamic magnocellular neurons secreting oxytocin and vasopressin. *Neuroscience*, 7: 773 – 808.

Randle, J.C.R., Bourque, C.W. and Renaud, L.P. (1984) α-Adrenergic activation of rat hypothalamic supraoptic neurons maintained in vitro. *Brain Res.*, 307: 374 – 378.

Sawchenko, P.E. and Swanson, L.W. (1981) Central noradrenergic pathways for the integration of hypothalamic neuroendocrine and autonomic responses. *Science*, 214: 685 – 687.

Segal, M., Foote, S.L. and Aston-Jones, G. (1983) Physiological properties of ascending locus coeruleus axons in the squirrel monkey. *Brain Res.*, 274: 381 – 387.

Sklar, A.H. and Schrier, R.W. (1983) Central nervous system mediators of vasopressin release. *Physiol. Rev.*, 63: 1243 – 1280.

Smythe, G.A., Brandshaw, J.E. and Vining, R.F. (1983) Hypothalamic monoamine control of stress-induced adrenocorticotropin release in the rat. *Endocrinology*, 113: 1062 – 1071.

Spyer, K.M. (1982) Central nervous integration of cardiovascular control. *J. Exp. Biol.*, 100: 109 – 128.

Swanson, L.W. and Sawchenko, P.E. (1983) Hypothalamic integration: organization of the paraventricular and supraoptic nuclei. *Annu. Rev. Neurosci.*, 6: 269 – 324.

Swanson, L.W., Sawchenko, P.E., Berod, A., Hartman, B.K., Helle, K.B. and Vanorden, D.E. (1981) An immunohistochemical study of the organization of catecholaminergic cells and terminal fields in the paraventricular and supraoptic nuclei of the hypothalamus. *J. Comp. Neurol.*, 196: 271 – 285.

Swanson, L.W., Sawchenko, P.E., Rivier, J. and Vale, W.W. (1983) Organization of ovine corticotropin-releasing factor immunoreactive cells and fibers in the rat brain: an immunohistochemical study. *Neuroendocrinology*, 36: 165 – 186.

Tapia-Arancibia, L., Arancibia, S. and Astier, H. (1985) Evidence for α_1-adrenergic stimulatory control of in vitro release of immunoreactive thyrotropin-releasing hormone from rat median eminence: in vivo corroboration. *Endocrinology*, 116: 2314 – 2319.

Tribollet, E. and Dreifuss, J.J. (1981) Localization of neurones projecting to the hypothalamic paraventricular nucleus area of the rat: a horseradish peroxidase study. *Neuroscience*, 6: 1315 – 1328.

Weiner, R.I. and Ganong, W. (1978) Role of brain monoamines and histamine in regulation of anterior pituitary secretion. *Physiol. Rev.*, 58: 905 – 976.

J. Ciriello, M.M. Caverson and C. Polosa (Eds.)
Progress in Brain Research, Vol. 81
© 1989 Elsevier Science Publishers B.V. (Biomedical Division)

CHAPTER 24

Control of neurosecretory vasopressin cells by noradrenergic projections of the caudal ventrolateral medulla

Trevor A. Day

Department of Physiology and the Neuroscience Centre, University of Otago Medical School, Dunedin, New Zealand

Introduction

While the autonomic nervous system is recognized as the most rapidly acting extrinsic regulator of the circulation, humoral mechanisms also play an essential role in circulatory control. The manner in which autonomic, humoral and local autoregulatory control systems overlap and interact forms the basis for cardiovascular homeostasis, but has also served to obscure the significance of the less dramatic humoral contribution. This is particularly true in the case of the neurohypophysial hormone arginine vasopressin (AVP). Better known for its antidiuretic actions, the vasomotor effects of AVP were long considered of limited importance as supraphysiological concentrations are generally required to elevate arterial pressure in intact, normotensive animals. AVP is now known to be an extremely potent vasoconstrictor, however, an attribute masked by this peptide's unique ability to enhance baroreflex buffering to its own pressor actions (Cowley et al., 1983; Undesser et al., 1985).

Physiological stimuli capable of producing reflex alterations in AVP secretion, such as haemorrhage or pain, are well characterized. Much less certain, however, are the identities of the pathways by which relevant sensory information entering the central nervous system at the level of the medulla oblongata or spinal cord reaches neurosecretory AVP cells of the hypothalamus. Considerable attention has been devoted to the possible involvement of noradrenergic (NA) projections arising from the caudal ventrolateral medulla (McKellar and Loewy, 1981; Sawchenko and Swanson, 1981). Anatomical studies suggest that visceral afferent information is relayed to the ventrolateral medulla (VLM) via both ventrolaterally directed projections from the nucleus of the tractus solitarius (NTS) and ascending spinoreticular projections (Loewy and Burton, 1978; Ricardo and Koh, 1978; Sawchenko and Swanson, 1981; Menetrey et al., 1983; Perrin and Crousillat, 1983; Ross et al., 1985). These inputs are thought to contribute to circulatory regulation both by altering the activity of VLM efferent projections controlling autonomic outflow to the heart and vascular beds (Ciriello et al., 1986, for review) and by altering the NA output of the caudal VLM to the supraoptic (SON) and paraventricular (PVN) nuclei, those areas in which neurosecretory AVP synthesizing perikarya are concentrated.

Actions of noradrenaline and A1 projections

It has long been known that the SON and PVN are the recipients of perhaps the densest NA innervation of any region of the entire CNS (Fuxe, 1965). More recently, it has been demonstrated that the bulk of this innervation, particularly in the case of the SON and the magnocellular division of PVN, arises from the A1 cell group of the caudal VLM (McKellar and Loewy, 1981; Sawchenko and Swanson, 1981). While some earlier pharmacological data suggested that NA was inhibitory to neurosecretory cell activity, a sizable body of evidence has now accrued in support of the view that both NA itself, at low concentrations, and A1 afferent fibre activation, excites AVP cells and stimulates AVP secretion (Day et al., 1985c; Day, 1987).

In keeping with the preferential termination of noradrenergic terminal fibres in the region of AVP rather than oxytocin (OXY) immunoreactive perikarya (McNeill and Sladek, 1980; Sawchenko and Swanson, 1981), the excitatory effects of the A1 input generally appear to be preferentially directed at AVP rather than OXY neurosecretory cells (Day and Renaud, 1984; Day et al., 1984; see also Kannan et al., 1984). This effect may also arise in part from a differential sensitivity of AVP and OXY cells to the effects of NA, as NA has been noted to have a brisker action on functionally identified AVP than OXY cells (Day et al., 1985c), and stimulates the release of considerably greater quantities of AVP than OXY from perfused hypothalamic explants (Randle et al., 1986a).

The excitatory effects of applied NA on AVP cell activity and AVP secretion are mimicked by the application of α_1-adrenoreceptor agonists and blocked by α_1-adrenoreceptor antagonists (Randle et al., 1984; Day et al., 1985c; Armstrong et al., 1986; Willoughby et al., 1987; Yamashita et al., 1987), prompting the conclusion that the stimulatory effects of A1 afferents are mediated via the actions of NA upon post-synaptic α_1-adrenoreceptors. We have observed, however, that SON cell responses to A1 stimulation are unaltered by systemic, intracerebroventricular, or direct SON application of α-adrenoreceptor antagonists in doses 100 – 1500 times that required to block excitatory effects of locally applied NA (Fig. 1) (Day, 1987; Day and Sibbald, 1989). It must be conceded, although it seems unlikely in view of the doses

used, that this finding may simply reflect a failure of the antagonist to access intra-synaptic post-junctional receptors. Such an explanation would be in line with the "intimacy theory" first proposed by Dale and Gaddum (1930) to explain the failure of atropine to block some of the effects of parasympathetic nerve activation; consistent with this scenario, NA afferents have now been shown to make true synaptic contacts with neurosecretory cells (Alonso and Assenmacher, 1984; Silverman et al., 1985), rather than the type of loose contacts previously reported in some CNS regions (Descarries and Lapierre, 1973). On the other hand, it is pertinent to note that while A1 stimulation elicits quite brief changes in neurosecretory cell discharge probability (30 – 50 msec; see Fig. 1) which are

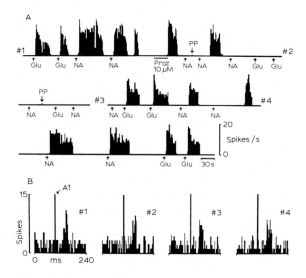

Fig. 1. In vivo extracellular recordings demonstrating responses of a phasically active, putative AVP-secreting SON cell to local pressure application of drugs (A) and stimulation of the A1 cell group region of the caudal VLM (B). This unit was excited by both glutamate (Glu) and NA (both at 100 μM for 10 sec). Local application of a high concentration of the α_1-antagonist prazosin (Praz; 10 μM, 30 sec) initially blocked both NA and glutamate effects, suggesting a lack of specificity at this dose. Glutamate responses recovered first, NA responses later. Time between ratemeter segments: 15, 35 and 20 min. PP = posterior pituitary stimulation for verification of antidromic spike. The response of this unit to A1 region stimulation (100 μA, 0.5 msec pulse) was essentially unaltered throughout, as indicated by the series of peristimulus histograms in (B) (timing of collection shown by corresponding numbers in A).

consistent with the occurrence of a "fast" excitatory post-synaptic potential (PSP), a review of the relevant literature suggests that neurally released NA, acting via α- or β-adrenoreceptors, is incapable of producing PSPs of less than hundreds of milliseconds in duration, at the very least (e.g. see Egan et al., 1983; Yoshimura et al., 1987). Those studies which have investigated the mode of action of exogenously applied NA on neurosecretory cells indicate that while NA depolarizes membrane potential via α_1-adrenoreceptor activation, it does so in a relatively unconventional fashion involving the inhibition of a resting outward K^+ current (Randle et al., 1986b). This mechanism seems unlikely to be compatible with the generation of a "fast" PSP. In general, it is noteworthy that the only instances where neurally released NA has been argued to be capable of eliciting "fast" post-synaptic events is in certain sympathetically innervated tissues such as arteriolar smooth muscle where the existence of specialized intra-synaptic "γ"-adrenoreceptors has been postulated (Hirst et al., 1985, for review). If the situation in SON were analogous, then the excitatory effects of applied NA would be explained on the basis of an extra-synaptic population of α_1-adrenoreceptors, pharmacologically distinct from the intra-synaptic γ-adrenoreceptor population which would primarily, and perhaps exclusively, be accessed by neurally released NA.

Possible A1 afferent co-transmitters

Neuropeptide Y

The difficulties experienced in blocking the excitatory effects of A1 afferents on AVP cell discharge led naturally to a consideration of the possible involvement of a novel co-transmitter in the expression of A1 input effects. Immunohistochemical studies have demonstrated the existence of neuropeptide Y (NPY) in A1 cells (Everitt et al., 1984) and the application of this peptide has been shown to excite a small proportion of SON AVP cells and to stimulate AVP

release (Day et al., 1985b; Willoughby and Blessing, 1987). In recent in vitro studies we have confirmed that the direct excitatory effects of NPY on SON cells are usually exceedingly modest (Wilson et al., 1988; see Fig. 2). This suggests that NPY is unlikely to be the primary neurotransmitter utilized by A1 afferents and indeed, as was discussed above with respect to NA, there is yet to be a demonstration in any system that any neuropeptide is capable of mediating fast synaptic events of the type apparently involved in the interaction between A1 afferents and SON AVP cells. Thus, in the two cases where probably the strongest evidence has been provided for the involvement of a neuropeptide in the process of neurotransmission, substance P and LHRH-like peptide, evoked events range from seconds to minutes in duration (Dun, 1985; Jan and Jan, 1985).

In these same in vitro studies on the actions of NPY, however, evidence was obtained of facilitatory NA/NPY interactions which appear to be very similar to that reported for NA and NPY on vascular smooth muscle when co-released from sympathetic post-ganglionic fibres (Edvinsson et al., 1987). Thus, while NPY at concentrations up to 10^{-6} M had unreliable direct effects on AVP cell discharge, NPY at concentrations down to

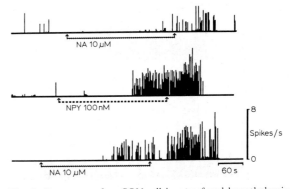

Fig. 2. Responses of an SON cell in a perfused hypothalamic slice to bath application of NA and NPY. This unit, which displayed occasional, brief burst discharges at rest, was mildly excited by NA and showed an unusually pronounced response to NPY. Re-application of NA shortly after NPY elicited a much greater response than previously, suggesting a potentiation of NA effects.

10^{-8} M markedly potentiated the excitatory effects of low doses of NA (Fig. 2) (Wilson et al., 1988).

Excitatory amino acids

A recent report that application of a broad-spectrum excitatory amino acid (EAA) antagonist abolishes spontaneous excitatory PSPs in SON cells examined in vitro has resulted in the suggestion that EAAs may be the major type of excitatory transmitter utilized by SON afferents (Gribkoff and Dudek, 1988). We have now examined this suggestion in vivo with respect to the A1 input to SON cells (Day and Sibbald, 1989). Brief applications of the EAA antagonist kynurenic acid inhibited spontaneous discharge in all SON AVP cells tested, an effect which usually endured for at least several minutes beyond termination of application. During this period of inhibition the excitability of all cells tested appeared to be non-specifically depressed, applications of NA or carbachol, as well as glutamate, failing to excite cells in the usual manner. During periods of prolonged (> 10 min) exposure to kynurate, however, a slow recovery of excitability was evidenced by the reappearance of spontaneous activity and a return of NA and carbachol evoked burst discharges. These findings were interpreted as being consistent with kynurenate application initially hyperpolarizing cells albeit indirectly by reducing the ongoing level of excitatory input, and cell membrane potential then gradually recovering and reapproaching the threshold for action potential initiation. Such effects would be analogous to the sequelae of synaptic isolation on SON neurosecretory cells observed in vitro: an initial cessation of spontaneous activity followed by a slow return (Andrew, 1987). Of particular significance, however, was the observation that, following spontaneous recovery of excitability during extended kynurenate application, the excitatory

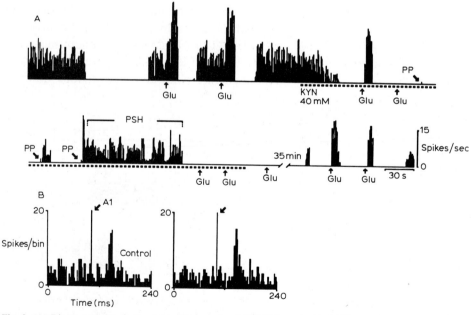

Fig. 3. (A) Direct pressure application of kynurenic acid (KYN) on to this SON putative AVP cell suppressed spontaneous discharge and blocked the excitatory effects of locally applied glutamate (Glu, 100 μM, 10 sec). After an initial period of quiescence (5 min between upper and lower ratemeter segments) activity could be evoked by a single antidromic invasion from posterior pituitary (PP; see Andrew and Dudek, 1984, for discussion of rationale), allowing PSH collection. Responses to glutamate did not recover until approximately 30 min after cessation of kynurenate application. (B) Comparison of peristimulus histograms collected before (control) and during kynurenate application indicated no change in response to A1 region stimulation (100 μA, 0.5 msec pulse).

effects of A1 stimulation on SON cells remained intact, despite the persistence of a total blockade of glutamate excitations (Fig. 3). As was noted with respect to the failure of α-adrenoreceptor antagonists to block A1 excitations, it may be argued that the inability of kynurenate to block A1 inputs simply reflects a failure of the antagonist to access intra-synaptic post-junctional receptors; if this were the case it would seem necessary to postulate that the inhibitory actions of kynurenate on spontaneous activity were due to elimination of antagonist accessible synaptic inputs to SON cells, whereas A1 inputs were in a special category having inaccessible synaptic clefts.

Noradrenergic projections from the A2 group of NTS

Tracing studies and effects of NTS stimulation on SON cells

Investigations of the role of NA afferents in the control of AVP secretion progressed rapidly following the demonstration that the A1 cell group is the primary source of NA projections to the SON and the magnocellular division of PVN (McKellar and Loewy, 1981; Sawchenko and Swanson, 1981). Subsequent tracing studies, however, have demonstrated that the NTS also provides direct, albeit sparse projections to both SON and PVN neurosecretory cells and that a significant proportion of this projection arises from the A2 NA cell group (Fig. 4) (Tribollet et al., 1985; Cunningham and Sawchenko, 1988; Day and Sibbald, 1988a). In contrast to the preferential termination of A1 projection fibres in the region of AVP perikarya, NTS projections have been reported to be distributed amongst both AVP and OXY cells (Cunningham and Sawchenko, 1988), although subsequent work suggests that non-aminergic subcomponent projections may selectively target those regions in which OXY perikarya are concentrated (Sawchenko et al., 1988a,b).

On the basis of these anatomical data one would anticipate that NTS stimulation might influence the activity of both AVP and OXY cells. Indeed,

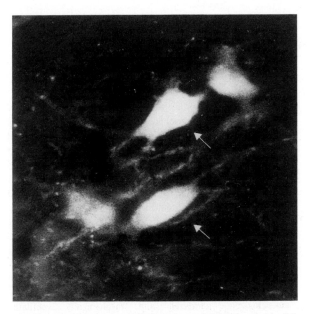 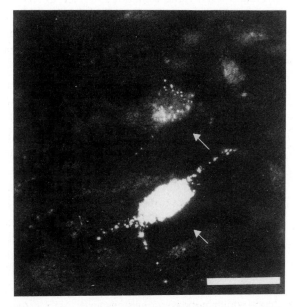

Fig. 4. A2 catecholamine cells (left) in medial NTS at level of the caudal aspect of the area postrema, two of which are retrogradely labelled (right) 24 h after injection of rhodamine-labelled microspheres into ipsilateral SON; on average just over half of all NTS cells labelled by SON injections of retrograde tracer were found to be catecholaminergic (see Day and Sibbald, 1988a for details of methodology).

308

this has previously been demonstrated in the case of PVN neurosecretory neurons (Day et al., 1984; see below for discussion) and a preliminary report from Raby and Renaud (1987; see also chapter by Renaud and Raby, this volume) indicates that they have made similar observations with respect to SON. We, however, have recently reported that NTS stimulation predominantly excites AVP rather than OXY SON cells (Day and Sibbald, 1988b). This discrepancy is difficult to understand, although part of the explanation may lie in the fact that our studies were confined primarily to the caudal SON, where AVP perikarya are concentrated. Thus, if direct NTS to SON projections primarily influence the rostral, OXY-rich component of SON as suggested by some work (Sawchenko et al., 1988a,b), then those relatively few OXY cells located in the caudal SON may lie outside the sphere of influence of the NTS projection.

The similarity which we observed (Day and Sibbald, 1988b) between the effects of NTS stimulation and those previously reported following A1 stimulation (Day and Renaud, 1984) led us to consider the possibility that, despite the existence of a direct projection, the effects of NTS stimulation on SON AVP cell activity might be attributable to activation of a relay projection through the A1 cell group. Such a possibility would also be consistent with anatomical evidence of an NTS projection to the A1 region (Loewy and Burton, 1978; Ricardo and Koh, 1978; Sawchenko and Swanson, 1981; Ross et al., 1985). Direct comparison of NTS and A1 region activation effects in animals with stimulating electrodes simultaneously positioned at both locations have now shown that 90% of AVP cells respond identically to stimulation of either NTS or the A1 region (Day and Sibbald, 1988c). Moreover, the mean latency to onset of excitation was 51 ± 1 msec following NTS stimulation and 38 ± 1 msec following A1 region stimulation, a delay which appears consistent with NTS effects involving a relay through some other region such as the VLM. This suggestion receives strong support from our additional finding that interruption

of A1 region neuronal function, either by electrolytic lesions or microinjection of the inhibitory neurotransmitter γ-aminobutyric acid, abolished the excitatory effects of NTS stimulation on putative AVP cells (Fig. 5). These data are most readily interpreted as indicating that NTS effects on SON AVP cells are relayed specifically via the A1 cell group. Such an arrangement would also serve to explain a previous report that AVP-induced pressor effects elicited in cord-sectioned animals by NTS injections of the excito-toxin

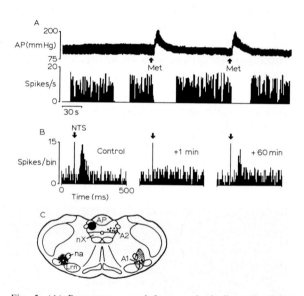

Fig. 5. (A) Ratemeter record from a phasically active SON neurosecretory cell; arterial baroreceptor activation, which was achieved by i.v. injection of the vasoconstrictor metaraminol (Met), inhibited cell discharge. (B) Stimulation of the ipsilateral NTS (100 µA, 0.5 msec) excited this unit, an effect which was reversibly blocked by inhibition of neuronal function in the A1 region, as indicated by peristimulus histograms collected 1 and 60 min after ipsilateral caudal VLM injection of γ-aminobutyric acid (50 nmol in 100 nl). (C) Diagrammatic representation of coronal section through the caudal medulla, illustrating location of NTS stimulation site, ipsilateral VLM injection site marked by inclusion of Alcian Blue in the injectate, and the extent of a contralaterally positioned VLM electrolytic lesion made at the commencement of the experiment. Animal was anaesthetized, paralyzed and mechanically ventilated throughout. Note that the ratemeter sequence in (A) was collected immediately after the "1 min" PSH in (B), suggesting that A1 region function does not contribute to the baroreceptor inhibition of AVP cells.

kainic acid were blocked by prior injection of kainic acid into the caudal VLM (Kubo et al., 1985).

Comparison of NTS activation effects on SON and PVN cells

Evidence that the NTS projects onto both OXY and AVP neurosecretory cells (Cunningham and Sawchenko, 1988) would appear to explain an earlier report that NTS stimulation excites both neurosecretory cell types in PVN, whereas A1 stimulation preferentially excites AVP cells (Day et al., 1984). In view of the findings discussed above with respect to SON, however, could the effects of NTS stimulation on PVN neurosecretory AVP cells also be mediated by the A1 cell group? While this possibility cannot be eliminated without direct testing, the available data suggests that it is unlikely. Firstly, there was no difference in PVN cell response latencies following NTS versus A1 stimulation (Day et al., 1984); secondly, while SON AVP cells respond only to NTS stimulation at levels which give rise to A1-directed projections (Day and Sibbald, 1988b), effects on PVN AVP cells could readily be elicited by stimulation at all levels of NTS where A2 catecholamine cells were present (Day et al., 1984).

If both SON and PVN neurosecretory AVP cells receive a direct projection from NTS, why are the effects of NTS stimulation relayed via the A1 cell group in the case of SON cells but not in the case of PVN cells? A plausible explanation for the effectiveness of the NTS direct projection in the case of PVN AVP cells may lie in the fact that the NTS projects not only to the magnocellular division of PVN, but also to the immediately adjacent parvocellular division (Sawchenko and Swanson, 1981; Cunningham and Sawchenko, 1988). Thus, NTS projections to SON and PVN neurosecretory AVP cell perikarya may be so sparse as to be of little functional significance, but in the case of PVN neurosecretory cells NTS projection fibres could make significant direct contacts with dendrites which are known to extend well into the adjacent

parvocellular region (van den Pol, 1982). Consistent with this possibility, Silverman and coworkers (1985) have provided evidence at the ultrastructural level that AVP-immunoreactive neurosecretory cell dendrites in the parvocellular PVN do receive synaptic contacts from afferent NA fibres.

Physiological role of A1 projections to AVP cells

Much attention has already been devoted to what one might have assumed to be the simple question of whether NA afferents generally, and the A1 projection in particular, are excitatory or inhibitory to neurosecretory AVP cell discharge and thus AVP secretion. From the preceding discussion it is apparent that investigation of this question has been unexpectedly complicated by issues such as whether NA is even the primary neurotransmitter in this pathway. Ultimately, however, this work must constitute little more than a necessary preamble to determining the physiological role of the A1 cell group in the control of AVP secretion. In this regard it seems necessary for us to eventually be able to define precisely what type of sensory information is provided to A1 cells and, even more importantly, precisely which of these types of information are passed on to AVP cells solely or at least primarily via the A1 projection. To date, with but one or two notable exceptions (e.g. Blessing and Willoughby, 1985), the role of the A1 input to AVP cells has largely been inferred from anatomical studies demonstrating certain key projections to the A1 region, such as that from the NTS, and from electrophysiological studies in which the responses of putative A1 cells to certain stimuli have been tested. With respect to the latter, a particular concern is the tendency to construe A1 cell responsiveness to an input as evidence of a role in relaying that information to AVP cells. Clearly a careful distinction must be drawn between receiving information and being the primary conduit for that information. A further concern is the need to carefully specify the sensory inputs being investigated. Thus, while stimuli such as haemorrhage, common carotid occlusion and cardiac buffer nerve sectioning or stimulation have all been demonstrated to alter AVP cell discharge, AVP secretion, and in some instances even putative A1 cell discharge, the precise identity of the sensory receptors involved is uncertain, rendering the significance of these observations difficult to assess.

Circulatory pressure receptor inputs

Activation of arterial baroreceptors or atrial stretch receptors inhibits AVP secretion and cell discharge (Koizumi and Yamashita, 1978; Harris, 1979; Ledsome, 1985) and it has been shown that vasoconstrictor-induced increases in arterial pressure (Kannan et al., 1986) or constriction of the descending aorta (McAllen and Blessing, 1987) inhibits putative A1 cells. Consequently, it has been postulated that a withdrawal of stimulatory A1 input activity may underlie the inhibitory effects of baroreceptor activation on AVP cell discharge (McAllen and Blessing, 1987). Such a suggestion, however, would require that A1 cells provide a tonic excitatory drive to AVP cells and ignores evidence that baroreceptor inhibition of AVP cells is not prevented by destruction of SON and PVN NA afferents (Day and Renaud, 1984; Day et al., 1984). Although VLM lesions sometimes block baroreceptor inhibition of AVP cells (Banks and Harris, 1984), this may stem from the fact that a proportion of ascending NTS fibres first pass through the VLM (Sawchenko and Swanson, 1982); in accord with this interpretation we have recently noted in the course of other work that pharmacological blockade of A1 region function does not alter the effects of baroreceptor activation on AVP cells (Fig. 5) (Day and Sibbald, 1988c). Indeed, rather than A1 projection fibres relaying inhibitory baroreceptor information to neurosecretory AVP cells, current evidence favours the involvement of a polysynaptic pathway which passes through both locus coeruleus and diagonal band of Broca and which uses γ-aminobutyric acid as the final neurotransmitter

(Banks and Harris, 1984; Jhamandas and Renaud, 1986, 1987).

Whereas arterial baroreceptor or atrial stretch receptor activation inhibits AVP release, stimuli commonly thought to act by unloading these receptors, such as haemorrhage, have the converse effect (Ledsome, 1985). With respect to the central pathways underlying this inverse relationship between circulatory pressure receptor activity and AVP plasma levels, the simplest circuit imaginable would involve one tonically active input to AVP cells, the activity of which could be increased or decreased as appropriate. While such a scheme appears to have generally dominated thinking on this issue, it now seems increasingly unlikely to be accurate. For example, while blockade of local γ-aminobutyric acid receptors prevents baroreceptor inhibition of SON AVP cells, it does not generally increase their basal discharge rate as would be expected if this pathway was tonically active (Jhamandas and Renaud, 1987). Admittedly this input may be more active in an unanaesthetized preparation, but it is clear that consideration should be given to the possibility that the effects of pressure receptor unloading on AVP cells may depend upon the activation of different or additional central pathways to those whose activity changes in response to activation of these same receptors. In particular, while it is unlikely that A1 afferents feature in the inhibitory effects of baroreceptor and atrial stretch receptor activation on neurosecretory AVP cells, they may participate in the stimulatory effects elicited by the unloading of these receptors. Consistent with this possibility it has been demonstrated that acute reduction of venous return by constriction of the vena cava excites putative A1 cells (McAllen and Blessing, 1987), that blockade of neuronal function in the A1 region abolishes the stimulatory effects of both caval constriction and haemorrhage on AVP secretion (Blessing and Willoughby, 1985), and that haemorrhage stimulates the release of NA in the SON (Kendrick and Leng, 1988). Collectively these findings appear to offer the clearest information yet available on the physiological role of the A1 cell group in the control of AVP cells and secretion, although even here certain questions remain.

Unfortunately, it is by no means certain that caval constriction and haemorrhage actually exert their influence on AVP cells exclusively or even primarily by unloading arterial baroreceptors and/or atrial stretch receptors. It has been noted that haemorrhage invariably elicits a considerably larger rise in AVP secretion than complete interruption of sino-aortic and vagal afferents, leading to the suggestion that the effects of haemorrhage on AVP release may not be due so much to unloading arterial baroreceptors and/or atrial stretch receptors as to the activation of other receptors (Bishop et al., 1984; Ledsome, 1985). Possible candidates for this role include chemoreceptors, which might be activated by ischaemia-induced metabolic acidosis, and cardiac ventricular mechanoreceptors, whose firing increases in response to falls in ventricular pressure (Oberg and Thoren, 1972; Wang et al., 1988). Consistent with the existence of cardiac receptors whose activation might stimulate AVP release via an A1 projection, it has been shown that stimulation of the central cut end of the cervical vagus stimulates neurosecretory cell discharge and AVP secretion (Dyball, 1968; Dyball and Koizumi, 1969), and excites putative A1 cells (Kannan et al., 1986). This pathway seems likely to correspond to that which is activated by NTS stimulation (Day and Sibbald, 1988c).

Arterial chemoreceptor inputs

Selective activation of arterial chemoreceptors excites SON AVP cells and stimulates the secretion of AVP into the circulation (Share and Levy, 1966; Harris, 1979), but evidence concerning a role in this effect for the VLM, and the A1 cell group in particular, is largely equivocal. While it has been demonstrated that application of inhibitory neurotransmitters to the ventral surface of the caudal VLM blocks the release of AVP normally elicited by carotid occlusion (Feldberg and Rocha e Silva, 1981), it is uncertain whether the effects of

this particular stimulus are attributable to chemoreceptor activation or baroreceptor unloading, or whether the site of neurochemical blockade is the A1 group. Banks and Harris (1984) report that VLM lesions frequently block chemoreceptor activation of SON AVP cells, although in every case where such lesions blocked chemoreceptor responses the effects of baroreceptor activation were also blocked, raising again the question of whether these lesions interrupted NTS ascending projections rather than specifically disrupting A1 projections (see above). Perhaps the most intriguing evidence relating to this question are reports, again from Harris and coworkers (Harris et al., 1984, 1987; Banks and Harris, 1988), that carotid chemoreceptor activation excites ipsilateral SON AVP cells, but not PVN or contralateral SON cells, and that the pathway via which chemoreceptor afferent information ascends passes through the rostromedial hypothalamus before reaching SON. These details do not fit with the known projection pattern of the A1 cell group, which innervates both SON and PVN (McKellar and Loewy, 1981; Sawchenko and Swanson, 1981), nor the excitatory effect of A1 stimulation on neurosecretory AVP cells of PVN as well as SON (Day and Renaud, 1983; Day et al., 1984). Finally, in recent preliminary studies we found that bilateral lesions of the A1 region which blocked the excitatory effect of NTS stimulation on SON AVP cells (Day and Sibbald, 1988c) failed to affect the responses of such cells to chemoreceptor activation. This finding is seemingly at variance with the observations of Banks and Harris (1984), as discussed above, but may be explained by the lesions being situated somewhat caudoventral to theirs, thus eliminating A1 cells while avoiding interruption of ascending NTS projections.

Spinal afferent inputs

To date, relatively little attention has been given to the role of spinal afferent information in the control of AVP release, or the pathways by which such information might access SON and PVN AVP cells. Activation of hepato-portal osmoreceptors or renal sensory nerves, both of which convey information to the CNS via spinal afferents (Vallet and Baertschi, 1982; Ciriello and Calaresu, 1983), preferentially excites SON AVP cells (Baertschi and Vallet, 1981; Day and Ciriello, 1985), a pattern reminiscent of the AVP selective effects of A1 stimulation. With respect to renal afferent information, subsequent work revealed that SON AVP cells responded to renal infusion of the algesic substances capsaicin and bradykinin, but not to manoeuvres known to activate established renal receptor types (Day and Ciriello, 1987). It seems reasonable to suggest then that the renal afferents prompting AVP cell activation only do so in response to noxious stimuli, whether these afferents are solely nociceptive or respond to other stimuli as well and only in effect signal noxious events at higher levels of activation, as suggested for some intestinal sensory afferents (Blumberg et

al., 1983), remains to be determined. Noxious stimuli have certainly been shown to excite neurosecretory cells and enhance AVP secretion (Tata and Buzalkov, 1966; Hamamura et al., 1984), perhaps as part of an "early warning" system to allow circulatory adjustments appropriate to tissue damage likely to entail subsequent blood loss. Consistent with a role for the A1 cell group in the nociceptive activation of AVP cells it is clear that the caudal VLM receives spinoreticular projections conveying nociceptive information (Menetrey et al., 1983; Perrin and Crousillat, 1983; Sotgiu, 1986) and preliminary evidence has been obtained that neurons in the A1 region are involved in the excitation of AVP cells following nociceptor activation (Fig. 6).

Role of A1 projections in the control of other functions

Investigations of the physiological role of the A1 cell group have invariably focussed on the control of a specific function, and a number of studies have been directed at determining whether certain critical information that is perceived as being important in the regulation of that function, such as baroreceptor or chemoreceptor activity in the case of AVP control, is relayed via the A1 projection. Although valid, such an approach may ultimately prove too narrow, ignoring as it does the probable diversity of function of the A1 group. Thus it is well established that the A1 group projects to areas other than SON and the magnocellular division of the PVN (e.g. Day et al., 1980; McKellar and Loewy, 1982; Saper et al., 1983), and that A1 stimulation affects the activity of a variety of other cell types, such as septal, preoptic, and tuberoinfundibular neurons (e.g. Day et al., 1984; Kannan et al., 1987; Kim et al., 1987). In some cases the widespread distribution of A1 projection fibres may serve to co-ordinate related responses. For example, involvement of a NA mechanism in the control of adrenocorticotrophin secretion is well established (Carlson and Gann, 1987; Plotsky, 1987) and a common input to neurosecretory AVP

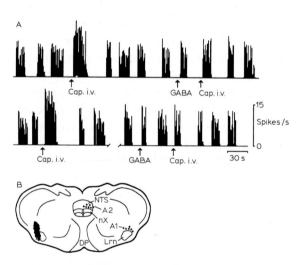

Fig. 6. (A) Injection of the algesic substance capsaicin (4 μg in 0.1 ml) into the femoral artery while occluding the femoral vein excited this contralaterally located, phasically active SON neurosecretory cell. Microinjection of γ-aminobutyric acid (80 nmol in 100 nl) into the caudal ventrolateral medulla reversibly blocked this effect. (B) Diagrammatic representation of coronal section through the caudal medulla, illustrating location of VLM injection site as marked by inclusion of Alcian Blue in the injectate. Note correspondence between injection site and A1 cell group position.

and tuberoinfundibular corticotrophin-releasing factor neurons from A1 neurons might well serve to explain the parallel shifts frequently observed in neurohypophysial AVP secretion and pituitary-adrenal axis activity (Raff et al., 1983; Lee et al., 1986).

One issue of particular interest has been the question of A1 cell group involvement in the autonomic as opposed to humoral control of the circulation. Evidence presented by Coote and MacLeod (1974a,b) originally suggested that A1 cells might provide an inhibitory projection to spinal sympathetic neurons. The majority of relevant anatomical studies have since shown that the A1 cell group does not provide any significant descending projections (McKellar and Loewy, 1982), but nevertheless it has been established that stimulation of neuronal perikarya within the caudal VLM lowers arterial pressure by inhibiting sympathetic outflow (Blessing and Reis, 1982). Although evidence was presented at an early stage that the caudal VLM depressor area did not correspond to the A1 cell group, at least in the rat (Day et al., 1983), it was still considered likely by some workers that this depressor effect might be mediated by an inhibitory projection from the A1 cell group to sympathoexcitatory neurons of the rostral VLM (Willette et al., 1984; Granata et al., 1986). This proposal of course is difficult to reconcile with evidence that A1 projection fibres excite neurosecretory AVP cells, as this would suggest that A1 activation would tend to increase vasomotor tone by humoral means while simultaneously reducing it via neural means. More recently, it has been established that A1 cells do not project to the rostral VLM (Sun and Guyenet, 1986; Blessing et al., 1988) and separation of the depressor area and the A1 group has recently been confirmed in the rabbit by Li and Blessing (1988).

Summary

Activation of noradrenergic afferents arising from the A1 cell group of the caudal VLM excites neurosecretory AVP cells of both the supraoptic and paraventricular nuclei, thus stimulating the release of this potent vasoconstrictor into the circulation. Although this effect is mimicked by application of α_1-adrenoreceptor agonists to AVP cells, the excitatory effects of A1 afferents may not be mediated by activation of post-synaptic α_1-receptors. Evidence has also been obtained that the actions of A1 afferents are not dependent upon the release of excitatory amino acids or NPY, although the latter is co-stored with NA in A1 cells and potentiates the actions of low concentrations of NA on AVP cells.

Although a projection to AVP and OXY neurosecretory cells from the A2 NA cell group of the NTS has been established, this projection does not appear to contribute directly to the control of SON AVP cell activity. Rather, NTS stimulation excites SON AVP cells via a relay projection through the A1 cell group. This pathway is likely to correspond to that involved in the stimulatory effects of haemorrhage and caval constriction on AVP secretion, although it is uncertain whether the effects of these particular stimuli are contingent upon unloading of arterial baroreceptors and atrial stretch receptors, as commonly presumed, or upon the activation of other receptors such as ventricular mechanoreceptors or chemoreceptors. On balance, current evidence suggests that the A1 projection is unlikely to be critically involved in mediating the effects of arterial baroreceptor, arterial chemoreceptor, or atrial stretch receptor activation on AVP cells.

Acknowledgements

The contributions of J. Sibbald and B. Wilson to this work are gratefully acknowledged, as is the technical assistance provided by N. Still and D. Shieffelbien. Studies conducted in the author's laboratory were supported by grants from the Medical Research Council of New Zealand, the New Zealand Neurological Foundation, the National Heart Foundation of New Zealand, and the New Zealand Lottery Board.

314

References

Alonso, G. and Assenmacher, I. (1984) Ultrastructural analysis of the noradrenergic innervation of rat supraoptic nucleus. *Neurosc. Lett.*, 49: 45 – 50.

Andrew, R.D. (1987) Endogenous bursting by rat supraoptic neuroendcocrine cells is calcium dependent. *J. Physiol. (Lond.)*, 384: 451 – 465.

Andrew, R.D. and Dudek, F.E. (1984) Analysis of intracellularly recorded phasic bursting by mammalian neuroendocrine cells. *J. Neurophysiol.*, 51: 552 – 566.

Armstrong, W.E., Gallagher, M.J. and Sladek, C.D. (1986) Noradrenergic stimulation of supraoptic neuronal activity and vasopressin release in vitro: mediation by an α_1-receptor. *Brain Res.*, 365: 192 – 197.

Baertschi, A.J. and Vallet, P.G. (1981) Osmosensitivity of the hepatic portal vein area and vasopressin release in rats. *J. Physiol. (Lond.)*, 315: 217 – 230.

Banks, D. and Harris, M.C. (1984) Lesions of the locus coeruleus abolish baroreceptor-induced depression of supraoptic neurones in the rat. *J. Physiol. (Lond.)*, 355: 383 – 398.

Banks, D. and Harris, M.C. (1988) Activation of hypothalamic arcuate but not paraventricular neurons following carotid body chemoreceptor stimulation in the rat. *Neuroscience*, 24: 967 – 976.

Bishop, V.S., Thames, M.D. and Schmid, P.G. (1984) Effects of bilateral vagal cold block on vasopressin in conscious dogs. *Am. J. Physiol.*, 246: R566 – R569.

Blessing, W.W. and Reis, D.J. (1982) Inhibitory cardiovascular function of neurons in the caudal ventrolateral medulla of the rabbit: relationship to the area containing A1 noradrenergic cells. *Brain Res.*, 253: 161 – 171.

Blessing, W.W. and Willoughby, J.O. (1985) Inhibiting the rabbit caudal ventrolateral medulla prevents baroreceptor-initiated secretion of vasopressin. *J. Physiol. (Lond.)*, 367: 253 – 265.

Blessing, W.W., Hedger, S.C., Joh, T.H. and Willoughby, J.O. (1987) Neurons in the area postrema are the only catecholamine-synthesizing cells in the medulla or pons with projections to the rostral ventrolateral medulla (C_1 area) in the rabbit. *Brain Res.*, 419: 336 – 340.

Blumberg, H., Haupt, P., Jänig, W. and Kohler, W. (1983) Encoding of visceral noxious stimuli in the discharge patterns of visceral afferent fibres from the colon. *Pflügers Arch.*, 398: 33 – 40.

Carlson, D.E. and Gann, D.S. (1987) Responses of adrenocorticotropin and vasopressin to hemorrhage after lesions of the caudal ventrolateral medulla in rats. *Brain Res.*, 406: 385 – 390.

Ciriello, J. and Calaresu, F.R. (1983) Central projections of afferent renal fibers in the rat: an anterograde transport study of horseradish peroxidase. *J. Auton. Nerv. Syst.*, 8: 273 – 285.

Ciriello, J., Caverson, M.M. and Polosa, C. (1986) Function of the ventrolateral medulla in the control of the circulation. *Brain Res. Rev.*, 11: 359 – 391.

Coote, J.H. and Macleod, V.H. (1974a) The influence of bulbospinal monoaminergic pathways on sympathetic nerve activity. *J. Physiol. (Lond.)*, 241: 453 – 475.

Coote, J.H. and Macleod, V.H. (1974b) Evidence for the involvement in the baroreceptor reflex of a descending inhibitory pathway. *J. Physiol. (Lond.)*, 241: 477 – 496.

Cowley, A.W., Quillen, E.W. and Skelton, M.M. (1983) Role of vasopressin in cardiovascular regulation. *Fed. Proc.*, 42: 3170 – 3176.

Cunningham, E.T., Jr. and Sawchenko, P.E. (1988) Anatomical specificity of noradrenergic inputs to the paraventricular and supraoptic nuclei of the rat hypothalamus. *J. Comp. Neurol.*, 274: 60 – 76.

Dale, H.H. and Gaddum, J.H. (1930) Reactions of denervated voluntary muscle, and their bearing on the mode of action of parasympathetic and related nerves. *J. Physiol. (Lond.)*, 70: 109 – 144.

Day, T.A. (1987) Role of A1 noradrenergic afferents in the control of vasopressin secretion: in vivo electrophysiological studies. In J. Ciriello, F.R. Calaresu, L.P. Renaud and C. Polosa (Eds.), *Organization of the Autonomic Nervous System: Central and Peripheral Mechanisms*, Alan Liss, New York, pp. 425 – 434.

Day, T.A. and Ciriello, J. (1985) Afferent renal nerve stimulation excites supraoptic vasopressin neurons. *Am. J. Physiol.*, 249: R368 – R371.

Day, T.A. and Ciriello, J. (1987) Effects of renal receptor activation on neurosecretory vasopressin cells. *Am. J. Physiol.*, 253: R234 – R241.

Day, T.A. and Renaud, L.P. (1984) Electrophysiological evidence that noradrenergic afferents selectively facilitate the activity of supraoptic vasopressin neurons. *Brain Res.*, 303: 233 – 240.

Day, T.A. and Sibbald, J.R. (1988a) Direct catecholaminergic projection from nucleus tractus solitarius to supraoptic nucleus. *Brain Res.*, 454: 387 – 392.

Day, T.A. and Sibbald, J.R. (1988b) Solitary nucleus excitation of supraoptic vasopressin cells via adrenergic afferents. *Am. J. Physiol.*, 254: R711 – R716.

Day, T.A. and Sibbald, J.R. (1988c) Supraoptic vasopressin cell excitation following solitary nucleus stimulation is mediated via the A1 noradrenaline cell group. *Soc. Neurosci. Abstr.*, 14: 256.3.

Day, T.A. and Sibbald, J.R. (1989) Noradrenergic afferent excitation of supraoptic vasopressin cells: failure to demonstrate role for α-adrenergic or amino acid receptors. *Neurosci. Lett. Suppl.*, 34: S75.

Day, T.A., Blessing, W.W. and Willoughby, J.O. (1980) Noradrenergic and dopaminergic projections to the medial preoptic area of the rat. A combined horseradish peroxidase/catecholamine fluorescence study. *Brain Res.*, 193:

543 – 548.

Day, T.A., Ro, A. and Renaud, L.P. (1983) Depressor area within caudal ventrolateral medulla of the rat does not correspond to the A1 catecholamine cell group. *Brain Res.*, 279: 299 – 302.

Day, T.A., Ferguson, A.V. and Renaud, L.P. (1984) Facilitatory influence of noradrenergic afferents on the excitability of rat paraventricular nucleus neurosecretory cells. *J. Physiol. (Lond.)*, 355: 237 – 249.

Day, T.A., Ferguson, A.V. and Renaud, L.P. (1985a) Noradrenergic afferents facilitate the activity of tuberoinfundibular neurons of the hypothalamic paraventricular nucleus. *Neuroendocrinology*, 41: 17 – 22.

Day, T.A., Jhamandas, J.H. and Renaud, L.P. (1985b) Comparison between the actions of avian pancreatic polypeptide, neuropeptide Y and noradrenaline on rat supraoptic vasopressin neurons. *Neurosci. Lett.*, 62: 181 – 185.

Day, T.A., Randle, J.C.R. and Renaud, L.P. (1985c) Opposing α- and β-adrenergic mechanisms mediate dose-dependent actions of noradrenaline on supraoptic vasopressin neurons in vivo. *Brain Res.*, 358: 171 – 179.

Descarries, L. and Lapierre, Y. (1973) Noradrenergic axon terminals in the cerebral cortex of the rat. I. Radioautographic visualization after topical application of DL-[^{3}H]norepinephrine. *Brain Res.*, 51: 141 – 160.

Dun, N.P. (1985) Substance P. In M.A. Rogawski and J.L. Barker (Eds.), *Neurotransmitter Actions in the Vertebrate Nervous System*, Plenum Press, New York, pp. 459 – 478.

Dyball, R.E.J. (1968) Stimuli for the release of neurohypophysial hormones. *Br. J. Pharmacol. Chemother.*, 33: 319 – 328.

Dyball, R.E.J. and Koizumi, K. (1969) Electrical activity in the supraoptic and paraventricular nuclei associated with neurohypophysial hormone release. *J. Physiol.*, 201: 711 – 722.

Edvinsson, L., Hakanson, R., Wahlestedt, C. and Uddman, R. (1987) Effects of neuropeptide Y on the cardiovascular system. *Trends Pharmacol. Sci.*, 8: 4631 – 4635.

Egan, T.M., Henderson, G., North, R.A. and Williams, J.T. (1983) Noradrenaline-mediated synaptic inhibition in rat locus coeruleus neurones. *J. Physiol.*, 345: 477 – 488.

Everitt, B.J., Hökfelt, T., Terenius, L., Tatemoto, K., Mutt, V. and Goldstein, M. (1984) Differential co-existence of neuropeptide Y (NPY)-like immunoreactivity with catecholamines in the central nervous system of the rat. *Neuroscience*, 11: 443 – 462.

Feldberg, W. and Rocha e Silva, M., Jr. (1981) Inhibition of vasopressin release to carotid occlusion by γ-aminobutyric acid and glycine. *Br. J. Pharmac.*, 72: 17 – 24.

Fuxe, K. (1965) Evidence for the existence of monoamine neurons in the central nervous system. IV The distribution of monoamine nerve terminals in the central nervous system. *Acta Physiol. Scand., Suppl.*, 64: 247: 37 – 85.

Granata, A.R., Numao, Y., Kumada, M. and Reis, D.J. (1986) A1 noradrenergic neurons tonically inhibit sympathoexcitatory neurons of C1 area in rat brainstem. *Brain Res.*, 377: 127 – 146.

Gribkoff, V.K. and Dudek, F.E. (1988) The effects of the excitatory amino acid antagonist kynurenic acid on synaptic transmission to supraoptic neuroendocrine cells. *Brain Res.*, 442: 152 – 156.

Hamamura, M., Shibuki, K. and Yagi, K. (1984) Noxious inputs to supraoptic neurosecretory cells in the rat. *Neurosci. Res.*, 2: 49 – 61.

Harris, M.C. (1979) Effects of chemoreceptor and baroreceptor stimulation on the discharge of hypothalamic supraoptic neurones in rats. *J. Endocrinol.*, 82: 115 – 125.

Harris, M.C., Banks, D., Stokes, W.N. and Jamieson, S.M. (1987) Carotid body chemoreceptors and forebrain activation. In J. Ciriello, F.R. Calaresu, L.P. Renaud and C. Polosa (Eds.), *Organization of the Autonomic Nervous System: Central and Peripheral Mechanisms*, Alan Liss, New York, pp. 337 – 345.

Harris, M.C., Ferguson, A.V. and Banks, D. (1984) The afferent pathway for carotid body chemoreceptor input to the hypothalamic supraoptic nucleus in the rat. *Pflügers Arch.*, 400: 80 – 87.

Hirst, G.D.S., De Gleria, S. and van Helden, D.F. (1985) Neuromuscular transmission in arterioles. *Experientia*, 41: 874 – 879.

Jan, Y.N. and Jan, L.Y. (1985) Luteinizing hormone-releasing hormone. In M.A. Rogawski and J.L. Barker (Eds.), *Neurotransmitter Actions in the Vertebrate Nervous System*, Plenum Press, New York, pp. 459 – 478.

Jhamandas, J.H. and Renaud, L.P. (1986) Diagonal band neurons may mediate arterial baroreceptor input to hypothalamic vasopressin-secreting neurons. *Neurosci. Lett.*, 65: 214 – 218.

Jhamandas, J.H. and Renaud, L.P. (1987) Bicuculline blocks an inhibitory baroreflex input to supraoptic vasopressin neurons. *Am. J. Physiol.*, 252: R947 – R952.

Kannan, H., Yamashita, H. and Osaka, T. (1984) Paraventricular neurosecretory neurons: synaptic inputs from the ventrolateral medulla in rats. *Neurosci. Lett.*, 51: 183 – 188.

Kannan, H., Osaka, T., Kasai, M., Okuya, S. and Yamashita, H. (1986) Electrophysiological properties of neurons in the caudal ventrolateral medulla projecting to the paraventricular nucleus of the hypothalamus in rats. *Brain Res.*, 376: 342 – 350.

Kannan, H., Kasai, M., Osaka, T. and Yamashita, H. (1987) Neurons in the paraventricular nucleus projecting to the median eminence: a study of their afferent connections from peripheral baroreceptors, and from the A$_1$-catecholaminergic area in the ventrolateral medulla. *Brain Res.*, 409: 358 – 363.

Kendrick, K.M. and Leng, G. (1988) Haemorrhage-induced release of noradrenaline, 5-hydroxytryptamine and uric acid in the supraoptic nucleus of the rat, measured by microdialysis. *Brain Res.*, 440: 402–406.

Kim, Y.I., Dudley, C.A. and Moss, R.L. (1987) A1 noradrenergic input to medial preoptic-medial septal area: an electrophysiological study. *Neuroendocrinology*, 45: 77–85.

Koizumi, K. and Yamashita, H. (1978) Influence of atrial stretch receptors on hypothalamic neurosecretory neurones. *J. Physiol.*, 285: 341–358.

Kubo, T., Amano, H. and Misu, Y. (1985) Caudal ventrolateral medulla. A region responsible for the mediation of vasopressin-induced pressor responses. *Naunyn-Schmiedeberg's Arch. Pharmacol.*, 328: 368–372.

Ledsome, J.R. (1985) Atrial receptors, vasopressin and blood volume in the dog. *Life Sci.*, 36: 1315–1330.

Lee, M.-E., Thrasher, T.N., Keil, L.C. and Ramsay, D.J. (1986) Cardiac receptors, vasopressin, and corticosteroid release during arterial hypotension in dogs. *Am. J. Physiol.*, 251: R614–R620.

Li, Y.-W. and Blessing, W.W. (1988) Precise localization of vasodepressor neurones in the caudal ventrolateral medulla of the rabbit. *Proc. Austr. Physiol. Pharmacol. Soc.*, 19: 198P.

Loewy, A.D. and Burton, H. (1978) Nuclei of the solitary tract: efferent projections to the lower brainstem and spinal cord of the cat. *J. Comp. Neurol.*, 181: 421–450.

McAllen, R.M. and Blessing, W.W. (1987) Neurons (presumably A1-cells) projecting from the caudal ventrolateral medulla to the region of the supraoptic nucleus respond to baroreceptor inputs in the rabbit. *Neurosci. Lett.*, 73: 247–252.

McKellar, S. and Loewy, A.D. (1981) Organization of some brain stem afferents to the paraventricular nucleus of the hypothalamus in the rat. *Brain Res.*, 217: 351–357.

McKellar, S. and Loewy, A.D. (1982) Efferent projections of the A1 catecholamine cell group in the rat: an autoradiographic study. *Brain Res.*, 241: 11–19.

McNeill, T.H. and Sladek, J.R. Jr. (1980) Simultaneous monoamine histofluorescence and neuropeptide immunocytochemistry: correlative distribution of catecholamine varicosities and magnocellular neurosecretory neurons in the rat supraoptic and paraventricular nuclei. *J. Comp. Neurol.*, 193: 1023–1033.

Menetrey, D., Roudier, F. and Besson, J.M. (1983) Spinal neurons reaching the lateral reticular nucleus as studied in the rat by retrograde transport of horseradish peroxidase. *J. Comp. Neurol.*, 220: 439–452.

Oberg, B. and Thoren, P. (1972) Increased activity in left ventricular receptors during haemorrhage or occlusion of caval veins in the cat: a possible cause of the vaso-vagal reaction. *Acta Physiol. Scand.*, 85: 164–173.

Perrin, J. and Crousillat, J. (1983) Splanchnic afferent input to the lateral reticular nucleus of the cat. *J. Auton. Nerv. Syst.*, 8: 383–393.

Plotsky, P.M. (1987) Facilitation of immunoreactive corticotropin-releasing factor secretion into the hypophysial-portal circulation after activation of catecholaminergic pathways or central norepinephrine injection. *Endocrinology*, 121: 924–930.

Raby, W.N. and Renaud, L.P. (1987) Characterization of a noradrenergic pathway from the dorsomedial medulla (A2) to the hypothalamic supraoptic nucleus (SON) in the rat. *Soc. Neurosci. Abstr.*, 13: 711.10.

Raff, H., Shinsako, J., Keil, L.C. and Dallman, M.F. (1983) Vasopressin, ACTH, and corticosteroids during hypercapnia and graded hypoxia in dogs. *Am. J. Physiol.*, 244: E453–E458.

Randle, J.C.R., Bourque, C.W. and Renaud, L.P. (1984) α-Adrenergic activation of rat hypothalamic supraoptic neurons maintained in vitro. *Brain Res.*, 307: 374–378.

Randle, J.C.R., Bourque, C.W. and Renaud, L.P. (1986a) α_1-Adrenergic receptor activation depolarizes rat supraoptic neurosecretory neurons in vitro. *Am. J. Physiol.*, 251: R569–R574.

Randle, J.C.R., Mazurek, M., Kneifel, D., Dufresne, J. and Renaud, L.P. (1986b) α_1-Adrenergic receptor activation releases vasopressin and oxytocin from perfused rat hypothalamic explants. *Neurosci. Lett.*, 65: 219–223.

Ricardo, J.A. and Koh, E.T. (1978) Anatomical evidence of direct projections from the nucleus of the solitary tract to the hypothalamus, amygdala and other forebrain structures in the rat. *Brain Res.*, 153: 1–26.

Ross, C.A., Ruggiero, D.A. and Reis, D.J. (1985) Projections from the nucleus tractus solitarii to the rostral ventrolateral medulla. *J. Comp. Neurol.*, 242: 511–534.

Saper, C.B., Reis, D.J. and Joh, T. (1983) Medullary catecholamine inputs to the anteroventral third ventricular cardiovascular regulatory region in the rat. *Neurosci. Lett.*, 42: 285–291.

Sawchenko, P.E. and Swanson, L.W. (1981) Central noradrenergic pathways for the integration of hypothalamic neuroendocrine and autonomic responses. *Science*, 214: 685–687.

Sawchenko, P.E. and Swanson, L.W. (1982) The organization of noradrenergic pathways from the brainstem to the paraventricular and supraoptic nuclei in the rat. *Brain Res. Rev.*, 4: 275–325.

Sawchenko, P.E., Benoit, R. and Brown, M.R. (1988a) Somatostatin-28 immunoreactive inputs to the paraventricular and supraoptic nuclei: principal origin from non-aminergic neurons in the nucleus of the solitary tract. *J. Chem. Neuroanat.* (in press).

Sawchenko, P.E., Plotsky, P.M., Pfeiffer, S.W., Cunningham, E.T., Jr., Vaughan, J., Rivier, J. and Vale, W. (1988b) Inhibin β in central neural pathways involved in the control of oxytocin secretion. *Nature*, 334: 615–617.

Share, L. and Levy, M.N. (1966) Effect of carotid chemoreceptor stimulation plasma antidiuretic hormone titre. *Am. J. Physiol.*, 210: 157–161.

Silverman, A.-J., Oldfield, B., Hou-Yu, A. and Zimmerman,

E.A. (1985) The noradrenergic innervation of vasopressin neurons in the paraventricular nucleus of the hypothalamus: an ultrastructural study using radioautography and immunocytochemistry. *Brain Res.*, 325: 215 – 229.

Sotgiu, M.L. (1986) Effects of noxious stimuli on neurons of the lateral reticular nucleus region in rabbits. *Brain Res.*, 375: 169 – 171.

Sun, M.-K. and Guyenet, P.G. (1986) Effect of clonidine and γ-aminobutyric acid on the discharges of medullo-spinal sympathoexcitatory neurons in the rat. *Brain Res.*, 368: 1 – 17.

Tata, P.S. and Buzalkov, R. (1966) Vasopressin studies in the rat. III. Inability of ethanol anaesthesia to prevent ADH secretion due to pain and haemorrhage. *Pflügers Arch.*, 290: 294 – 297.

Tribollet, E., Armstrong, W.E., Dubois-Dauphin, M. and Dreifuss, J.J. (1985) Extra-hypothalamic afferent inputs to the supraoptic nucleus area of the rat as determined by retrograde and anterograde tracing techniques. *Neuroscience*, 15: 135 – 148.

Undesser, K.P., Hasser, E.M., Haywood, J.R., Johnson, A.K. and Bishop, V.S. (1985) Interactions of vasopressin with the area postrema in arterial baroreflex function in conscious rabbits. *Circ. Res.*, 56: 410 – 417.

Vallet, P.G. and Baertschi, A.J. (1982) Spinal afferents for peripheral osmoreceptors in the rat. *Brain Res.*, 239: 271 – 274.

Wang, B.C., Flora-Ginter, G., Leadley, R.J., Jr. and Goetz, K.L. (1988) Ventricular receptors stimulate vasopressin release during hemorrhage. *Am. J. Physiol.*, 254: R204 – R211.

Willette, R.N., Punnen, S., Krieger, A.J. and Sapru, H.N. (1984) Interdependence of rostral and caudal ventrolateral medullary areas in the control of blood pressure. *Brain Res.*, 321: 169 – 174.

Willoughby, J.O. and Blessing, W.W. (1987) Neuropeptide Y injected into the supraoptic nucleus causes secretion of vasopressin in the unanesthetized rat. *Neurosci. Lett.*, 75: 17 – 22.

Willoughby, J.O., Jervois, P.M., Menadue, M.F. and Blessing, W.W. (1987) Noradrenaline, by activation of alpha-1-adrenoceptors in the region of the supraoptic nucleus, causes secretion of vasopressin in the unanaesthetized rat. *Neuroendocrinology*, 45: 219 – 226.

Wilson, B.K.J., Sibbald, J.R. and Day, T.A. (1988) Neuropeptide Y potentiates excitatory actions of noradrenaline on supraoptic neurosecretory cells. *Soc. Neurosci. Abstr.*, 14: 256.18.

Yamashita, H., Inenaga, K. and Kannan, H. (1987) Depolarizing effect of noradrenaline on neurons of the rat supraoptic nucleus in vitro. *Brain Res.*, 405: 348 – 352.

Yoshimura, M., Polosa, C. and Nishi, S. (1987) Slow EPSP and the depolarizing action of noradrenaline on sympathetic preganglionic neurons. *Brain Res.*, 414: 138 – 142.

J. Ciriello, M.M. Caverson and C. Polosa (Eds.)
Progress in Brain Research, Vol. 81
© 1989 Elsevier Science Publishers B.V. (Biomedical Division)

CHAPTER 25

Nucleus tractus solitarius innervation of supraoptic nucleus: anatomical and electrophysiological studies in the rat suggest differential innervation of oxytocin and vasopressin neurons

Wilfrid N. Raby and Leo P. Renaud[*]

Neurosciences Unit, Montreal General Hospital Research Institute and McGill University, 1650 Cedar Avenue, Montreal, Quebec, Canada H3G 1A4

Introduction

It is almost five decades since Chang and colleagues (Chang et al., 1940) reported a pressor response to electrical stimulation in the dorsomedial medulla in cordotomized dogs. Recent functional studies in various species (e.g. rat; Nakai et al., 1982; Yamane et al., 1984) have determined more precisely the participation of vasopressin in this response and have supported a growing body of evidence (e.g. Day and Renaud, 1984; Day et al., 1984; Lightman et al., 1984; Kannan et al., 1984; Tanaka et al., 1985; Head et al., 1987) in favor of a facilitatory role of ascending catecholaminergic projections from the caudal medulla on hypothalamic vasopressin-secreting neurons. There is now substantial anatomical documentation of projections to the hypothalamic *paraventricular* nucleus from the caudal ventrolateral and dorsomedial medulla (Norgren, 1978; Ricardo and Koh, 1978; Sawchenko and Swanson, 1981, 1982; Swanson et al., 1981; McKellar and Loewy, 1982). Moreover, electrophysiological data do indeed indicate that electrical stimulation in the caudal ventrolateral medulla (cVLM) and the caudal nucleus tractus

solitarius (cNTS) is facilitatory to paraventricular vasopressin-secreting magnocellular neurosecretory neurons (Day et al., 1984; Kannan et al., 1984; Tanaka et al., 1985). Also apparent from the studies of Day et al. (1984) is a difference in the input to paraventricular neurosecretory neurons from these two areas: cVLM stimulation is selectively excitatory to vasopressin-secreting neurons whereas cNTS stimulation excites *both* oxytocin and vasopressin-secreting neurons. Data from *supraoptic* nucleus, which is composed almost exclusively of magnocellular neurons projecting to the neurohypophysis, also support a selective excitatory input from the A1 ventrolateral medulla cells to the vasopressin-secreting neurons (Day and Renaud, 1984). In contrast, preliminary observations indicate that electrical stimulation in cNTS excites *both* vasopressin- and oxytocin-secreting supraoptic neurons (Raby and Renaud, 1987). We therefore undertook a more detailed anatomical and electrophysiological study of their input from dorsomedial medulla.

Anatomical tracer studies

Studies using both anterograde and retrograde tracers (see Sawchenko and Swanson, 1981, 1982; McKellar and Loewy, 1982; Tribollet et al., 1985;

---

[*]*To whom correspondence should be addressed.*

Cunningham and Sawchenko, 1988) have determined that catecholaminergic neurons in the cVLM A1 cell group and in the cNTS A2 cell group project to the supraoptic nucleus. Efforts to provide more detailed descriptions of these connections using retrograde tracers are hampered by the small dimension, irregular contour and inaccessible location of the supraoptic nucleus itself, and the need to use a tracer that will not diffuse from its site of deposition. In the studies reported here, we exposed one supraoptic nucleus via a ventral transpharyngeal approach (thereby allowing direct access to the nucleus) in pentobarbital anesthetized Long-Evans rats and used pressure ejection through a micropipette (20–40 μm diameter tip) to instill a small quantity (0.05–0.2 μl) of a suspension of rhodamine conjugated latex microspheres (Katz et al., 1984; Lumaflor, New York City) into the nucleus. Animals were then maintained under anesthesia for 18–24 h and sacrificed by transcardiac perfusion with 4% formaldehyde–0.5% glutaraldehyde for visualization of catecholamine histofluorescence (Furness et al., 1978). Brains from six animals were sectioned at 40 μm and examined for neurons demonstrating rhodamine and/or catecholamine fluorescence. Two injections confined to the anatomical boundaries of the supraoptic nucleus (Fig. 1) labelled neurons in several forebrain areas including the immediate perinuclear zone, organum vasculosum of the lamina terminalis, median preoptic nucleus and subfornical organ. In the caudal brainstem, labelled neurons were present in both ipsilateral and contralateral cVLM (Fig. 2) and cNTS. Table I il-

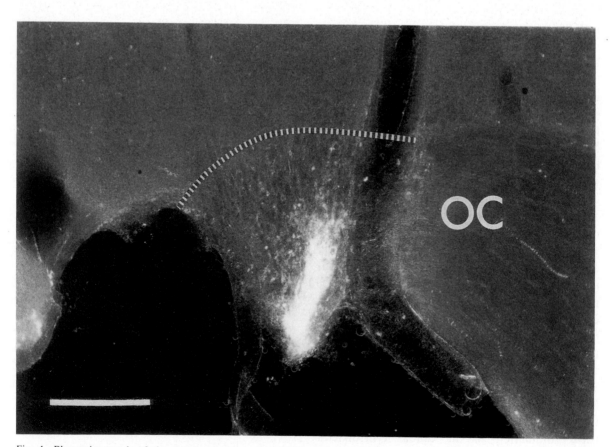

Fig. 1. Photomicrograph of the rat supraoptic nucleus illustrating the location of a small injection of rhodamine labelled microspheres. Note that the microspheres are confined to the anatomical boundaries of the nucleus. OC = optic chiasm.

lustrates that these small injections labelled only a small proportion of the catecholaminergic neurons caudal to the obex. However, nearly all ipsilateral and most contralateral rhodamine labelled cells in the cVLM were catecholaminergic indicating that most of the supraoptic input from cVLM arises from the A1 noradrenergic cells. In the cNTS, where approximately 1/2 to 1/3 as many cells contained rhodamine label (compared to cVLM), a larger percentage were non-catecholaminergic.

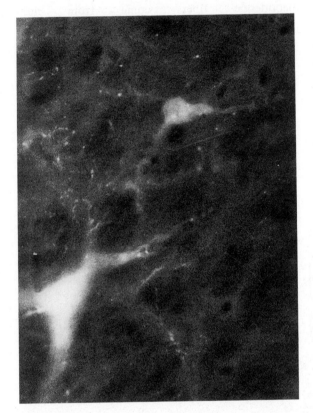 

Fig. 2. Photomicrograph on the right illustrates rhodamine fluorescent neurons in the caudal ventrolateral medulla; on the left, the same section is visualized for catecholamine fluorescence. Note that the rhodamine cell is also catecholaminergic.

TABLE I

Distribution of neurons in the caudal ventrolateral medulla (cVLM) and nucleus tractus solitarius (cNTS) that display fluorescence for rhodamine (Rho) and/or catecholamines (CAT) in two cases with rhodamine latex microsphere injections into the supraoptic nucleus

Site	Ipsilateral			Contralateral		
	Cat	Rho	Cat + Rho	Cat	Rho	Cat + Rho
cVLM	415	0	28	407	8	17
	417	1	27	382	0	6
cNTS	310	4	10	300	2	2
	270	2	13	305	6	0

Most rhodamine labelled neurons were located in the medial subnucleus and nucleus commissuralis of the NTS.

An examination of the anatomical location of vasopressin and oxytocin cells in the supraoptic nucleus relative to the chemical neuroanatomy of certain supraoptic afferent fibers provides the following interesting and possibly important correlations. First, the catecholamine terminal plexus in supraoptic is most dense in the ventral part of the nucleus, where the majority of vasopressin neurons are located (McNeill and Sladek, 1980; Swanson et al., 1981; Cunningham and Sawchenko, 1988); this input arises primarily from the cVLM A1 noradrenergic cell group (Sawchenko and Swanson, 1981, 1982, 1983). Second,

recent immunocytochemical studies have revealed the presence of fibers containing two peptides, β-inhibin and somatostatin 28, innervating the dorsal portion of the supraoptic nucleus, where the majority of oxytocin cells are situated; many of these peptidergic fibers come from non-catecholaminergic cNTS neurons (Sawchenko et al., 1988a,b).

Electrophysiology of NTS supraoptic connections

In vivo extracellular recordings from rat supraoptic neurons are characterized not only by their antidromic activation from the neurohypophysis but also by the ability to distinguish between putative

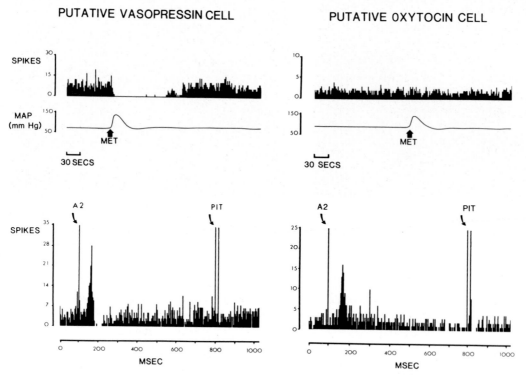

Fig. 3. The upper part of each column illustrates ratemeter recordings from two different supraoptic neurosecretory neurons and simultaneous mean arterial blood pressure tracings during a transient increase in blood pressure consequent to intravenous metaraminol (2 – 5 µg). Note that the cell on the left ceases activity during the rise in blood pressure, thus defining it as a vasopressin-secreting neuron. The cell on the right is not responsive to blood pressure elevation and is therefore defined as oxytocin secreting. Below are peristimulus time histograms (resolution 4 msec per bin; 300 sweeps) for each neuron illustrating a transient increase in excitability following a stimulus to the caudal nucleus tractus solitarius (cNTS). The second stimulus (PIT) is delivered to the posterior pituitary and illustrates the constant latency antidromic response.

vasopressin- and oxytocin-secreting neurons on the basis of firing patterns and sensitivity to baroreceptor activation (Fig. 3; see Renaud, 1988 for review). In order to determine whether the excitability of these supraoptic neurons could be influenced by cNTS stimulation and thereby obtain some insight into the possible function of the cNTS input to supraoptic nucleus, we again utilized a transpharyngeal approach in male Long-Evans rats anesthetized with urethane (1.25 g/kg) or pentobarbital (50 mg/kg i.p. with subsequent i.v. supplements). Following exposure of the ventral surface of the hypothalamus and caudal brainstem, a bipolar stimulating electrode was positioned in the neurohypophysis to antidromically activate supraoptic neurons, and a monopolar (glass-coated) tungsten electrode (tip exposure 50 μm, tip diameter 25 μm) was inserted into the NTS area. Stimulation of the cNTS was achieved with cathodal pulses (20 – 80 μA). In seven experiments, similar monopolar stimulation was also applied to an electrode positioned in the cVLM.

Observations obtained from 56 putative vasopressin-secreting neurons and 14 putative

TABLE II

Tabulation of data from electrophysiological studies of rat supraoptic nucleus neurons tested with single shock stimulation in the ipsilateral caudal nucleus tractus solitarius (cNTS), classified according to cell type and response pattern in peristimulus histograms: (+) excitation, (−) inhibition, (0) no response. For comparison below are data from caudal ventrolateral medullarly (cVLM) stimulation obtained here and in earlier studies (Day and Renaud, 1984)

cNTS stimulation		Response (%)		
Cell type	Number	(+)	(−)	(0)
Vasopressin	56	73	7	20
Oxytocin	14	64	6	30
cVLM stimulation				
Vasopressin	35	98	2	0
Oxytocin	28	2	8	90

oxytocin-secreting cells indicated that a majority of neurons in both categories displayed a transient excitation following cNTS stimulation at intensities as low as 20 μA (Table II). The peristimulus time histograms in Fig. 3 illustrate that these responses have latencies of 40 – 60 msec and durations of 30 – 50 msec for neurons in both categories. Most effective stimulation sites, identified by histological verification of the tip of the stimulation electrode, coincided with the location of the catecholaminergic neurons in the A2 cell group. Similar data were obtained from six supraoptic cells recorded after contralateral cNTS stimulation.

Different responses to cNTS versus cVLM stimulation

The data presented above reveal distinct differences between the inputs to supraoptic neurons from cVLM and cNTS. Results from an earlier study (Day and Renaud, 1984) confirmed here on 12 neurons indicated that cVLM stimulation selectively excites vasopressin- (but not oxytocin)-secreting supraoptic neurons. Retrograde tracer data (Table I) support earlier evidence (Sawchenko and Swanson, 1981, 1982, 1983) that afferents from the cVLM arise almost exclusively from the A1 noradrenergic cell group. Hence, the sensitivity to 6-hydroxydopamine pretreatment of the excitatory responses of supraoptic vasopressin neurons to a cVLM stimulus (Day and Renaud, 1984) supports the notion that they are mediated through ascending catecholaminergic fibers. However, despite evidence for an α_1-mediated excitation of supraoptic vasopressin-secreting cells (Randle et al., 1984, 1986a; Day et al., 1985; Inenaga et al., 1986; Yamashita et al., 1987) and release of vasopressin (Armstrong et al., 1986; Randle et al., 1986b; Willoughby et al., 1987) by exogenously applied noradrenaline, the inability to block synaptically-evoked excitation with adrenergic blocking agents raises questions as to the role of noradrenaline in mediating this particular transient excitation (see chapter by Day, this volume).

Whatever the synaptic mechanism for its generation, a similar pattern of transient excitation is obtained from a majority of *both* vasopressin- and oxytocin-secreting neurons, at comparable latencies, following a cNTS stimulus (Fig. 3). However, when vasopressin neurons were tested with sequential stimulation of cNTS and cVLM, the latency to the latter stimulus was found to be consistently shorter by 5 – 7 msec (Fig. 4). This observation along with anatomical evidence for projections from the NTS to VLM (Loewy and Burton, 1978; Sawchenko et al., 1987) might indicate that the cNTS-evoked responses to vasopressin-secreting neurons are relayed via the VLM. Hence, we prepared 12 animals in a manner similar to those outlined earlier but included an injection (0.2 – 0.4 μl) of 50 μM kainic acid into the contralateral VLM to destroy the A1 cell group. Once a cNTS-evoked response was established from a characterized supraoptic neuron, the effects of transient synaptic interruption in the ipsilateral VLM (by injections of either 20 μM muscimol or γ-aminobutyrate) were evaluated. Eosin Y was added to the infused solutions to facilitate the histological reconstruc-

tion of the extent of the lesions and infusions (Fig. 5).

The outcome of these experiments is illustrated in Fig. 6. In 8 of 9 vasopressin-secreting neurons, injections of muscimol or γ-aminobutyrate reversibly attenuated or blocked the cNTS-evoked response. In contrast, similar treatment had no influence on the cNTS-evoked response of any of five oxytocin-secreting neurons. Evidently the cNTS-evoked excitation of supraoptic (and probably paraventricular) vasopressin-secreting neurons involves a relay in the ventrolateral

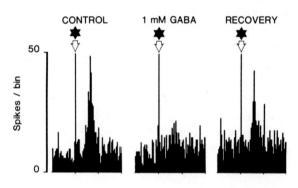

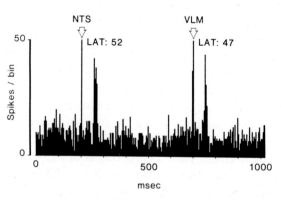

Fig. 4. Peristimulus histogram illustrates a similar pattern of excitatory response of the same supraoptic vasopressin-secreting neuron to stimulation in the caudal nucleus tractus solitarius (NTS) and caudal ventrolateral medulla (VLM). Analysis of sequential bins at a 1 msec resolution for each of 7 neurons revealed a consistent 5 – 7 msec shorter latency to the VLM stimulus.

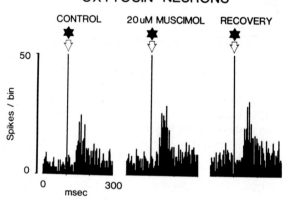

Fig. 5. Sequential peristimulus histograms from a vasopressin-secreting (top) and an oxytocin-secreting neuron (bottom) illustrate the effects of injections of muscimol or GABA into the ipsilateral VLM on the cNTS-evoked response (see text). Note that only the vasopressin cell response is abolished by this procedure.

medulla, whereas oxytocin-secreting neurons are activated through a direct pathway. These connections are schematically illustrated in their ultimate simplicity in Fig. 7. Possible transmitter(s) in the direct cNTS-supraoptic projection include a comparatively small catecholamine innervation that has recently been re-examined in detail (Cunningham and Sawchenko, 1988), and a novel non-catecholamine peptidergic innervation that contain neurons and fibers immunoreactive for somatostatin-28 (SS-28) (Sawchenko et al., 1988a) or β-inhibin (Sawchenko et al., 1988b). Interestingly, SS-28 administered i.c.v. produces an elevation in both vasopressin (Brown et al., 1988b) and oxytocin (Brown et al., 1988a) secretion in the rat, while the original tetradecapeptide (somatostatin 1 – 14) given into the lateral ventricle

of sheep inhibits the elevation in plasma vasopressin induced by hemorrhage (Wang et al., 1987). Our preliminary observations indicate that SS-28 applied to rat supraoptic neurons maintained in vitro produces a prolonged hyperpolarization and suppression of activity in concentrations of 10^{-8} to 10^{-6} M (Raby et al., 1988). Activin (or β-inhibin), on the other hand, enhances plasma oxytocin levels when injected into the rat paraventricular nucleus (Sawchenko et al., 1988b). There is yet no information on its actions at the cellular level.

Concluding comments

Inputs to the NTS arriving in glossopharyngeal and vagal afferents have at least two pathways whereby they can influence hypothalamic magnocellular neurosecretory neurons. Information destined to enhance the activity of vasopressinergic neurons, e.g. through unloading of peripheral baroreceptors consequent to hemorrhage or loss of blood volume (see Blessing and Willoughby, 1985a,b; McAllen and Blessing, 1987), seems to be preferentially channeled through the A1 neurons of the caudal ventrolateral medulla. Other visceral inputs to NTS from gastric mechano- and chemoreceptors (Raybould et al., 1985; Banks and Harris, 1987) as well as hepatic osmoreceptors (Baertschi and Vallet, 1981) and of

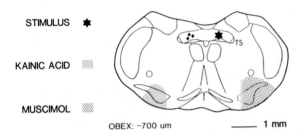

Fig. 6. Schematic diagram of the caudal medulla to illustrate the site and extent of the kainic acid lesion in the contralateral ventral medulla, and extent of GABA/muscimol spread on the side ipsilateral to the stimulus in the caudal solitary nucleus.

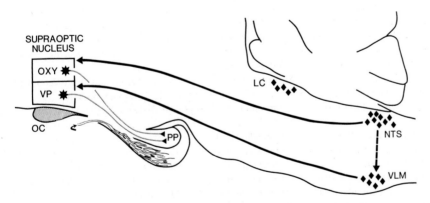

Fig. 7. Schematic representation of proposed pathways between the dorsomedial and ventral medulla, and the vasopressin and oxytocin neurons in supraoptic nucleus to explain the observations reported in the text.

somatosensory origin (Rossi and Brodal, 1956; Menétrey and Basbaum et al., 1987) may have a more select action directed towards the oxytocin-secreting neuronal population (for example, see Renaud et al., 1987) and may be relayed through a direct projection from NTS neurons. These suggestions provide the framework for further investigations.

Acknowledgements

This research is supported financially by the Medical Research Council of Canada and by the Quebec Heart Foundation. We thank Gwen Peard for typographical assistance.

References

Armstrong, W.E., Gallagher, M.J. and Sladek, C.D. (1986) Noradrenergic stimulation of supraoptic neuronal activity and vasopressin release in vitro: mediation by an α_1-receptor. Brain Res., 365: 192–197.

Baertschi, A.J. and Vallet, P.G. (1981) Osmosensitivity of the hepatic portal vein area and vasopressin release in rats. J. Physiol., 315: 217–230.

Banks, D. and Harris, M.C. (1987) Activation within dorsal medullary nuclei following stimulation in the hypothalamic paraventricular nucleus in rats. Pflügers Arch., 408: 619–627.

Blessing, W.W. and Willoughby, J.O. (1985a) Excitation of neuronal function in rabbit caudal ventrolateral medulla elevates plasma vasopressin. Neurosci. Lett., 58: 189–194.

Blessing, W.W. and Willoughby, J.O. (1985b) Inhibiting the rabbit caudal ventrolateral medulla prevents baroreceptor-initiated secretion of vasopressin. J. Physiol., 367: 253–265.

Brown, M.R., Crum, R. and Sawchenko, P. (1988a) Somatostatin-28 (SS-28) stimulation of vasopressin (AVP) and oxytocin (OT) secretion. Proc. Endocrinol. Soc. Abst., 660.

Brown, M.R., Mortrud, M., Crum, R. and Sawchenko, P. (1988b) Role of somatostatin in the regulation of vasopressin secretion. Brain Res., 452: 212–218.

Chang, H., Huang, J.J., Lu, Y.M. and Tsang, Y.C. (1940) A vagus-postpituitary reflex. IX. General locus of the vagus-supraoptic tract. Chin. J. Physiol., 15: 445–464.

Cunningham, E.T. and Sawchenko, P.E. (1988) Anatomical specificity of noradrenergic inputs to the paraventricular and supraoptic nuclei of the rat hypothalamus. J. Comp. Neurol., 274: 60–74.

Day, T.A. and Renaud, L.P. (1984) Electrophysiological

evidence that noradrenergic afferents selectively facilitate the activity of supraoptic vasopressin neurons. Brain Res., 303: 233–240.

Day, T.A., Ferguson, A.V. and Renaud, L.P. (1984) Facilitatory influence of noradrenergic afferents on the excitability of rat paraventricular nucleus neurosecretory cells. J. Physiol., 355: 237–249.

Day, T.A., Randle, J.C.R. and Renaud, L.P. (1985) Opposing α and β-adrenergic mechanisms mediate dose-dependent actions of noradrenaline on supraoptic vasopressin neurones in vivo. Brain Res., 358: 171–179.

Furness, J.B., Heath, J.W. and Costa, M. (1978) Aqueous aldehyde (Faglu) methods for the fluorescence histochemical localization of catecholamines and for ultrastructural studies of central nervous tissue. Histochemistry, 57: 285–295.

Head, G.A., Quail, A.W. and Woods, R.L. (1987) Lesions of A1 noradrenergic cells affect AVP release and heart rate during hemorrhage. Am. J. Physiol., 253: H1012–H1017.

Inenaga, K., Dyball, R.E.J., Okuya, S. and Yamashita, H. (1986) Characterization of hypothalamic noradrenaline receptors in the supraoptic nucleus and periventricular region of the paraventricular nucleus of mice in vitro. Brain Res., 369: 37–47.

Kannan, H., Yamashita, H. and Osaka, T. (1984) Paraventricular neurosecretory neurons: synaptic inputs from the ventrolateral medulla in rats. Neurosci. Lett., 51: 183–188.

Katz, L.C., Burkhalter, A. and Dreyer, W.J. (1984) Fluorescent latex microspheres as a retrograde neuronal marker for in vivo and in vitro studies of visual cortex. Nature, 310: 498–500.

Lightman, S.L., Todd, K. and Everitt, B.J. (1984) Ascending noradrenergic projections from the brainstem: evidence for a major role in the regulation of blood pressure and vasopressin secretion. Exp. Brain Res., 55: 145–151.

Loewy, A.D. and Burton, H. (1978) Nuclei of the solitary tract: efferent projections to lower brain stem and spinal cord of the cat. J. Comp. Neurol., 181: 421–450.

McAllen, R.M. and Blessing, W.W. (1987) Neurons (presumably A1-cells) projecting from the caudal ventrolateral medulla to the region of the supraoptic nucleus respond to baroreceptor inputs in the rabbit. Neurosci. Lett., 73: 247–252.

McKellar, S. and Loewy, A.D. (1982) Efferent projections of the A1 catecholamine cell group in the rat: an autoradiographic study. Brain Res., 241: 11–29.

McNeill, T.H. and Sladek, Jr. J.R. (1980) Simultaneous monoamine histofluorescence and neuropeptide immunocytochemistry. II. Correlative distribution of catecholamine varicosities and magnocellular neurosecretory neurons in the rat supraoptic and paraventricular nuclei. J. Comp. Neurol., 193: 1023–1033.

Menétrey, D. and Basbaum, A.I. (1987) Spinal and trigeminal projections to the nucleus of the solitary tract: a possible substrate for somatovisceral and viscerovisceral reflex activation. *J. Comp. Neurol.*, 255: 439–450.

Nakai, M., Yamane, Y., Umeda, Y. and Ogino, K. (1982) Vasopressin-induced pressor response elicited by electrical stimulation of solitary nucleus and dorsal motor nucleus of vagus of rat. *Brain Res.*, 251: 164–168.

Norgren, R. (1978) Projections from the nucleus of the solitary tract in the rat. *Neuroscience*, 3: 207–218.

Raby, W.N. and Renaud, L.P. (1987) Characterization of a noradrenergic pathway from the dorsomedial medulla (A2) to the hypothalamic supraoptic nucleus (SON) in the rat. *Soc. Neurosci. Abstr.*, 13: 1130.

Raby, W.N., Bourque, C.W., Benoit, R.A. and Renaud, L.P. (1988) Effects of somatostatin-28 on supraoptic magnocellular neurons in the rat. *Soc. Neurosci. Abstr.*, 14: 666.

Randle, J.C.R., Bourque, C.W. and Renaud, L.P. (1984) α-adrenergic activation of rat hypothalamic supraoptic neurons maintained in vitro. *Brain Res.*, 307: 374–378.

Randle, J.C.R., Bourque, C.W. and Renaud, L.P. (1986a) α_1-adrenergic receptor activation depolarizes rat supraoptic neurosecretory neurons in vitro. *Am. J. Physiol.*, 251: R569–R574.

Randle, J.C.R., Mazurek, M., Kneifel, D., Dufresne, J. and Renaud, L.P. (1986b) α_1-Adrenergic receptor activation releases vasopressin and oxytocin from perfused rat hypothalamic explants. *Neurosci. Lett.*, 65: 219–223.

Raybould, H.E., Gayton, R.J. and Dockray, G.J. (1985) CNS effects of circulating CCK-8: involvement of brainstem neurones responding to gastric distention. *Brain Res.*, 342: 187–190.

Renaud, L.P. (1988) Electrophysiology of a peptidergic neuron: The hypothalamic magnocellular neurosecretory cell. In M. Avoli, T.A. Reader, R.O. Dykes and P. Gloor (Eds.), *Neurotransmitters and Cortical Function*, Plenum, New York, pp. 495–515.

Renaud, L.P., Tang, J., McCann, M.J., Stricker, E.M. and Verbalis, J.G. (1987) Cholecystokinin and gastric distention activate oxytocinergic cells in rat hypothalamus. *Am. J. Physiol.*, 253: R661–R665.

Ricardo, J.A. and Koh, E.T. (1978) Anatomical evidence of direct projections from the nucleus of the solitary tract to the hypothalamus, amygdala and other forebrain structures in the rat. *Brain Res.*, 153: 1–26.

Rossi, G.F. and Brodal, A. (1956) Spinal afferents to the trigeminal sensory nuclei and the nucleus of the solitary tract. *Confin. Neurol.*, 16: 321–332.

Sawchenko, P.E. and Swanson, L.W. (1981) Central noradrenergic pathways for the integration of hypothalamic neuroendocrine and autonomic responses. *Science*, 214: 683–685.

Sawchenko, P.E. and Swanson, L.W. (1982) The organization of noradrenergic pathways from the brainstem to the paraventricular and supraoptic nuclei in the rat. *Brain Res. Rev.*, 4: 275–325.

Sawchenko, P.E. and Swanson, L.W. (1983) The organization of forebrain afferents to the paraventricular and supraoptic nuclei of the rat. *J. Comp. Neurol.*, 218: 121–144.

Sawchenko, P.E., Cunningham, Jr. E.T. and Levin, M.C. (1987) Anatomic and biochemical specificity in central autonomic pathways. In J. Ciriello, F.R. Calaresu, L.P. Renaud and C. Polosa (Eds.), *Organization of the Autonomic Nervous System: Central and Peripheral Mechanisms*, Alan R. Liss Inc., New York, pp. 267–281.

Sawchenko, P.E., Benoit, R. and Brown, M.R. (1988a) Somatostatin 28-immunoreactive in-puts to the paraventricular and supraoptic nuclei: principal origin from non-aminergic neurons in the nucleus of the solitary tract. *J. Chem. Neuroanat.*, 1: 81–94.

Sawchenko, P.E., Plotsky, P.M., Pfeiffer, S.W., Cunningham, E.T., Jr., Vaughn, J., Rivier, J. and Vale, W. (1988b) Inhibin β in central neural pathways involved in the control of oxytocin secretion. *Nature*, 334: 615–617.

Swanson, L.W., Sawchenko, P.E., Berod, A., Hartman, B.K., Helle, K.B. and Van Orden, D.E. (1981) An immunohistochemical study of the organization of catecholaminergic cells and terminal fields in the paraventricular and supraoptic nuclei of the hypothalamus. *J. Comp. Neurol.*, 196: 271–285.

Tanaka, J., Kaba, H., Saito, H. and Seto, K. (1985) Inputs from the A1 noradrenergic region to hypothalamic paraventricular neurons in the rat. *Brain Res.*, 335: 368–371.

Tribollet, E., Armstrong, W.E., Dubois-Dauphin, M. and Dreifuss, J.J. (1985) Extrahypothalamic afferent inputs to the supraoptic nucleus area of the rat as determined by retrograde and anterograde tracing techniques. *Neuroscience*, 15: 135–148.

Wang, X., Tresham, J.J., Congiv, M., Goghlan, J.P. and Scoggins, B.A. (1987) Somatostatin centrally inhibits vasopressin secretion during hemorrhage. *Brain Res.*, 436: 199–203.

Willoughby, J.O., Jervois, P.M., Menadue, M.F. and Blessing, W.W. (1987) Noradrenaline, by activation of alpha-1 adrenoreceptors in the region of the supraoptic nucleus, causes secretion of vasopressin in the unanesthetized rat. *Neuroendocrinology*, 45: 219–226.

Yamane, Y., Nakai, M., Yamamoto, J., Nemeda, Y. and Ogino, K. (1984) Release of vasopressin by electrical stimulation of the intermediate portion of the nucleus of the tractus solitarius in rats with cervical spinal cordotomy and vagotomy. *Brain Res.*, 324: 358–360.

Yamashita, H., Inenaga, K. and Kannan, H. (1987) Depolarizing effect of noradrenaline on neurons of the rat supraoptic nucleus in vitro. *Brain Res.*, 405: 348–352.

Subject Index

of horseradish peroxidase, 29, 54, 235
of rhodamine-labelled latex microspheres, 18,
    87, 108, 320
Rhodamine-labelled latex microspheres
combined with immunohistochemistry, 18, 88,
    108
injections into CVL, 87
injections into IML, 18, 108
injections into SON, 320
Rostral ventrolateral reticular nucleus, *see* RVL,
    49
Rostral ventromedial medulla, *see* RVM, 99
RVL
afferent inputs, 60, 89, 90, 105, 108, 109, 123,
    132, 143, 227
and baroreceptor reflex, 108, 226
and respiration, 100, 193, 208, 215
control of sympathetic nerve activity, 101,
    105, 118, 131, 159, 193
control of vascular resistance, 100, 207
cytoarchitecture in rat, 49, 105
effect of stimulation, 58, 159, 224, 266
in defense reaction, 58
kainic acid lesions in conscious animals, 267
lidocaine microinjections, 101
neuropharmacology, 71
pacemaker neurons, 106
pontine collaterals, 110
projections to spinal cord, 22, 29, 50, 105,
    117, 121, 132, 159
role in exercise pressor reflex, 257
role in vasomotor tone, 57, 99, 105, 159, 215,
    275
role of L-glutamate, 111, 159
RVM
and respiration, 100, 195
control of arterial pressure, 99, 195
control of sympathetic nerve activity, 101, 195
control of vascular resistance, 100, 101
immunoreactive neurons, 99, 100
in the rat, 99
lidocaine microinjections, 101
projections to spinal cord, 99

Serotonin
binding sites in parapyramidal region, 22
coexistence with CCK, 19–25
coexistence with ENK, 19–25
coexistence with substance P, 19–25
coexistence with TRH, 19–25
effect of lesions on substance P in IML, 21
effect of lesions on TRH in IML, 21
immunoreactive neurons in cat VLM, 12
immunoreactive neurons in rat VLM, 17, 70,
    99
microinjections in RVL, 229
neurotoxin-induced lesions, 21
projections from medulla to IML, 17–25
projections from parapyramidal region to
    NTS, 19
Somatostatin
coexistence with ENK, 20–25
immunoreactive neurons in cat VLM, 12
projections from medulla to spinal cord, 18
Somatosympathetic reflexes
anatomical substrates, 69
RVL control, 224
Spike-triggered average, 118, 132
SPN
adrenergic terminals on, 33
and pacemaker neurons, 112, 113
and RVL, 105, 112, 143, 159
effect of CVL on, 143, 149
effect of noradrenaline, 181
electrophysiological characteristics, 136, 143,
    149, 151, 161, 182–184
glutamate terminals on, 33
Subretrofacial nucleus (SRF)
location, 233
neurophysiological differentiation of neurons,
    238
topography, 237
vasomotor actions of, 233
Substance P
coexistence with 5-HT, 19–25
coexistence with ENK, 19–25
coexistence with TRH, 19–25